Quality Spine Care

John Ratliff • Todd J. Albert
Joseph Cheng • Jack Knightly
Editors

Quality Spine Care

Healthcare Systems, Quality Reporting, and Risk Adjustment

Springer

Editors
John Ratliff
Department of Neurosurgery
Stanford University
Stanford, CA
USA

Joseph Cheng
University of Cincinnati
Cincinnati, OH
USA

Todd J. Albert
Hospital for Special Surgery
New York, NY
USA

Jack Knightly
Atlantic Neurosurgical Specialists
Morristown, NJ
USA

ISBN 978-3-030-07433-3 ISBN 978-3-319-97990-8 (eBook)
https://doi.org/10.1007/978-3-319-97990-8

This Springer imprint is published by the registered company Springer Nature Switzerland AG
The registered company address is: Gewerbestrasse 11, 6330 Cham, Switzerland

To my wife, Carla Carvalho, and my children Maya and Jessica. Their patience throughout this process and the many, many other commitments that have taken me sometimes far from home has made everything I have accomplished possible. I owe it all to them.

John Ratliff

To my children Stuart, Elliot, and Emily who have taught me the Quality of Life and Love.

Todd J. Albert

I dedicate this work to my wife Rebecca and my son Josh. Their love and support means the world to me.

Joe Cheng

I would like to dedicate my work in this effort to my wife Sharon and my children Jake, Kieran, Carlie, and Anna for the time and encouragement they gave me to pursue this project.

Jack Knightly

Foreword

The provision of quality care is often assumed but infrequently delivered. Such is perhaps more evident in the spine arena than in any other in clinical medicine. The assumption of quality is a dangerous assumption indeed. The documentation of the study of quality, on the other hand, provides a grounding, if you will, that provides a foundation for the study quality and the palpable achievement of high quality.

Ratliff, Cheng, Albert, and Knightly have pieced together a masterful work that addresses the many facets of quality spine care. They pursue the past, looking to learn from prior experiences. They present metrics, methodologies, and strategies that can be used to objectivize the assessment of quality. They go on to present and analyze existing healthcare systems, in order to assess the current status quo and to provide a spring board for continuous improvement via quality reporting, the coordination and alignment of the variety of healthcare systems, and the operationalization of systems on a single institution, as well as national, basis.

In the pages that follow, the keys to quality spine care optimization lie. The more we all work with the same goal in mind, in an organized manner, the faster we will achieve optimal value in the spine arena. Please read with an open mind and apply with enthusiasm.

Cleveland, OH, USA — Mike Steinmetz
Cleveland, OH, USA — Ed Benzel

Preface

I have always been fascinated by the business aspects of healthcare. It may come from having spent the vast majority of my adult life working at academic medical centers, where many of the day-to-day challenges of running an enterprise are kept at arm's length. Even in academics, though, practitioners face daily reminders of the impact of insurance coverage, or lack thereof, on the capacity of patients to enjoy high-value care. Coverage policies and restrictions on beneficiary hospital access based upon whether or not a center meets a payer's distinction as a "center of excellence" all limit patient choices and influence patient care.

These soft approaches to rationing healthcare, through restricting choice and controlling access, may have profound effects on our patients. Maintaining patient access to care should be the primary goal of physician advocates in this space.

I learned the US system of healthcare finance through tutelage at the American Medical Association's Resource-Based Relative Value Scale (RBRVS) Update Committee (RUC), with the mentorship of giants like Greg Przybylski, Rick Boop, and John Wilson, after a supportive nudge from James Bean. Over many years, I developed the skill set necessary to navigate the arcana of the RUC and to advocate for neurosurgical patients. Concomitant with volunteering at the RUC, I was fortunate enough to have two mentors who join me as co-editors on this text. Joe Cheng contributed vastly to my understanding of coding and reimbursement and to my ability to teach these topics to others. Jack Knightly, following in the footsteps of thought leaders like Robert Harbaugh and Dan Resnick, helped me understand the separate, equally arcane system of quality improvement and quality reporting. Borrowing from Eisenhower, Knightly refers to it as the "quality-industrial complex." Last but certainly not least, my other co-editor Todd J. Albert, with Alex Vaccaro and others at Thomas Jefferson University, taught me the value of integrated systems and the strength that orthopedic and neurosurgical physicians can wield when working together.

I saw, as I started volunteering in both the RUC and neurosurgery's Quality Improvement Workgroup, how these two systems were coming together and how quality would take a greater and greater role in healthcare finance and access.

Hence the impetus of this text. There are many textbooks that cover the technical aspects of operative spine care. I know of none that provide surgeons with insight into the equally challenging aspects of healthcare delivery and quality assessment.

I hope this volume will provide a succinct overview of a variety of aspects of quality as applied to spine care.

I am especially indebted to my international authors, who provide insights into healthcare in China, Japan, England, Australasia, and India, and how quality is assessed within their systems. I sought international authors to see how the challenges of quality assessment and healthcare finance are met in other countries—I wondered if anyone else had come any closer than the USA to having this "figured out." I learned so much from reading their chapters and from reviewing the challenges faced in these disparate healthcare environments.

I hope you enjoy this text as much as my co-editors and I have enjoyed compiling it. Our authors have done a phenomenal job of compacting a tremendous volume of information into a concise 24 chapters. We hope you enjoy it.

Stanford, CA, USA John Ratliff

Acknowledgments

I would like to acknowledge first and foremost the contributions of my co-editors. Their guidance and mentoring throughout my career has been invaluable. I would also like to thank Dr. Iwasaki, for completing the Japan chapter with an unacceptably short lead time. His dedication to spine care is exemplary. Finally I would like to thank Alex Vaccaro for his friendship and guidance. Our authors have made this textbook possible, and we are in their debt.

John Ratliff

Contents

Contributors

Owoicho Adogwa, MD, MPH Rush University Medical Center, Chicago, IL, USA

Deepak Venkatesh Agarkhed, BEng, MBA Sakra World Hospital, Bangalore, Karnataka, India

Todd J. Albert, MD Hospital for Special Surgery, New York, NY, USA

Weill Cornell Medical School, New York, NY, USA

Mohammed Ali Alvi, MBBS Mayo Clinic Neuro-Informatics Laboratory, Mayo Clinic, Rochester, MN, USA

Department of Neurologic Surgery, Mayo Clinic, Rochester, MN, USA

Christopher P. Ames, MD Department of Neurosurgery, University of California, San Francisco, San Francisco, CA, USA

Brian L. Anderson, MD, MHA Department of Neurosurgery, Penn State University, Milton S. Hershey Medical Center, Hershey, PA, USA

Bryan Ashman, MBBS, MsurgEd, FRACS Division of Surgery, Canberra Hospital, Garran, ACT, Australia

Johannes A. Bernbeck, MD Orthopedics-Spine, Southern California Permanente Medical Group, Downey, CA, USA

Erica F. Bisson, MD, MPH Department of Neurosurgery, Clinical Neurosciences Center, University of Utah, Salt Lake City, UT, USA

Harsimran S. Brara, MD, FAANS Neurosurgery, Southern California Permanente Medical Group, Los Angeles, CA, USA

Lee M. Breakwell, MBChB, MSc, FRCS(Tr&Orth) Sheffield Children's Hospital, Sheffield, UK

Daniel Burkett, MD Department of Neurosurgery, University of Wisconsin School of Medicine and Public Health, Madison, WI, USA

Mohamad Bydon, MD Mayo Clinic Neuro-Informatics Laboratory, Mayo Clinic, Rochester, MN, USA

Department of Neurologic Surgery, Mayo Clinic, Rochester, MN, USA

John Chen Li Tat, MBBS(NUI), BAO, LRCSI, FRCS(Ed) Department of Orthopaedic Surgery, Singapore General Hospital, Singapore, Singapore

Joseph Cheng, MD, MS Department of Neurosurgery, University of Cincinnati College of Medicine, Cincinnati, OH, USA

Xiongying Chen, MD, PhD Jackson Hospitalist Program, Jackson Hospital, Montgomery, AL, USA

Ashley A. Cole, BMedSci, FRCS, DM Sheffield Children's Hospital, Sheffield, UK

Chad M. Craig, MD, FACP Spine Service, Department of Orthopaedic Surgery and Department of Medicine, Hospital for Special Surgery, New York, NY, USA

Atman M. Desai, MD Department of Neurosurgery, Stanford University School of Medicine, Stanford, CA, USA

Melissa R. Dunbar, MPH Department of Neurosurgery, Lahey Hospital & Medical Center, Burlington, MA, USA

Mohamed Elminawy, MBBCh Mayo Clinic Neuro-Informatics Laboratory, Mayo Clinic, Rochester, MN, USA

Department of Neurologic Surgery, Mayo Clinic, Rochester, MN, USA

Eric J. Feuchtbaum, MD Spine Center, Hospital for Special Surgery, New York, NY, USA

T. J. Florence, PhD Columbia College of Physicians and Surgeons, New York, NY, USA

Takahito Fujimori, MD, PhD Department of Orthopedic Surgery, Japan Community Healthcare Organization, Osaka Hospital, Osaka, Japan

Julian L. Gendreau, BS Mercer University School of Medicine, Macon, GA, USA

Department of Neurosurgery, Stanford University School of Medicine, Stanford, CA, USA

Zoher Ghogawala, MD, FACS Department of Neurosurgery, Lahey Hospital & Medical Center, Burlington, MA, USA

Department of Neurosurgery, Tufts University School of Medicine, Boston, MA, USA

Jonathan N. Grauer, MD Department of Orthopaedics and Rehabilitation, Yale University School of Medicine, New Haven, CT, USA

Kern H. Guppy, MD, PhD Neurosurgery, The Kaiser Permanente Medical Group, Sacramento, CA, USA

Michael Gutman, BA Rothman Institute, Philadelphia, PA, USA

Clayton Haldeman, MD Department of Neurosurgery, University of Wisconsin School of Medicine and Public Health, Madison, WI, USA

Robert E. Harbaugh, MD, FAANS, FACS, FAHA Department of Neurosurgery, Penn State University, Milton S. Hershey Medical Center, Hershey, PA, USA

Omid R. Hariri, DO, MSc Department of Neurosurgery, Stanford University School of Medicine, Stanford, CA, USA

Jessica Harris, MS, RD Surgical Outcomes and Analysis, Southern California Permanente Medical Group, San Diego, CA, USA

Allen L. Ho, MD Department of Neurosurgery, Stanford University School of Medicine, Stanford, CA, USA

Michael James Hutton, MBBS, BSc, FRCS Princess Elisabeth Orthopaedic Centre, Royal Devon & Exeter Hospital, Exeter, UK

Motoki Iwasaki, MD, PhD Department of Orthopaedic Surgery, Osaka Rosai Hospital, Osaka University Graduate School of Medicine, Sakai, Japan

David A. Janiec, MBA Rothman Institute, Philadelphia, PA, USA

Kareem J. Kebaish, BA Department of Orthopaedics and Rehabilitation, Yale University School of Medicine, New Haven, CT, USA

Jack Knightly, MD Atlantic Neurosurgical Specialists, Morristown, NJ, USA

Sandro M. Krieg, MD, MBA Department of Neurosurgery, Universitätsklinikum rechts der Isar der Technischen Universität München, Munich, Germany

Virginie Lafage, PhD Hospital for Special Surgery, New York, NY, USA

Mayan Lendner, BS Rothman Institute, Philadelphia, PA, USA

Catherine H. MacLean, MD, PhD Center for the Advancement of Value in Musculoskeletal Care, Hospital for Special Surgery, New York, NY, USA

Gabriel S. Makar, BS Rothman Institute, Philadelphia, PA, USA

Bernhard Meyer, MD Department of Neurosurgery, Universitätsklinikum rechts der Isar der Technischen Universität München, Munich, Germany

John E. O'Toole, MD, MS Rush University Medical Center, Chicago, IL, USA

Griffin H. Olsen, MD Surgical Services Clinical Program, Intermountain Healthcare, Murray, UT, USA

Taylor D. Ottesen, BS Department of Orthopaedics and Rehabilitation, Yale University School of Medicine, New Haven, CT, USA

Mark J. Ott, MD Central Region Administration, Intermountain Healthcare, Murray, UT, USA

Paul Samuel Page, MD Department of Neurosurgery, University of Wisconsin School of Medicine and Public Health, Madison, WI, USA

Tejbir Singh Pannu, MD, MS Hospital for Special Surgery, New York, NY, USA

Arjun Vivek Pendharkar, MD Department of Neurosurgery, Stanford University School of Medicine, Stanford, CA, USA

Zach Pennington, BS Department of Neurosurgery, Johns Hopkins Hospital, Baltimore, MD, USA

Xiang Qian, MD, PhD Anesthesiology, Preoperative and Pain Medicine, Stanford University School of Medicine, Stanford, CA, USA

John Ratliff, MD Department of Neurosurgery, Stanford University, Stanford, CA, USA

Daniel K. Resnick, MD, MS Department of Neurosurgery, University of Wisconsin School of Medicine and Public Health, Madison, WI, USA

Pratik Rohatgi, MD Department of Neurosurgery, Penn State University, Milton S. Hershey Medical Center, Hershey, PA, USA

Satish Rudrappa, MCh, FASS, FRCS Neurosciences Department, Sakra World Hospital, Bangalore, Karnataka, India

Clemens M. Schirmer, MD, PhD Comprehensive Stroke Center, Department of Neurosurgery and Neuroscience Institute, Geisinger, Danville, PA, USA

Frank J. Schwab, MD Hospital for Special Surgery, New York, NY, USA

Jonathan P. Scoville, MD Department of Neurosurgery, Clinical Neurosciences Center, University of Utah, Salt Lake City, UT, USA

Ehab Shiban, PD Dr. med. Department of Neurosurgery, Universitätsklinikum rechts der Isar der Technischen Universität München, Munich, Germany

Eric S. Sussman, MD Department of Neurosurgery, Stanford University School of Medicine, Stanford, CA, USA

Ariel Takayanagi, DO Department of Neurosurgery, Riverside University Health Systems, Moreno Valley, CA, USA

Luis M. Tumialán, MD Department of Neurosurgery, Barrow Neurological Institute, St. Joseph's Hospital and Medical Center, Phoenix, AZ, USA

Alexander R. Vaccaro, MD, PhD, MBA Rothman Institute, Philadelphia, PA, USA

Sushrut S. Vaidya, BA Economics Department, International College of Liberal Arts (iCLA), Kofu, Yamanashi Prefecture, Japan

Christina Vannello, BSN Rothman Institute, Philadelphia, PA, USA

Arvin R. Wali, MD Department of Neurosurgery, University of California San Diego, San Diego, CA, USA

Michael E. West, BBA, CPA, MBA Rothman Institute, Philadelphia, PA, USA

Corinna C. Zygourakis, MD Department of Neurosurgery, Johns Hopkins Hospital, Baltimore, MD, USA

Part I

Historical Aspects

Historical Aspects of Quality in Healthcare

1

Omid R. Hariri, Ariel Takayanagi, T. J. Florence, and Arvin R. Wali

Introduction: Quality in Healthcare

Quality. 1. [noun] the standard of something as measured against other things of a similar kind; the degree of excellence of something. [1]

Optimization of patient value should be at the center of any successful healthcare system [2]. This can be achieved by maximizing the quality of care while minimizing costs. This is demonstrated in Michael Porter's healthcare value equation (value = quality/cost) in which value is a function of benefit and cost.

In a patient-centered healthcare system, the numerator, quality, should be measured in terms of outcomes that matter to patients [3]. The most widely used clinical measures for quality, such as the Physician Quality Reporting System, are process measures. Although process measures are easier to obtain than outcomes measures and are valuable in assessing diagnostic and procedural practices, they do not necessarily correlate with outcomes [4]. In order to create treatment algorithms based on outcomes rather than process, the Patient Protection and Affordable Care Act has created provisions such as the Patient-Centered Outcomes Research Institute to identify the most effective forms of treatment [4, 5].

O. R. Hariri (✉)
Department of Neurosurgery, Stanford University School of Medicine, Stanford, CA, USA
e-mail: ohariri@stanford.edu

A. Takayanagi
Department of Neurosurgery, Riverside University Health Systems, Moreno Valley, CA, USA

T. J. Florence
Columbia College of Physicians and Surgeons, New York, NY, USA

A. R. Wali
Department of Neurosurgery, University of California San Diego, San Diego, CA, USA

J. Ratliff et al. (eds.), *Quality Spine Care*,
https://doi.org/10.1007/978-3-319-97990-8_1

The International Consortium for Health Outcomes Measurement (ICHOM) was founded on the principles described in Michael Porter's and Elizabeth Teisburg's *Redefining Healthcare* principles. ICHOM works with physicians, patients, and registries, to create a global standard for outcome measures according to medical condition.

Porter stratifies outcomes that matter to patients into a tier system to better define healthcare quality for patients. This comprehensive assessment of quality includes the direct outcomes (mortality and degree of recovery from the medical condition), failures in the treatment process, time of recovery, and long-term outcomes [3]. Improving quality in any of these realms can reduce cost and increase the value of care. A recent version of the equation has incorporated "service," or patient satisfaction (value = (quality+service)/cost), to include the patient's evaluation of the care received [6].

Many approaches exist to reduce cost, the denominator in the value equation. One approach is to focus on reducing costs in the highest-cost patients [5]. Porter and ICHOM's approach is to measure cost as the total expense incurred for the full cycle of care for the specific medical condition across specialties, rather than dividing cost by specialty or type of service. This allows for a patient-centered measurement of cost [7].

Although patient value should be at the center of the healthcare system, it is important to consider the impact that quality of care has on other stakeholders as well.

Stakeholders in Quality of Care

Quality of care can be considered in terms of three stakeholders: the patient, the payer, and society.

The Patient

Quality of healthcare is determined by the system's ability to meet the patient's individual needs. Most important is the ability to provide well-planned care and manage a patient's medical condition by providing necessary treatment options. For example, a patient who suffers from severe back pain due to metastatic spinal disease may not be able to sustain open back surgery but may benefit from minimally invasive techniques such as cement augmentation or separation surgery [8]. The availability of such options helps to meet a patient's needs and increase the quality of provided care.

Another patient interest to consider is functional status. Not only does it affect a patient's autonomy and quality of life but also his or her ability to earn wages and provide for one's family [9].

Although providing service that leads to patient satisfaction is important, the patient's perception of quality of care does not necessarily correlate with health status. In a study that examined the relationship between quality of surgical spine care and patient satisfaction, improvement in quality of life and improvement in general health were not associated with patient satisfaction [10]. In addition, perception of quality of care may be influenced by socioeconomic status, educational, and cultural backgrounds [11].

The Payer

In short, payers foot the proximal costs of health treatments – the literal common denominator of the Utah value equation. Naively, one expects payers to work to minimize costs. Yet payers in the United States represent a heterogenous group: the American healthcare system is an amalgam of different payer entities. Thus what constitutes cost minimization, and therefore value maximization, for payers in practice is a nuanced question affected by incentives unique to each group. Here we will consider three views of the payer perspective of value in spine care: from large government agencies like Medicare, from private insurance companies, and from society as a whole.

Government Agencies

The US government runs two massive healthcare payer agencies in Medicare and Medicaid. Across all programs, the government is responsible for paying for the care of roughly 107 million people at a total cost of $1.2 trillion/year [12]. Several factors make government agencies particularly sensitive to emphasizing high-value, high-quality procedures. Foremost is the dual challenge of rising enrollment and rising medical costs in the setting of the political impossibility of significant budget expansion. Moreover, Medicare patients represent an elder segment of the US population; medical expenditures for those 65 and older are roughly three times higher than someone closer to the median US citizen ($18,988 vs $6632) [13]. Finally, Medicare cares for patients over the long term – essentially from enrollment to the grave. These pressures likely account for the recent heavy focus on quality assessment with the Performance Quality Rating System (PQRS). From a neurosurgical perspective, PQRS is notable for its emphasis on measuring and explicitly improving functional outcomes after treatment along the neuraxis. In effect, the Centers for Medicare and Medicaid Services (CMS) has challenged spine surgeons to demonstrate the value of their procedures.

Private Health Insurance

Private health insurance remains the majority payment model in the US health system. Estimates vary, but roughly two thirds of Americans are covered by private health insurance plans at a total cost of $1.1 trillion dollars per year. Probability of private coverage is associated with both income and full-versus-part-time working status; thus the privately insured population tends to be wealthier (and therefore healthier) than the publicly insured. Moreover, insurance is closely tied to one's employment: around 80% of all private insurance policies are employer-provided policies.

This has interesting consequences for the incentive structure of private insurance companies. The customers of private insurance companies are most often not patients themselves but their employers. For publicly traded companies, ultimate responsibility lies with creating value for shareholders. Moreover, in the modern economy, employment durations may be brief; loss of employment leads to loss of coverage. Indeed, in a 3-year period from January 2009 to December 2012, 35.1 percent of Americans were uninsured for at least 1 month. The average period without insurance was 17.4 months, or more than half of that period. Thus a single private insurance company is relatively decoupled from the long-term consequences of a given procedure. An efficacious procedure from the perspective of private insurance is one with minimal operative costs for a given indication, short recovery time, and proven efficacy in the near-to-middle term. All told, private insurance companies wield significant influence in shaping current practices via selective reimbursement of procedures. These factors likely shape the apparent arbitrariness with which these decisions are reached [14].

Society

Ultimately, society bears the cost of all healthcare expenditures. Every dollar spent on healthcare is one not spent on infrastructure, science, or education. All told, the United States spent $3.3 trillion on healthcare expenditures in 2016. This represents outlays of roughly $10,350 per person, or 17% of gross domestic product. These numbers are only projected to grow. It is a tired fact by now that on a per-dollar basis, health outcomes in the United States are significantly worse than similar western industrialized countries.

As political and economic pressure builds to address these disparities, surgeons can play a leading role in ensuring system-wide quality. The public requires surgeons who offer validated, reliable procedures only when indicated. We must continue our efforts to minimize complications and prevent reoperations. While these are characteristics common to good surgeons, perhaps less appreciated are their cumulative effects on the health system as a whole.

Society

The interest of the entire population must be considered when evaluating quality of care in terms of society as a whole [15]. Because society spans across more than one generation, the goals for achieving high-quality care are long term [16]. For example, a society may invest in preventative care to decrease healthcare expenses of preventable diseases.

Clear guidelines on patient selection for treatment are beneficial to prevent unnecessary costs to society. In a study of elderly patients who underwent surgery for lumbar spinal stenosis, comorbid disease and increasing age were shown to be associated with an increased risk of major complications, rehospitalization, and discharge to skilled nursing facility; all of which are costly to society [17].

In addition to reducing direct medical care expenses, careful patient selection may prevent loss of productivity. A study examining risk factors for loss of work productivity after surgery for lumbar disc herniation revealed that patients with severe disability and poor motivation to work were more likely to require an extended time off work [18]. The study suggests that patients who are at risk of a poor outcome should receive vocational counseling and early rehabilitation in order to prevent a loss of employment. Incorporating measures to prevent unemployment into healthcare may help patients return to work sooner and continue to contribute to society.

Historical Perspectives on Assessing Quality in Spinal Surgery

Introduction

Over the years, surgeons care deeply about providing their patients high-quality procedures; patients themselves must trust their surgeons to provide high-quality care. Ongoing assessment of quality in spinal surgery remains fundamental to ensuring acceptable outcomes, solidifying trust between patient and provider, and improving the practice altogether. Toward these goals, spine surgeons require tools to assess current practices and new procedures. Ideally, such measures should be objective, easy to administer, and standardized to facilitate comparison.

While today discussions of quality of care may be dominated by the Centers for Medicare and Medicaid Services' Physician Quality Reporting System (CMS PQRS), physicians have been interested in the objective assessment of the effectiveness of their interventions throughout the history of modern medicine. In this section, we will trace the evolution of objective quality assessment in spinal surgery from the twentieth century to the present. As we will see, this development occurred in a saltatory fashion. It remains interesting to consider societal and resource constraints driving development.

Early Period (1930s–1980s)

The earliest modern tool for assessing outcome quality in bony surgery is the Massachusetts General Hospital Anatomic Economic Functional Rating System (MGHAEF) [19]. Developed in the late 1920s by the Fracture Service at MGH, it was popularized during the early 1930s during the height of the Great Depression. Originally applied to measure outcomes of reduction of compound fracture of the lower limb, this scale is remarkably modern. Authors of MGHAEF recognized the need to report the multidimensional outcomes of surgical treatment, both on the bone itself and on the life of the patient.

The scale consists of three dimensions, each scored from zero to four. The anatomic limb exploited the then-recent proliferation of medical X-ray imaging to evaluate the success of intervention on bone healing, with aligned healing as the

Table 1.1 The Massachusetts General Hospital Anatomic Economic Functional Rating System as applied to spinal fusion surgery

Anatomic		Economic		Functional	
A0	Pseudarthrosis	E0	Completely invalid	F0	Pain worse than before surgery
A1	Unilateral pseudarthrosis	E1	No gainful occupation	F1	Pain the same as before surgery; can perform daily tasks of living
A2	Insufficient unilateral fusion mass	E2	Able to work but did not return to previous occupation	F2	Low level of pain; able to perform all activities except sport
A3	Contiguous fusion mass without hypertrophy	E3	Returned to previous occupation in limited status	F3	Rare, brief recurrences of pain or sciatica
A4	Solid fusion with hypertrophy	E4	Returned to previous occupation without restriction	F4	No pain even during sport

Data from Vanti et al. [20]

best outcome and pseudarthrosis as the worst. The economic outcome dimension evaluated a patient's capacity to return to work at >1 year, with return to work without restriction as the desired outcome and completely invalid as the least desirable. The functional limb concerned a patient's pain. On this scale, highest scores were awarded to pain-free patients, and lowest scores were assigned to patients whose pain increased following surgery. Complete scores were recorded in compound notation: thus a patient with a perfect outcome would be reported as $A_4E_4F_4$, a convention that would carry forward.

Over decades, this scale was modified ad hoc to suit the needs of inquiring surgeons on their area of expertise. A complete, modern version of MGHAEF applied to spine fusion surgery is demonstrated in Table 1.1 [20].

Modern Assessments (1980s–Present)

During the 1980s, as aging baby boomers began to experience the consequences of spine degeneration, spine surgery quality metric assessments were revisited. The first conceptually significant example is work done by Dawson et al. [21] in a case series of 58 patients undergoing lumbar arthrodesis via autologous bone graft. Patients were graded via a modified MGHAEF scale both pre- and postoperatively; as the goal of surgery was not to achieve normal preoperative anatomy, the anatomic scale was dropped from preoperative assessment. Importantly, though successful fusion was observed in 92% of cases, economic and functional improvements were noted in only 70–80%.

To critics of the MGHAEF method, this suggested that ultimate impact on the patient may be a more salient feature of quality assessment, even as surgeons strive for technical perfection. This idea was likely at the forefront of the mind of Donald

Table 1.2 The Prolo scale

Economic		Functional	
E1	Completely invalid	F1	Total incapacity (or worse than before operation)
E2	No gainful occupation (including housework or retirement activities)	F2	Mild-moderate level of low back pain and/or sciatica (or pain the same as before but able to perform ADLs)
E3	Able to work not at previous occupation	F3	Low level of pain; able to perform all activities except sport
E4	Working at previous occupation at part time or limited status	F4	Rare, brief recurrences of pain or sciatica
E5	Able to work at previous occupation without restriction	F5	No pain even during sport

Data from Vanti et al. [20] and Prolo et al. [22]

J. Prolo, MD, as he developed his eponymous scale for quantitative assessment of lumbar surgery outcomes [20]. Originally outlined in a case series of 34 patients undergoing posterior laminar interbody fusion (PLIF), the Prolo scale is bidimensional: only economic and functional outcomes contribute to a patient's score. Explicit rating of anatomical outcome is dropped completely. Along the remaining dimensions, outcomes are classified along a scale from 1 to 5. Along the economic axis, these outcomes range from E1 (complete invalid) to E5 (able to return to work without restriction). Along the functional axis, outcome rage from F1 (total incapacity, or worse than before surgery) to F5 (complete recovery, no pain even with sport). Outcomes are also noted in compound notation; thus the best possible score on the Prolo scale would be reported E_5F_5.

This approach has distinct advantages. First, it is aligned with clinical reasoning: mild anatomic imperfections not causing symptoms are by definition clinically insignificant; conversely, a patient presenting with pain would only have anatomy evaluated secondarily. Moreover, without an imaging requirement, the scale is significantly cheaper and easier to administer. It is robust to retroactive application even in the face of incomplete records. Third, without specific anatomical scoring, the scale is easily generalizable to multiple regions of the body. Finally, non-zero integer notation allows for ratiometric comparison of functional status before and after surgery within single patients. The complete Prolo scale is demonstrated in Table 1.2.

Legislative Assessments of Quality

The development of spine-specific metrics for quality assessment occurred in parallel to an evolving social and legal framework for evaluating quality of medical care more generally. As these considerations tend to dominate discussions of quality, it is worth briefly discussing their development here.

The creation of Medicare and Medicaid in 1965 led to a need to ensure basic measures of quality and consistency of medical care. To this end, Congress created a set of "Conditions of Participation" or requirements hospitals must meet to receive payments from these programs. Such requirements included round-the-clock nursing and complete staff credentialing and submission to utilization review. This practice review was performed by a rotation of several official bodies: In 1972, the task fell to Utilization Review Committees (URCs), which were widely seen as ineffective due to absence of formal evaluation criteria. Soon after, URCs gave way to Professional Standards Review Organizations (PSROs), networks of physician-run nonprofits mandated to evaluate provided quality of care. Unable to contain costs, PSROs were replaced Peer Review Organizations (PROs) in 1983. These new PROs had a more specific mission to reduce complication, readmission, and mortality; moreover, they were given authority to implement solutions. The PRO model is generally accepted to be more successful than prior review bodies and continues to play a role under Centers for Medicare and Medicaid Services. These efforts by Congress to ensure care quality via legislation are supplemented by nonprofit organizations, including the Joint Commission on Accreditation of Hospitals (JCAH) and the National Academy of Medicine (formerly the Institute of Medicine).

Contemporary efforts toward quality improvement have trended toward incentivized public reporting. Surgical teams lead this trend with the establishment of the Surgical Care Improvement Program (SCIP) in 2003. Aimed at reducing surgical complications and mortality, SCIP constituted a voluntary reporting database with payments provided by Medicare for participation. The SCIP blueprint was used to develop the Physician Quality Reporting System (PQRS) created by Congress with the passage of the Affordable Care Act (ACA) in 2010 [4].

Future of Quality Assessment

Current Quality Assessment Metrics

Several methods are available to assess the quality of life of patients. These quality assessments may be collected at any point during a patient's medical or surgical treatment plan. Metrics typically utilized for quality assessment include patient questionnaires such as the SF-36, EuroQol, or Oswestry Disability Index [23–25]. These metrics serve as markers of efficacy for clinical interventions or may be mathematically converted into health utility scores such as quality-adjusted life years (QALYs) providing a more robust means of measuring clinical outcome than with longevity alone.

Given the diversity of terminology and metrics used in quality-of-life questionnaires, the National Institutes of Health (NIH) in 2004 led a multicenter initiative to develop the Patient-Reported Outcomes Measurement Information System (PROMIS) to further standardize, validate, and enhance patient-reported outcomes (PROs) across multiple medical conditions [26]. Embracing the electronical health record (EHR), PROMIS utilizes computer adaptive tests (CATs) to assess for severity of numerous symptoms such as pain, fatigue, depression, anxiety, and physical functionality for patients with diverse medical conditions [26, 27]. PROMIS has the potential to unify PROs in an efficient, computerized manner with consistent recorded values and terminology to serve as a universal quality assessment for all patients [28].

Integration of Quality Metrics into EHR Systems

The future of quality assessment lies in the capacity of the EHR to serve as a data repository for PROs to capture quality-of-life information for millions of patients at different intervals of their treatment. Efforts such as PROMIS offer the possibility of creating a universal quality assessment language to describe patient quality of life during any treatment plan for any medical condition in any healthcare setting. As clinicians become more familiar with quality assessment, these metrics and questionnaires will become routinely collected clinical variables similar to the collection of vital signs or physical exam findings. Prior investigations have demonstrated the feasibility of collecting quality assessment data utilizing the EHR as part of routine clinical work flow without prolonging average visit time for each patient [29]. Big data analytics of this large volume of clinical data will provide greater validity and public access to these clinical parameters and will bring greater insight into nuances in treatment plans that may enhance quality of life for particular patient groups.

Cost-Utility and Cost-Effectiveness Research

As patient quality-of-life information becomes increasingly available to clinicians and health professionals, utilization of this data will lead to greater quality-driven care. Health utility models and cost-effectiveness studies are already increasingly utilized to capture the cost-efficacy of neurosurgical interventions and provide quantification of the quality of life impact as well as social cost implications of surgical interventions [30]. Investigations in cost-effectiveness of interventions allow for mathematical modeling to determine if the gains in quality of life after medical or surgical interventions justify the individual or social costs incurred by that treatment [31, 32]. Through having consistent, high-quality data that captures quality of life before and after interventions, quality of cost-effectiveness studies will further guide patient management and health policy.

Conclusion

It is evident that in the new era of medicine, assessment of quality will continue to be vital in patient counseling and the overall care provided. Profound understanding of quality should be emphasized early on during medical education. Moreover, better integration of quality metrics into clinical practice will improve overall patient care and outcomes.

Creation of a more comprehensive quality measure will require more perspectives from other healthcare systems to be obtained. Understanding the architecture, success, and challenges faced by other systems will aid in assessing scalability of quality assessment internationally.

References

1. Quality | Definition of quality in English by Oxford dictionaries [Internet]. Oxf Dictionaries Engl [cited 2018 Jun 7]. Available from: https://en.oxforddictionaries.com/definition/quality
2. Porter ME, Thomas H, Lee MD. The strategy that will fix health care. Harv Bus Rev [Internet]. 2013 [cited 2018 Jun 8]. Available from: https://hbr.org/2013/10/the-strategy-that-will-fix-health-care
3. Porter ME. What is value in health care? N Engl J Med. 2010;363:2477–81.
4. Marjoua Y, Bozic KJ. Brief history of quality movement in US healthcare. Curr Rev Musculoskelet Med. 2012;5:265–73.
5. Parekh AK. Revisiting health care's value equation. Milbank Q [Internet]. 2015 [cited 2018 Jun 7]. Available from: https://www.milbank.org/quarterly/articles/revisiting-health-cares-value-equation/
6. Makadon HJ, Bharucha F, Gavin M, Oliveira J, Wietecha M. Value management: optimizing quality, service, and cost. J Healthc Qual. 32:29–34.
7. Measuring outcomes – Institute for strategy and competitiveness – Harvard Business School [Internet]. [cited 2018 Jun 8]. Available from: https://www.isc.hbs.edu/health-care/vbhcd/Pages/measuring-outcomes.aspx
8. Hariri O, Takayanagi A, Miulli DE, Siddiqi J, Vrionis F. Minimally invasive surgical techniques for management of painful metastatic and primary spinal tumors. Cureus. 2017;9:e1114.
9. Nuckols TK, Escarce JJ, Asch SM. The effects of quality of care on costs: a conceptual framework. Milbank Q. 2013;91:316–53.
10. Godil SS, Parker SL, Zuckerman SL, Mendenhall SK, Devin CJ, Asher AL, et al. Determining the quality and effectiveness of surgical spine care: patient satisfaction is not a valid proxy. Spine J. 2013;13:1006–12.
11. Cleary PD, Edgman-Levitan S. Health care quality. Incorporating consumer perspectives. JAMA. 1997;278:1608–12.
12. Smith J, Medalia C. Health Insurance Coverage in the United States: 2014 [Internet]. Census.gov. [cited 2018 Jun 10]. Available from: https://www.census.gov/library/publications/2015/demo/p60-253.html
13. Medicare C for, Baltimore MS 7500 SB, Usa M. NHE-Fact-Sheet [Internet]. 2018 [cited 2018 Jun 10]. Available from: https://www.cms.gov/research-statistics-data-and-systems/statistics-trends-and-reports/nationalhealthexpenddata/nhe-fact-sheet.html
14. Vaccaro AR, Bono CM. The future direction of minimally invasive surgery: is its fate controlled by the physician, patient, industry, or insurance? Minim Invasive Spine Surg. CRC Press; 2007.
15. Campbell SM, Roland MO, Buetow SA. Defining quality of care. Soc Sci Med. 2000;51:1611–25.
16. Caveats to consider when calculating healthcare value – The American Journal of Medicine [Internet]. [cited 2018 Jun 8]. Available from: https://www.amjmed.com/article/S0002-9343(14)01087-0/fulltext
17. Deyo RA, Mirza SK, Martin BI, Kreuter W, Goodman DC, Jarvik JG. Trends, major medical complications, and charges associated with surgery for lumbar spinal stenosis in older adults. JAMA. 2010;303:1259–65.
18. Puolakka K, Ylinen J, Neva MH, Kautiainen H, Häkkinen A. Risk factors for back pain-related loss of working time after surgery for lumbar disc herniation: a 5-year follow-up study. Eur Spine J. 2008;17:386–92.
19. Kennedy RH. Fracture of the shaft of both bones of the leg. Ann Surg. 1931;93:563–86.
20. Vanti C, Prosperi D, Boschi M. The Prolo Scale: history, evolution and psychometric properties. J Orthop Traumatol. 2013;14:235–45.
21. Dawson EG, Lotysch M, Urist MR. Intertransverse process lumbar arthrodesis with autogenous bone graft. Clin Orthop. 1981:90–6.

22. Prolo DJ, Oklund SA, Butcher M. Toward uniformity in evaluating results of lumbar spine operations. A paradigm applied to posterior lumbar interbody fusions. Spine. 1986;11:601–6.
23. Brazier JE, Roberts J. The estimation of a preference-based measure of health from the SF-12. Med Care. 2004;42:851–9.
24. Fairbank JC, Pynsent PB. The Oswestry disability index. Spine. 2000;25:2940–52. discussion 2952
25. Williams A. The role of the Euroqol instrument in QALY calculations [Internet]. Centre for Health Economics, University of York; 1995 Mar. Report No.: 130chedp. Available from: https://ideas.repec.org/p/chy/respap/130chedp.html
26. Gershon RC, Rothrock N, Hanrahan R, Bass M, Cella D. The use of PROMIS and assessment center to deliver patient-reported outcome measures in clinical research. J Appl Meas. 2010;11:304–14.
27. Wagner LI, Schink J, Bass M, Patel S, Diaz MV, Rothrock N, et al. Bringing PROMIS to practice: brief and precise symptom screening in ambulatory cancer care. Cancer. 2015;121:927–34.
28. Alonso J, Bartlett SJ, Rose M, Aaronson NK, Chaplin JE, Efficace F, et al. The case for an international patient-reported outcomes measurement information system (PROMIS®) initiative. Health Qual Life Outcomes. 2013, 11:210.
29. Azad TD, Kalani M, Wolf T, Kearney A, Lee Y, Flannery L, et al. Building an electronic health record integrated quality of life outcomes registry for spine surgery. J Neurosurg Spine. 2016;24:176–85.
30. Wali AR, Brandel MG, Santiago-Dieppa DR, Rennert RC, Steinberg JA, Hirshman BR, et al. Markov modeling for the neurosurgeon: a review of the literature and an introduction to cost-effectiveness research. Neurosurg Focus. 2018;44:E20.
31. Shepard DS. Cost-effectiveness in health and medicine. In: Gold MR, Siegel JE, Russell LB, Weinstein MC, editors. New York: Oxford University Press; 1996. J Ment Health Policy Econ 2:91–2.
32. Weinstein MC, Stason WB. Foundations of cost-effectiveness analysis for health and medical practices. N Engl J Med. 1977;296:716–21.

Quality and Standardization of Medical Education

2

Jonathan P. Scoville and Erica F. Bisson

Abbreviations

AAMC	Association of American Medical Colleges
ACGME	Accreditation Council for Graduate Medical Education
AMA	American Medical Association
CACMS	Committee on Accreditation of Canadian Medical Schools
EMR	Electronic Medical Record
LCME	Liaison Committee on Medical Education
MSPE	Medical Student Performance Evaluation
SLOE	Standardized Letter of Evaluation
USN&WR	US News and World Report
USMLE	United States Medical Licensing Examination

Introduction

As medical schools in the United States and around the world attempt to balance the principles of standardization, modernization, and tradition, they may struggle to maintain focus on the core values of education while implementing more modern or at times more politically expedient methods of teaching. These goals of expediency and education are often paradoxical, because although the ultimate goal of medical education should be to create a physician and lifelong learner with the tools necessary to succeed in a chosen specialty, medical students and residency programs alike feel that student preparation at times falls short [1]. Whereas the aim for medical

J. P. Scoville · E. F. Bisson (✉)
Department of Neurosurgery, Clinical Neurosciences Center, University of Utah, Salt Lake City, UT, USA
e-mail: erica.bisson@hsc.utah.edu

J. Ratliff et al. (eds.), *Quality Spine Care*,
https://doi.org/10.1007/978-3-319-97990-8_2

schools has been to train a practitioner with the requisite medical skill set, a residency program expects to receive incoming students with the knowledge to apply the principles of medicine to dynamic disease processes [2]. Therefore, the quality of a medical school education is reflected in its ability to produce resident physicians that have not only the basic knowledge but also the correct resources for learning their respective craft. Thus, the true measure of the quality of medical education that students receive is directly correlated with their success or graduation from residency training programs [3].

Throughout this chapter, we will explore the status of medical education today and attempt to measure its quality overall. We will explore innovative curricula and the attitudes of students toward the changing paradigms in medical education. We will then look at the challenges that face medical schools as they endeavor to produce a high-quality product, including standards of accreditation and how the integration of technology has hindered or helped medical students. Lastly, we will address the questions of resident attrition and why it occurs. Quality measures in medical school education should be as stringent as those applied to medical practice; we cannot hold the future doctors of the world to standards that are either nontransparent or nonexistent.

Quality in Medical School Education

Quality in medical school education for schools leading to the MD degree is currently determined by the Liaison Committee on Medical Education (LCME), which is jointly sponsored by the American Medical Association (AMA) and the Association of American Medical Colleges (AAMC) and approved by the US Department of Education. MD programs in Canada are sponsored by the Committee on Accreditation of Canadian Medical Schools (CACMS). In the United States, the committee is made up of appointed representatives from parent organizations that include current medical students and educators. The purpose of this committee is to establish accreditation criteria and make site visits to schools that seek first-time or renewal accreditation by the LCME. The committee judges the quality of medical school education by developing and enforcing standards that are updated and published on a year-to-year basis as "The Functions and Structure of a Medical School." This document details 12 standards that cover diverse aspects of the structure of medical school education including curricular design and content, academic leadership, learning environments, and student selection (Table 2.1). The LCME states that its main mandate is to assure that medical schools "provide assurances that its graduates exhibit general professional competencies that are appropriate for entry to the next stage of their training and that serve as the foundation for lifelong learning and proficient medical care."

Table 2.1 Standards of medical education defined by the Liaison Committee on Medical Education (LCME)

Standard	Definition	Comments
1. Mission, planning, organization, and integrity	Requires that each school has a quality improvement committee and provides students with access to appropriate learning materials	There is no specified structure to quality improvement, except that the school must establish short- and long-term goals
2. Leadership and administration	States that each school must have enough staff with appropriate qualifications to provide quality instruction	Vague terminology about teaching qualifications left up to the school and LCME to define
3. Academic and learning environments	Promotes the role of resident-led education, diversity, respect, and professional standards	Only one clinical experience is required
4. Faculty preparation, productivity and policies	Focuses on faculty appointment and promotion, including continual scholarly pursuits	The appointment and promotion process is left up to the schools, with no specific milestones mentioned
5. Educational resources and infrastructure	Defines that each school must have the necessary funds to provide adequate buildings, study space, library, and technology support to its students	Specific language used to promote adequate infrastructure necessary to medical school education
6. Competencies, curricular objectives, and curricular design	States that all schools must provide detailed learning objectives, which must be met by each student, including clinical experiences in the out- and inpatient settings, with at least 130 weeks of instruction	No specifics on how learning objectives are to be met, leaving the requirements and method by which they are accomplished up to the respective faculty
7. Curricular content	Ensures that medical curriculum includes content from biomedical, behavioral, and socioeconomic sciences, including content and clinical experiences from each organ system. Schools must include teaching on medical ethics, communication skills, and problem-solving skills	While this is the most complete and specific section, the responsibility for defining how these principles are taught and how the students accomplish them is left up to the faculty of the school
8. Curricular management, evaluation and enhancement	Establishes a faculty committee to ensure that there is continual review and enrichment of learning objectives. Programs must be continually and internally evaluated by using outcome data to compare themselves with the national norms	The use of outcome data including national norms is important for medical schools to be held accountable to a national quality level; however, there is no mention of at what point a change must be made or what is included in the outcome data

(continued)

Table 2.1 (continued)

Standard	Definition	Comments
9. Teaching, supervision, assessment, and student and patient safety	Establishes centralized system for assuring adequate assessment of medical student achievement, including clinical skills, and medical knowledge, with formative feedback, in a fair and timely manner	All formative feedback must be provided within 6 weeks. Although a manner for student feedback and assessment is set up, the determination of actual student achievement is left up to the faculty
10. Medical student selection, assignment, and progress	Details standards for medical student selection, such as technical skills and the intelligence, integrity, and personal and emotional characteristics necessary for them to become competent physicians	Although standards are promoted for medical school applicants, the ultimate decision for admission is left up to the admission committee
11. Medical student academic support, career advising, and educational records	Establishes the Medical Student Performance Evaluation (MSPE), a formal assessment meeting for residency preparation to be held in the 4th year, as well as career and academic advisement services including tutoring services	The qualifications of tutoring service are not discussed. The exact subject matter discussed in the MSPE is not detailed
12. Medical student health services, personal counseling, and financial aid services	Includes provisions for financial aid, health and disability insurance, and personal counseling programs	Provides standards for basic well-being of students

Although the 12 standards are comprehensive in their coverage of the various supplemental services needed in providing the necessary support for graduation, the establishment of curriculum is left entirely up to the respective medical schools and their faculty. This also includes the establishment of learning objectives and how each medical school assesses the adequate completion of each objective for each student. Therefore, although the LCME provides an outline of what a curriculum should include, the ultimate evaluation of medical education is left up to the individual institution. While emphasis is placed on the preparation of medical students for residency programs, there is only one mandated evaluation meeting designed to specifically address this question, and it occurs before October 1 of the student's final year. This single evaluation meeting may not be adequate to assess a student's preparedness, suggesting that there should be a more standardized timeline in which to evaluate students. Overall quality in medical school education as defined by the LCME is the level to which each school's graduates are prepared for residency, and while the 12 standards attempt to outline the necessary structure medical education must follow to achieve this, they are too vague in defining the manner in which they should be applied.

Medical Curriculum

Although the curriculum of each medical school is ultimately determined by the respective medical school's curriculum committee, the curriculum must include at least 130 weeks of medical student education that incorporates biomedical, behavioral, and socioeconomic sciences as well as content and clinical experiences related to "each organ system; each phase of the human life cycle; continuity of care; and preventive, acute, chronic, rehabilitative, end-of-life, and primary care." This training should enable students to reach certain defined goals. A graduating student should be able to "recognize wellness, determinants of health, and opportunities for health promotion and disease prevention; recognize and interpret symptoms and signs of disease; develop differential diagnoses and treatment plans; recognize the potential health-related impact on patients of behavioral and socioeconomic factors, [and] assist patients in addressing health-related issues involving all organ systems." It is up to the medical school curriculum committee, which should be made up of faculty and students, to translate this mandate into a 130-week program designed not only to cover the primary objectives as stated above but also to prepare students for their standardized tests. The only regulation of this curriculum is the LCME accreditation process, which requires review and approval by the LCME and site visits that are designed to assess its application. However, the primary end point of this approval process is to make sure that the curriculum covers all of the required material, rather than evaluating whether graduating students have actually learned from the curriculum. For instance, assessing the success of previous graduates may provide a more concrete assessment of a school's quality.

Since 1910, medical school education has been based on the principles proposed by Abraham Flexner in his original attempt to standardize the quality of medical school education. This standardization was called for by physicians of the time, because it was thought that too many medical schools focused too much on profit and graduated "ill-prepared medical men" [4]. Flexner's work helped create the now-traditional 4-year medical school curriculum that consists of the first 2 years of didactic training and the second 2 years of clinical work. Over the past 2 decades, however, Flexner's model has started to change, as medical schools across the country have started to incorporate clinical experiences earlier in the curriculum, with longitudinal clinical mentoring programs in which students dedicate time each week to clinical work throughout their first 2 years [5, 6]. Medical schools have also changed their didactic schedule from one based on the so-called "block" schedule, which focused more on one core subject at a time, to a "system-based" schedule, which incorporates the core subjects such as pharmacology, anatomy, and physiology into the corresponding organ systems [7]. The 4-year model has also been challenged, with medical school across the United States, including Duke University and Columbia University, finishing their entire didactic course within the first year, leaving the second and third for clinical experiences and the fourth for elective work and research [8]. This 3-year medical education experiment was also used during World War II as well as in the 1970s because of physician shortages and the need to train physicians quickly [2, 9, 10]. On the other end of the spectrum, some medical schools are offering an elective 5th year that allows the student to incorporate research or a master's degree with their traditional 4-year program. Finally, some medical schools have even proposed that there should be no time requirement at all but that the progression and graduation of each medical student should depend on the completion of necessary learning objectives and required skills [10, 11].

Ultimately, the duration of medical school education whether 3 years or 4 has made little difference in the preparation of medical students for residency and practice, but the integration of clinical experience earlier into medical student curriculum, as well as the focus on more system-based leaning, has produced more favorable results [12–14]. Variability still exists because the main determinant of curriculum is still the individual curriculum committee. Although most subject matter covered in medical schools is fairly similar, the manner of presentation and evaluation is school specific. The evaluation of medical student performance at this level may include weekly quizzes and a final exam or a more interactive grading method; evaluation is at its foundation subjective in nature and cannot be used to truly compare two students from separate schools.

Standardized testing is the main outcome measure by which medical students can be compared across schools. It begins after the completion of the didactic years and, in the MD degree-seeking programs, with the US Medical Licensing Examination (USMLE) step 1 examination. This is then followed by standardized tests given for every clinical block as well as completion of the USMLE step 2 examination prior to graduation. These standardized tests weigh heavily in the success of students' entry into residency, and although higher performance on these tests in medical school has been correlated with better performance on standardized licensing exams in residency, it has failed to correlate with overall resident success [1, 13, 15, 16].

Overall, the structure of the medical school curriculum has remained similar to those ideas first documented by Flexner in 1910, although changes are being made to ensure that medical education encompasses the necessary clinical and scientific knowledge to promote medical student success in residency. Standardized testing, while valuable as a safeguard against medical students not gaining the knowledge requisite of a graduating student, is a poor predictor of overall preparedness for residency and future clinical experience [16]. Other measures must be developed and maintained on a national and standardized level to aid medical schools in determining core learning objectives that must be met prior to medical school completion.

Challenges to Quality Improvement

Ensuring the quality of medical school education as defined by the written mandates of the LCME is an exceptional task for any curriculum committee, and it is made even more pronounced by challenges facing today's medical educators. One challenge is how to best integrate an ever-evolving technology landscape into medical education, while also keeping up with technological advances in medicine. Other challenges include how to best maintain accreditation given changing standards of achievement, how to best train medical educators through incorporating current research in medical education as well as incorporating changing standards for faculty, and how to best combat resident attrition rates. All these challenges are currently being overcome by medical schools in unique and innovative ways.

Technological Advances

Technology continues to have both positive and negative influences on medicine. For example, whereas recent advances in technology have allowed for safer and more efficient surgical techniques, technology has also led to a decrease in overall time spent with patients [17]. Medical schools are asked to constantly incorporate ever-changing technological advances into their educational curriculum while also focusing on teaching time-honored clinical skills and covering basic science topics.

Many medical schools are embracing technological advances by giving first-year students electronic tablets on which some have placed electronic versions of key textbooks [17]. For example, Yale medical school gives its first-year students an iPad and expects its students to use it throughout their 4-year course [17]. Another example of medical schools embracing technology is the online posting of daily lectures. The University of Cincinnati provides an electronic online calendar from which every student can access live video streaming of their daily lectures. These are also recorded for later viewing and can be combined with online documents such as the learning objectives from each lecture and hyperlinks to online book chapters that cover the topic in greater detail. This use of technology has numerous positives: students can listen to lectures in their own home while accessing other content such as textbook chapters, PowerPoint slide presentations, accompanying quizzes, and message boards meant to enrich their learning experience [18]. This type of learning is preferred by the rising generation [17, 19, 20]. The average young adult today spends 7 h accessing media from online content, but during that 7 h, they can assimilate 11 h worth of information [17, 21]. The use of these online formats allows students to spend less time in lectures and more time in small group discussions and clinical case reviews. These technological integrations are clearly vital in the appropriate education of today's physicians [22].

The trend away from traditional lecturing has seen a decrease in live participation; while some online lecturer platforms can include viewer participation, most either do not or students choose to view the lectures in their non-live recorded version [23]. Recent studies have shown that medical students do make consistent use of online materials, at times viewing them multiple times, especially when the information for the course is presented exclusively in an online format [17]. In head-to-head studies between similar student groups receiving either traditional live lectures or online recorded lectures, there has been no significant difference in program-administered test and standardized testing results [24–27]. It has been argued that the combination of multiple online viewings has essentially increased lecture attendance [17]. One of the main concerns of Australian medical students in a recently published article was the lack of anatomical lectures at their schools, which inspired the students to create extracurricular anatomy teaching sessions [28]. Anatomy courses have been one of the main core courses to be transitioned to online formats. Some have even suggested that practical learning in anatomy should also transition from hands-on cadaveric dissection to online modules. Although a recent study has shown that the general attitude toward online lecture formats in anatomy is positive [29], counterarguments suggest that the hands-on dissection experience should never be fully replaced by online modules [28].

The implementation of the electronic medical record (EMR) is arguably the widest application of technology in medicine in the past 10 years and has mostly been embraced by higher institutes of learning [21]. Medical students have earlier access to EMR, and, because of their higher level of computer skills, many are more facile than their predecessors at accessing the sea of patient information and data points available. Although the EMR is a wonderful tool for performing timely and accurate documentation as well as assimilating laboratory values and vital sign statistics in complex decisionmaking, there is concern that it is replacing face-to-face time with patients in history taking and physical examination. A recent study concluded that the average medical student will spend more time researching a patient on the EMR than they will spend in face-to-face consultation with the actual patient and his/her family [21].

Specialty Selection and Residency Attrition

The ultimate outcome measure of medical school achievement is determined by residency placement. This is one of the most highly touted and advertised parameters of a medical school's success; however, the methods by which medical schools advise their students on specialty selection and residency application are individual to the institution [30]. The only standardized evaluation that is performed is the Medical Student Performance Evaluation (MSPE), which is a standardized document sent to residency programs along with the student's application. The document replaced the previously written dean's letter. It includes an overview of the first 2 years of medical school education as well as the subjective evaluations from each clinical clerkship and the performance on standardized tests to date. The student is then summarized in what is supposed to be an objective manner, providing recommendations on what would make the student an acceptable residency candidate [31]. The MSPE, which is intended to serve as a readily available tool for selection by residency application committee, is the 3rd most used criterion cited when offering interviews but only the 14th most cited criterion when actually ranking a student [11, 12]. It is the only standardized summarization of a medical student's overall quality by the educators that should take some responsibility for overall training, but it is thought to be too inconsistent, lacking in objective measures, and too self-serving to be used as an objective measure of quality [12].

A task force was recently deployed by the LCME to remodel the MSPE. Their goal will be to establish a document that is more objective in its evaluation of the student. One of the current and potential problems of the MSPE is that it is completed by educators that act as both student advisors and evaluators. These individuals have an inherent conflict of interest, to present the medical student in the best manner and to provide a truthful and useful evaluation of the student's skill sets and qualification for the specialty into which they desire to match [12]. It has been proposed that the MSPE instead be written by faculty of the department into which the student desires to match [12]. This model has been implemented in emergency medicine residencies with the standardized letter of evaluation (SLOE) [11]. Studies have found that the SLOE better correlates to resident performance than the MSPE [11]. Other proposals suggest that the MSPE should also include other standards of quality more consistent with personality, such as professionalism grades. It has been noted that the promptness with which applicants submit their residency applications correlates with residency success, and peer assessments of work habits correlate with intern-year success. Requiring a more transparent evaluation document written by a more objective party will allow residency programs to better assess the quality of the applicant and will lead to more appropriate matches and lower attrition rates [31]. Most importantly, it should spawn an open and honest feedback dialogue between students and faculty about the true quality of student performance and thereby establish which changes are needed based on factors including which specialties the student should consider.

Attrition rates are remarkably high in some residency programs, with published annual rates ranging from 1.2% to 7.9% per year and a mean rate of 4.0% across all residencies with published attrition rates (Table 2.2) [32, 33]. Part of the attrition rate is most certainly made up of trainees that did not meet necessary program requirements; however, it is more difficult to find statistics about these trainees than those that voluntarily left their program, possibly because they are less likely to volunteer such information. The reasons why trainees voluntarily leave their programs have been studied and reportedly include scarcity of role models, need for more educational opportunities, negative interactions with faculty and coresidents, no safe space to voice personal concerns, and an undesirable work-life balance [33].

Table 2.2 Attrition rates for medical specialties [32, 33]

Specialty	Attrition rate (%/year)
Otolaryngology	1.2
Emergency medicine	1.5
Internal medicine	2.7
Neurology	2.9
Pediatrics	2.9
Anesthesiology	3.6
Obstetrics and gynecology	4.2
Family medicine	4.7
General surgery	5.1
Psychiatry	7.9

Most trainees that leave a program switch to a separate specialty; this trend has been reported in both surgical and nonsurgical specialties, with the majority changing to specialties that have a better perceived work-life balance (i.e., anesthesia and radiology). The next most common destination was a separate program within the same specialty [32].

Whether the trainee is asked to leave or withdraws voluntarily, the main question is "where did it go wrong?" Was it related to the quality of the medical student's education? Did the student not possess the technical skills and knowledge basis necessary to succeed in the chosen specialty? Or was it a failure in exposure to the demands of the particular field of medicine? Did the resident lack the necessary support system and mindfulness to avoid burn-out? And in both cases, was there open and honest communication between the medical educators and the student? If the main definition of quality medical education is the success of the student as a resident, then the LCME must provide provisions for monitoring attrition rates and seek amelioration when needed, including the incorporation of mindfulness teaching to students and faculty to minimize burn-out.

Educator Training and Accreditation Innovation

Any improvements in medical student education must first begin at the level of the medical educator. The LCME standard 4 dictates that the faculty of a medical school must be qualified through their education, training, experience, and continuing professional development. They must also have the time to deliver teaching, leadership, and service based on the goals of the medical school. Furthermore, they are expected to produce scholarly advances to their field. These appointments are made by the medical school, with clearly defined goals to advancement including tenure and regular feedback sessions with department heads and the dean of medical education. Although this standard provides a basic structure of what a medical educator is, it does little to standardize the type of education or experience necessary in teaching medical students. The didactic years of medical education are most often taught by professors trained in didactic teaching methods, those that have achieved doctoral or master's degrees in education or in their specific subject area [34, 35]. The majority of medical schools are able to promote rigorous course schedules designed to impart the necessary medical knowledge on students, but it is in the transition from medical knowledge to clinical practice that the largest gap in education is experienced [36]. Most clinical practitioners have little or no formal training in educational methods, and yet they are expected to be the main source of clinical and medical knowledge not only during the traditional third and fourth years but also increasingly during the first and second years [35]. Studies have shown not only that medical students prefer to receive medical education from clinical consultants but also that most clinical consultants at academic medical schools have a desire to teach more [37]. The problem occurs when they lack the requisite skills to best reach students and impart the necessary clinical knowledge for recognizing and treating various diseases. Fortunately, increasing numbers of clinical practitioners are pursuing higher degrees in medical education, and courses have become more readily available to train them in the skills necessary to be successful. As more and more clinicians develop teaching skills and become more familiar with innovative teaching techniques, quality in medical education will improve. Faculty appointment committees should not only endorse and promote teaching education among their current faculty but should show preference for advancement to those that have sought ways to increase their teaching capabilities [35].

The pursuit of scholarly advancement is also important for medical educators. Research interests have long been linked to medical educator success at academic institutions, and published research is often promoted as a major milestone in advancement in tenure tracks, as well as a major factor in dismissal [8]. Research promotes creative learning and thinking, and it produces introductions to expertise not normally found within the medical education curriculum. Not only should medical educators be expert researchers, but they should also promote medical student engagement in early research [8, 38]. This does not necessarily need to be biomedical research but can be clinical, socioeconomic, and educational research as well.

Excellence in research is a common determinant of the quality of medical schools in the public opinion. For example, the US News and World Report (USN&WR) provides the most recognized rank list of medical schools and significantly bases its rankings off research funding at a university [8]. Despite quality standards published by the LCME, the USN&WR remains the only way American medical schools are categorized [8]. Other countries have adopted tiered systems based on rigorous quality standards of medical student education and rank schools based on their adherence to these standards. Korea has adopted a three-tiered system that gives schools a grade of "Must," "Should," or "Excellent," which corresponds to grades of "C," "B," or "A," respectively [39]. Grading occurs during the initial and subsequent accreditation processes. The results are then made public. In European medical schools, the ASPIRE system was implemented by the Association for Medical Education in Europe. In this system, medical schools are awarded recognition for student assessment, student engagement, and social accountability [40]. This program was started to offset the unfair recognition of medical schools by various reporting agencies such as the USN&WR, which left out expertise and advances in medical education. Goldstein et al. have recently proposed a new algorithm for measuring medical school quality based on the successes of each school's graduates [8]. Using this method, they found that some highly ranked medical schools did not rank as highly as their USN&WR score might indicate, while other universities rose to higher rankings; for example, the University of California, San Francisco ranked #4 in the 2016 USN&WR ranking but fell to #14 when ranked by Goldstein et al. because most of the institution's research is done by current faculty and is not continued by their graduates [8].

The current accreditation process continues to leave learning objectives up to the individual curricular committee, but there is some thought that instead of course-dependent learning objectives, there should be standardized milestones that each medical student must meet prior to graduation [36]. This mirrors the recently released ACGME milestones necessary for completion of residency. These

Table 2.3 ACGME milestones for competency-based medical education

Core competencies					
Patient care and procedural skills	Medical knowledge	Practice-based learning and improvement	Interpersonal and communication skills	Professionalism	Systems-based practice
Milestones					
Level 1: Meets expectations for beginning resident	Level 2: Above beginning but below average for mid-level resident	Level 3: Appropriate for mid-level resident	Level 4: Appropriate level for graduating resident	Level 5: Exceeding expectations for graduating resident	

milestones are based on a paradigm called competency-based medical education, which relies on self-motivated completion of the milestones described in Table 2.3, and are complemented by twice-yearly competency meetings with the program director. There has been some interest in changing the medical school accreditation to include more competency-based medical education, which could also potentially eliminate a strict time period for graduation and would be dependent on the satisfactory completion of each milestone [35, 36]. This type of process would give the LCME more direct control over the quality of medical education as more specific benchmarks for graduation would be present.

Conclusion

The drive to improve the quality of medical school education in the United States began with the work of Abraham Flexner in 1910 [4]. It was the beginning of the accreditation process, which holds medical schools today responsible in preparing their students for the rigors of residency. With increased interest in quality outcome measures in medicine, attention should focus more on medical education as a process from which increased quality assurances should be developed [39]. The development and dissemination of the LCME's 12 standards of medical education is an important step in developing these assurances. These standards provide a necessary outline for how medical education should be built, but they lack standardized milestones for medical school graduation, such as those seen in graduate medical education. They also lack any grading system by which medical schools could be placed to differentiate them in terms of quality of research, medical education, and clinical experience. Although certain unique curriculum programs attempt to address the need to improve medical education, they also lack standardized checkpoints that would allow for quality outcome assessments. There is also no standardized manner in which medical educators can undergo more training if desired, and there are no standardized requirements for continual advancement of their teaching skills [35].

Overall, the quality of medical education is determined by each individual school's curriculum committee as overseen by the LCME, but this model allows large gaps among medical schools. Although the ultimate measure of a quality education should be calculated by the success of each medical school's graduates, there is no accepted standardized way of calculating quality outcomes based on this measure. Innovations in technology as well as positive attitudes toward medical education along with a more standardized measure of students' knowledge base and clinical competencies will all be important in the drive to improve medical education.

References

1. Reed S, Shell R, Kassis K, Tartaglia K, Wallihan R, Smith K, et al. Applying adult learning practices in medical education. Curr Probl Pediatr Adolesc Health Care. 2014;44(6):170–81.
2. David AK. Medical education on a collision course: sooner rather than later? Fam Med. 2013;45(3):159–63.
3. Lucey CR. Medical education: part of the problem and part of the solution. JAMA Int Med. 2013;173(17):1639–43.
4. Medical Education in the United States of America. Lancet 1910;176(4534):242–3.
5. Vinci LM, Oyler J, Arora VM. The quality and safety track: training future physician leaders. Am J Med Qual. 2014;29(4):277–83.
6. Duvivier RJ, Boulet JR, Opalek A, van Zanten M, Norcini J. Overview of the world's medical schools: an update. Med Educ. 2014;48(9):860–9.
7. Skochelak SE, Stack SJ. Creating the medical schools of the future. Acad Med. 2017;92(1):16–9.
8. Goldstein MJ, Lunn MR, Peng L. What makes a top research medical school? A call for a new model to evaluate academic physicians and medical school performance. Acad Med. 2015;90(5):603–8.
9. DeZee KJ, Artino AR, Elnicki DM, Hemmer PA, Durning SJ. Medical education in the United States of America. Med Teach. 2012;34(7):521–5.
10. Raymond JR Sr, Kerschner JE, Hueston WJ, Maurana CA. The merits and challenges of three-year medical school curricula: time for an evidence-based discussion. Acad Med. 2015;90(10):1318–23.
11. Andolsek KM. Improving the medical student performance evaluation to facilitate resident selection. Acad Med. 2016;91(11):1475–9.
12. Arawi T, Rosoff PM. Competing duties: medical educators, underperforming students, and social accountability. J Bioethical Inq. 2012;9(2):135–47.
13. George P, Park YS, Ip J, Gruppuso PA, Adashi EY. The association between premedical curricular and admission requirements and medical school performance and residency placement: a study of two admission routes. Acad Med. 2016;91(3):388–94.
14. Shannon SC, Buser BR, Hahn MB, Crosby JB, Cymet T, Mintz JS, et al. A new pathway for medical education. Health Aff. 2013;32(11):1899–905.
15. Stohl HE, Hueppchen NA, Bienstock JL. Can medical school performance predict residency performance? Resident selection and predictors of successful performance in obstetrics and gynecology. J Grad Med Educ. 2010;2(3):322–6.
16. Guffey RC, Rusin K, Chidiac EJ, Marsh HM. The utility of pre-residency standardized tests for anesthesiology resident selection: the place of United States Medical Licensing Examination scores. Anesth Analg. 2011;112(1):201–6.
17. Nieder GL, Borges NJ. An eight-year study of online lecture use in a medical gross anatomy and embryology course. Anat Sci Educ. 2012;5(6):311–20.
18. Bacro TR, Gebregziabher M, Fitzharris TP. Evaluation of a lecture recording system in a medical curriculum. Anat Sci Educ. 2010;3(6):300–8.

19. Reis LO, Ikari O, Taha-Neto KA, Gugliotta A, Denardi F. Delivery of a urology online course using Moodle versus didactic lectures methods. Int J Med Inform. 2015;84(2):149–54.
20. Adamczyk C, Holzer M, Putz R, Fischer MR. Student learning preferences and the impact of a multimedia learning tool in the dissection course at the University of Munich. Ann Anat. 2009;191(4):339–48.
21. Colbert JA, Chokshi DA. Technology in medical education-Osler meets Watson. J Gen Intern Med. 2014;29(12):1584–5.
22. Wang F. Continuing medical education via telemedicine and sustainable improvements to health. Int J Telemed Appl. 2016;2016:2424709.
23. Billings-Gagliardi S, Mazor KM. Student decisions about lecture attendance: do electronic course materials matter? Acad Med. 2007;82(10 Suppl):S73–6.
24. Davis J, Crabb S, Rogers E, Zamora J, Khan K. Computer-based teaching is as good as face to face lecture-based teaching of evidence based medicine: a randomized controlled trial. Med Teach. 2008;30(3):302–7.
25. Hale LS, Mirakian EA, Day DB. Online vs classroom instruction: student satisfaction and learning outcomes in an undergraduate Allied Health pharmacology course. J Allied Health. 2009;38(2):e36–42.
26. Schreiber BE, Fukuta J, Gordon F. Live lecture versus video podcast in undergraduate medical education: a randomised controlled trial. BMC Med Educ. 2010;10:68.
27. Solomon DJ, Ferenchick GS, Laird-Fick HS, Kavanaugh K. A randomized trial comparing digital and live lecture formats [ISRCTN40455708]. BMC Med Educ. 2004;4:27.
28. Farey JE, Sandeford JC, Evans-McKendry GD. Medical students call for national standards in anatomical education. ANZ J Surg. 2014;84(11):813–5.
29. Nieder GL, Nagy F. Analysis of medical students' use of web-based resources for a gross anatomy and embryology course. Clin Anat. 2002;15(6):409–18.
30. Borowitz SM, Saulsbury FT, Wilson WG. Information collected during the residency match process does not predict clinical performance. Arch Pediatr Adolesc Med. 2000;154(3):256–60.
31. Naidich JB, Grimaldi GM, Lombardi P, Davis LP, Naidich JJ. A program director's guide to the medical student performance evaluation (former dean's letter) with a database. J Am Coll Radiol. 2014;11(6):611–5.
32. Kennedy KA, Brennan MC, Rayburn WF, Brotherton SE. Attrition rates between residents in obstetrics and gynecology and other clinical specialties, 2000–2009. J Grad Med Educ. 2013;5(2):267–71.
33. Bongiovanni T, Yeo H, Sosa JA, Yoo PS, Long T, Rosenthal M, et al. Attrition from surgical residency training: perspectives from those who left. Am J Surg. 2015;210(4):648–54.
34. Wardley CS, Applegate EB, Van Rhee JA. A comparison of student knowledge acquisition by organ system and skills in parallel problem-based and lecture-based curricula. J Physician Assist Educ. 2013;24(1):5–14.
35. Berman JR, Aizer J, Bass AR, Cats-Baril WL, Parrish EJ, Robbins L, et al. Creating an academy of medical educators: how and where to start. HSS J. 2012;8(2):165–8.
36. Wilkinson TJ, Hudson JN, McColl GJ, Hu WCY, Jolly BC, Schuwirth LWT. Medical school benchmarking – from tools to programmes. Med Teach. 2015;37(2):146–52.
37. Darragh L, Baker R, Kirk S. Teaching medical students, what do consultants think? Ulster Med J. 2015;84(1):37–41.
38. Paolino ND, Artino AR Jr, Saguil A, Dong T, Durning SJ, DeZee KJ. Predicting medical school and internship success: does the quality of the research and clinical experience matter? Mil Med. 2015;180(4 Suppl):12–7.
39. Ahn E, Ahn D. Beyond accreditation: excellence in medical education. Med Teach. 2014;36(1):84–5.
40. Harden RM, Roberts TE. ASPIRE: international recognition of excellence in medical education. Lancet. 2015;385(9964):230.

The History of Quality Assessment in Spine Care

3

Eric J. Feuchtbaum, Catherine H. MacLean, and Todd J. Albert

Introduction

The understanding and definition of quality in spine surgery have undergone a dramatic change in the last several decades. Traditionally spine surgeons have utilized perioperative, objective data centered on the surgeon's point of view, to evaluate quality. These metrics include complication rate, readmission rates, estimated blood loss, deformity correction, or rates of fusion. These metrics provide a unique insight into the technical aspects of the surgery but do not provide information regarding improvement in patient function or pain. Although these metrics are of importance and should not be ignored when evaluating the quality of spine surgery, the current healthcare landscape demands a more multifaceted, patient-centered approach to quality evaluation.

With new technologies expanding surgical indications and an increasing aging population, there is an enormous amount of healthcare dollars being spent treating spine patients. Fusion procedures in the Medicare population increased 15-fold from 2002 to 2007 [1]. Much of this spine-related healthcare expenditure is utilized treating perioperative complications or paying for expensive 30-day readmissions. As such, the spine surgeon must ask if this large increase in healthcare expenditures correlates with improved patient health status. Recently there has been a shift toward

E. J. Feuchtbaum (✉)
Spine Center, Hospital for Special Surgery, New York, NY, USA

C. H. MacLean
Center for the Advancement of Value in Musculoskeletal Care, Hospital for Special Surgery, New York, NY, USA

T. J. Albert
Hospital for Special Surgery, New York, NY, USA

Weill Cornell Medical School, New York, NY, USA

J. Ratliff et al. (eds.), *Quality Spine Care*,
https://doi.org/10.1007/978-3-319-97990-8_3

incorporation of patient-reported outcome (PRO) measures through development of self-report questionnaires that evaluate key domains such as pain, general quality of life, and disease-specific metrics. With greater understanding of PRO measures, surgeons recently have shifted the evaluation of quality in spine surgery toward a value-based model which evaluates quality based on the provision of the most effective care with the least amount of healthcare dollars spent. The overall purpose of this chapter is to discuss the transition from clinician-centric quality evaluation to the current quality assessment based on patient-reported outcomes and value.

Quality Measurement Framework: The Donabedian Model

The conceptual model that provides the framework for quality assessment in health and spine care stems from the Donabedian model. In his 1966 article, Avedis Donabedian created a framework centered on three pillars from which to assess quality which are structure, process, and outcomes [2, 3]. It is from these pillars that spine care quality assessment has its roots and also its transitions into the current state.

Structure refers to all the factors required to be in place to allow healthcare to be delivered. This includes the actual infrastructure such as the hospital, the equipment to deliver care, and the healthcare organization and the staff who actually deliver care [4]. Structure provides the foundation in which healthcare is able to be delivered. Structural characteristics are easy to observe and measure as they are finite objects.

Process refers to the actions that define healthcare. These actions may include making a diagnosis, providing treatment or preventative care, or offering patient education. In essence, process measurement defines the actual deliverance of healthcare. Process data can be measured by querying the medical records, observing healthcare activities, and interviewing physicians, patients, and families.

Finally outcome refers to the actual effects of healthcare delivery on patients, such as overall health status. Outcome may also refer to patient satisfaction and health-related quality of life. As will be discussed in the rest of this chapter, the quality assessment of spine care has transitioned from each of these pillars over time, initially using structure and process data as the sole metrics for assessing quality and finally transitioning to the current state, in which outcome measures are paramount. Outcome measures are felt to be superior as they give the greatest insight to the impact of healthcare decisions on patients.

Clinician-Centered Metrics

Historically, outcomes of spinal surgery were evaluated from the perspective of the surgeon without a direct account of patient-related outcomes. These clinician-centered outcomes such as length of stay, blood loss, presence of complications, presence of fusion, and amount of deformity correction measure the technical success of the surgery and were based subjectively from the treating surgeon's point of view. These clinician-centered outcomes stem from structural and process data as defined in the Donabedian model. As mentioned previously, much of these clinician-centered measures are used because they are easy to collect and often exist in easily accessible databases such as the patient medical record. Often times non-validated scales were used by clinicians such as "excellent," "good," "average," or "bad" and were based on the surgeons overall singular evaluation of these metrics without checks or balances to with which to compare against. However sole reliance of clinician-generated measures of quality is shortsighted. The surgeon's perspectives and evaluations made from imaging studies and physical exam findings often do not correlate with patient satisfaction [5]. This point has been elucidated in several studies. Weber et al. evaluated if the severity of lumbar spinal stenosis on preoperative MRI correlated with preoperative PRO or surgical outcomes. Their analysis demonstrated no statistical significance between PRO and MRI grading of stenosis, and as a result, the authors recommend against overemphasis of radiographic findings as a proxy for patient perspectives [6]. Similarly, Righesso et al. followed 150 patients afflicted with sciatica secondary to lumbar disc herniation complicated by neurological impairment who underwent microdiscectomy. The authors observed the patients for 24 months postoperatively with the use of routine neurological exam and two validated PRO measures. Their results demonstrated that despite persistent sensory or motor neurological deficits present on exam 24 months after the index procedure, the PRO measures showed significant improvement and equivalence in comparison to patients without persistent neurological deficits. The results demonstrate how surgeon-specific evaluation by physical exam may result in an outcome grading much different from the patients' perspective [7]. Similarly, Herkowitz et al. prospectively evaluated patients undergoing decompression versus decompression and fusion for degenerative spondylolisthesis and demonstrated that 36% of non-instrumented fusions went on to develop pseudoarthrosis, but all had good to excellent result [8]. Finally, a study by Lamberg evaluating isthmic spondylolisthesis in the pediatric population did not find a correlation between radiographic fusion and patient-related functional outcome [9].

The results of these studies highlight the lack of correlation between the radiographic finding of fusion and clinical results, demonstrating how quality cannot be judged solely on clinician-centered metrics such as interpretation of imaging for determination of fusion [8]. It is evident that the evaluation of quality in spine surgery cannot be based solely on subjective assessments of clinician-centered data by the surgeon. This will lead to a poor understanding of the natural history of surgically addressed spinal diseases and overall worse long-term outcomes potentially associated with increased healthcare expenditures.

Despite the initial clinician-centered approach to quality assessment, spine surgeons realized the need for patient-related experiences to be incorporated into a multifaceted quality assessment model. Haefeli et al. performed a cross-sectional survey among spine patients and surgeons across Europe in an attempt to identify which factors were important to each group in determining what constitutes a good outcome [10]. Most surgeons and patients had considerable agreement on the factors found to be important for a good outcome following surgery. These factors included relief of pain, improvement of activities of daily living, mobility, and capacity to work. The same group of surgeons also identified criteria necessary for inclusion in an effective outcome tool which included domains that covered pain, disability, quality of life, and a reflection of patient expectations. Surgeons also commented on the necessity for tools administered to patients to be brief and easily understandable. None of the criteria mentioned by surgeons dealt with clinician-centered data and perioperative results such as length of stay, fusion success, blood loss, or deformity correction [10]. This study highlights the disconnect between the historical assessment of quality focused solely on the measurement of technical aspects of medical care and evolving measurement approaches that also incorporate the measurement of outcomes that matter to and more likely to be reported by patients such as pain relief, functional status, and quality of life.

Patient-Reported Outcome Measures

The goals of spinal surgery, as outlined by Haefeli et al. from assessment of patients and physicians, are to relieve pain, to restore function, and to improve the quality of life [10]. Given these factors, it is appropriate to utilize quality measures that incorporate the patient's perspective of their postoperative health state. There has been a shift within the last two decades to incorporate PRO measures in gauging quality. This change in the quality assessment point of view to focus on the patient demonstrates the transition to the Donabedian principle of outcome and away from structural and process measures that focus on the clinician.

PRO measures come in the form of patient self-administered questionnaires that cover several domains but typically include pain, general health, disease-specific disability, and overall function. PRO measures are taken directly from patients without interpretation by clinicians and therefore serve as an unbiased snapshot to patient progress at a singular instance in time. They are not only useful as a research tool but can also be an invaluable instrument to follow patient progress over time post-intervention. PRO questionnaires by design provide numerical scores for interpretation. Scores from the preoperative state can be compared to scores obtained at several time points in the post-intervention course.

Unfortunately, early experience with PRO questionnaires proved them to be too lengthy and too cumbersome for patients to complete, resulting in incomplete data and difficulty with interpretation. There was rapid increase in the use of numerous un-validated questionnaires that made interpretation and comparison among individual patients to normal standards difficult. In his 2005 thesis, Zanoli recognized the need for reliable, valid, and responsive studies to allow correlation between different populations in order to observe reproducible data [11]. Zanoli noted there was no consensus regarding outcome assessment tools for spine patients and recognized the need for standardization and normative data for specific diagnoses to allow comparison between different groups. He also recognized that the number of instruments used in the last 30 years was excessive, citing nearly 90 different instruments available in over 500 published articles on low back pain alone. Several of the instruments were not used more than once or by different authors without modifications. He concluded that the early adoption of PRO questionnaires was encouraging, but the methodological issues, including the lack of consensus measures and standardization of questionnaires, remained as an impedance to proper use. He recommended that rather than focus on the creation of new instruments, an effort should be made to provide comparative studies and systematic reviews to consolidate the number of instruments used to those most reproducible and valid [11]. Similarly, the updated work by Guzman and colleagues identified 1079 articles published from 2004 to 2013 which utilized 206 unique PRO tools [12]. Nearly 33% of the studies provided only a level of evidence of 4. The observations of the authors were similar to that of Zanoli and highlight the increasing creation of and utilization of PRO tools. They also concluded that there is currently no consensus regarding which PRO tools should be applied to specific disease states and recommended a standardization of these questionnaires for improved unification and transparency of patient outcome measure [12].

The work of Zanoli highlighted the need for unification in the PRO measures used in spine surgery. This effort led the way for validation of spine-specific PRO tools. Several studies have outlined appropriate methods for validation of PRO [13–16]. Aaronson et al. and the Scientific Advisory Committee of the Medical Outcomes Trust identified eight concepts for consideration in evaluating PRO measures: reliability, validity, responsiveness, cultural and language considerations, alternative methods, time burden of completion, and considerations regarding the concept and measurement of the model [17]. Of these eight, reliability, validity and responsiveness are most often cited and of utmost importance. Reliability refers to the consistency with which the questionnaire produces similar results across different scenarios and is a testament to the precision of the instrument [17]. It refers to the internal consistency of the tool and describes the measurement error [14]. Validity is the degree to which an instrument actually measures the variable of interest: its ability to measure what it is supposed to measure [14]. The validity of an instrument is questioned when floor or ceiling effects are noted or when greater than 15% of respondents score in the lowest or highest percentile. These effects indicate that the independent variable of interest in the study no longer has an effect on the dependent variable [18]. In clinical relevance, floor and ceiling effects prevent the clinician from distinguishing between patients suffering from a disease who have mild, moderate, or severe dysfunction. Finally responsiveness refers to the sensitivity of the test or its ability to detect changes in a disease state based on changes in scoring [14]. It is measured using the area under the receiver operating curve, which is a plot of sensitivity over 1-specificity. Values range from 0.5 (random chance) to 1.0 which indicates perfect correlation; a value of 0.7 is considered adequate [14, 18].

Studies validating PRO measures compare changes in numerical score with standard categorical scales and as a result have identified the minimal changes in scores that represent clinically significant changes in disease states [19, 20]. This concept is referred to as the minimum clinical important difference (MCID) and can be used to recognize a clinically significant treatment effect of an intervention. MCID refers to the minimum change in a PRO measure that equates to a clinical significant change to the patient. This concept lays the foundation to an additional critically important assumption which is that a statically significant change in PRO may not always be clinically relevant [21, 22]. It is imperative for the clinician to understand these concepts in order to not only choose an appropriate PRO tool but also to be able to interpret the data, identify meaningful changes in scores, and understand how they relate to a specific health state. Only then will the clinician be able to track these changes over time and have greater understanding of the overall progress for patients following specific spine interventions. Currently PRO tools have become the gold standard to measure clinical effectiveness of spine surgery. Below, this chapter will delve into the validated PRO questionnaires most commonly used in patients with spinal pathology.

History of Outcome Metrics: General Health Assessment

Short Form Questionnaire

The Medical Outcomes Study Short Form (SF) questionnaire including forms SF-6, SF-12, and SF-36 is the most widely used instruments for assessment of general quality of life. It is a generic questionnaire, covering several domains, and has been validated for use in several disease states. The SF-36 consists of 36 items across physical and mental components. Each of these components is further subcategorized into four domains including (physical) functional capacity, physical aspects, pain, and general health and (mental) vitality, social functioning, emotional aspects, and mental health. The score is scaled from 0 to 100. A score of 50 represents the average in the general population with a standard deviation of 10 and an MCID of 4.9 per component score [19]. Studies have validated the use of SF-36 for spine-specific disease states and have proven its ability to measure global functional status in a wide variety of patients across the spectrum spine pathology both preoperative and postoperatively [23–25]. The SF questionnaire can also be used to compare patients afflicted with disease across multiple organ systems such as a comparison of a patient with lumbar neurogenic claudication to a patient with congestive heart failure. The SF-6 and SF-12 represent shorter versions of the SF-36 and have been validated for use in several studies compared to the SF-36 [25–27].

EuroQol Five-Dimension Questionnaire (EQ-5D)

The EQ-5D was introduced by the EuroQol Group nearly three decades ago as a simple five-dimension measurement of general health status [28]. The questionnaire consists of 245 distinct health states subdivided among 5 domains and was initially graded among 3 levels: no problem, moderate problem, or severe problem. The five general health domains include anxiety and depression, pain and discomfort, mobility, self-care, and daily activities [29]. The questionnaire is designed to categorize patient responses into specific health states which are given utility (numerical) values ranging from 0 (death) to 1 (ideal health) [30]. Health state indices were initially calculated across a large, general population of a given country which factors in a specific regional societal perspective. Furthermore, the utility values obtained from the EQ-5D representing specific disease states can be used to supply a numerical representation of a patient's health state when performing economic analysis [30] (to be discussed later in this chapter). An MCID of 0.05 has been elucidated from several studies [31, 32]. The reliability, validity, and responsiveness of EQ-5D have been confirmed for use in spinal pathologies [33, 34]. Mueller et al. evaluated the behavior of the EQ-5D compared to the Oswestry Disability Index (ODI) for back and leg pain among 8385 patients and observed a strong and statistically significant correlation between EQ-5D and ODI ($r = -0.776$) and for back pain ($r = -0.648$) [35]. Moderate statistically significant correlation was made between EQ-5D and ODI for leg pain ($r = -0.538$). The authors concluded that the EQ-5D can serve as an effective tool for monitoring outcomes in patients with lumbar spine pathology [35]. With more widespread global use of the EQ-5D across numerous disease states, ceiling effects were noted which prompted a review by the EuroQol Group in 2005. The group concluded that a three-level response system was the cause of the ceiling, and as such, the questionnaire was amended to include five health state levels: no problem, slight problem, moderate problem, severe problem, and extreme problem.

Pain Outcome Measures

As demonstrated in the study by Haefeli, pain is a primary driver of outcome success for both spine surgeons and patients. Pain is highly subjective in nature and difficult to interpret across different patients [10]. Objective measures to quantify pain are typically used such as visual analog scale (VAS) or numerical rating scales (NRS) [36, 37]. Visual scales including the VAS come in several varieties including an analog of faces in which the patient identifies perceived pain based on the face that best represents current pain level. Other visual analog scales utilize the amount of liquid held in a glass or position along a 10 cm horizontal as a proxy for patient-perceived pain. The numerical rating scale (NRS) is an 11-point numeric rating system in which a score of "0" represents no pain, whereas a score of "10" represents the worst possible pain [29, 38]. Although these scales are simple in terms of use, as mentioned previously, the subjective nature of pain experienced by the individual user makes validating the use of these tools difficult [39]. The studies regarding this matter are conflicting. Ostelo and colleagues attempted to develop practical guidelines regarding the MCID for the VAS and NRS through current literature review and query of an expert panel. Their analysis demonstrated wide variation in the study designs utilized to estimate MCID for NRS and VAS leading to a very broad consensus MCID of 30% change. This was based on expert opinion and not on actual level I–III evidence [39].

Parker et al. prospectively studied the MCID of the VAS to measure leg and low back pain in patients undergoing transforaminal lumbar interbody fusion. Their analysis demonstrated a MCID of 2.1–5.3 for leg pain and 2.1–4.7 for back pain [40]. Several studies have attempted to analyze the responsiveness of NRS and VAS but failed to find statistically significant difference in the two scales [41]. Contrarily, a study of NRS rating in patients with low back pain undergoing physical therapy demonstrated improvement in NRS score at 1 and 4 weeks after therapy initiation, allowing the authors to conclude an MCID of two points for NRS [42]. Similarly, a systematic review of the responsiveness of several PRO measures including VAS among patients undergoing spinal surgery demonstrated only medium correlation with ODI ($r = 0.69$) [43]. The authors concluded that responsiveness of VAS was not strong and therefore should be used in tandem with a disease-specific PRO (such as ODI) to obtain appropriate response to intervention.

It is evident from the above studies that the perception of pain is specific to the individual and currently our scales may not most appropriately capture the unique perception of pain experienced by the individual patient. Despite this, the use of the VAS has increased significantly in the last decade and was included in over 47.5% of articles queried by Guzman and colleagues [12] regarding PRO measures. The clinician should pay special attention to the history presented by the patient and attempt to make correlations to the pain scale score reported by the patient.

Disease-Specific Outcome Measures

Disease-specific PRO instruments relate to certain regions of the body (cervical vs. lumbar) and the type of symptoms experienced (axial pain vs. radiculopathy vs. myelopathy). The rationale behind disease-specific PRO tools was to link specific spine pathology with the dysfunction experienced by the patient. The most common specific questionnaires include the Oswestry Disability Index (ODI), the Neck Disability Index (NDI), the Japanese Orthopedic Association (JOA) questionnaire, and the Scoliosis Research Society (SRS)-22 questionnaire [12].

Oswestry Disability Index (ODI)

As demonstrated by Guzman et al., ODI was the second most commonly utilized PRO, behind the VAS, and was found in 38.4% of articles queried [12]. First published in 1980 by O'Brien, the ODI has been modified several times by the American Academy of Orthopedic Surgeons from the original ODI publication [44, 45]. The ODI consists of ten domains each described by six statements of increasing disability. The domains include pain, personal care, lifting, walking, sitting, standing, sleeping, sexual function, social activity, and travel tolerance. Scoring of each domain is obtained from a scale of 0–5, and each domain score is doubled, expressed as a percentage of 100 in which a score of 100 indicates the most severe dysfunction [44–47]. Scores are categorized into various levels of dysfunction with a score of

0–20 indicating minimal dysfunction, 21–40 indicating moderate dysfunction, 41–60 indicating severe dysfunction, and 61–80 representing a bedbound state. Scores greater than 80 are often considered outliers and are not accounted for [45]. Several studies have validated the reliability and validity of the ODI in several lumbar spine/low back-specific conditions [19, 45, 48]. The responsiveness was evaluated by Copay et al., and their analysis demonstrated an MCID of 12.8 [19]. The questionnaire is both quickly administered to the patient and scored by the clinician. Several versions of the ODI exist, and the specific version is often not mentioned in publications and potentially not scrutinized with rigorous validation [12]. The use of the version ODIv2.1a is the recommendation by the original author [12, 49].

Neck Disability Index (NDI)

The NDI is one of the most widely used and most validated PRO tools for the cervical spine, specifically for neck pain [50]. According to Guzman et al., the NDI was the fifth most common overall PRO instrument and was cited in 7.9% of studies identified in their query [12]. The NDI consists of ten questions that relate to neck dysfunction as it applies to sleeping, driving, work, recreation, concentration, headaches, reading, lifting, self-care, and pain intensity. Each category is scored from 0 to 6 with higher scores indicating increasing levels of dysfunction. The total score is doubled and represented as a percentage. The NDI has been validated based on a systematic review by MacDermid and colleagues [51]. Their study concluded that there was sufficient evidence to support the reliability, validity, and usefulness of the NDI as the most commonly utilized self-report measure for neck pain. Their analysis confirmed an MCID of 5 out of 50 points for neck pain and 10/50 points for cervical radiculopathy [51]. Similarly, Young and Cleland evaluated the reliability and validity of the NDI among patients with cervical radiculopathy and concluded fair reliability and adequate responsiveness. The MCID determined from these two studies was 13.4 and 10.2, respectively, which is similar to the systematic review by McDermid [52, 53].

Japanese Orthopedic Association (JOA) Questionnaire

The JOA questionnaire was developed as a result of the need for a more sophisticated PRO tool to evaluate the specific findings seen in cervical myelopathy which was not specifically queried in other PRO instruments such as the NDI [54]. The JOA questionnaire consists of six categories including upper and lower extremity motor function, sensory function of the trunk, upper and lower extremities, and function of the bladder [55]. The degree of myelopathy was determined by calculating a score for each of the six categories. Scoring is from 0 to 17 with higher scores indicating a greater degree of normal function. Myelopathic dysfunction was subcategorized based on scoring with a score of less than 9 indicating severe myelopathy, 9–13 indicating moderate myelopathy, and a score of greater than 13 indicating mild myelopathic dysfunction. The JOA questionnaire has been validated in several studies. Yonenobu et al. evaluated the intra- and inter-observer reliability among 10 spine specialists, 10 orthopedic surgeons, and 13 orthopedic residents who examined 29 patients with cervical myelopathy [54]. The intra- and inter-observer reliabilities were observed to be high (correlation coefficient = 0.826) leading the authors to conclude that the JOA questionnaire is a useful tool for the assessment of cervical myelopathy. Recently the JOA questionnaire was modified and increased the scoring value of motor function of the hand to a maximum of 5 points (compared to the original scoring maximum of 4) and removed trunk and lower extremity sensation from the scoring. In addition, the modification addresses the patient's ability to button a shirt which was not included in the original version. Similarly the use of chopsticks was converted to use of a spoon to be more applicable to western societies [56]. Although the modified JOA was utilized less frequently than the original JOA questionnaire in the Guzman study, the modified tool has been extensively validated, and its use is increasing [57, 58].

Scoliosis Research Society (SRS)-22 Questionnaire

Other than the ODI, the SRS-22 is the most common PRO questionnaire utilized in the adult and pediatric spinal deformity population. It is validated for both populations through several studies start here [59–67] in the English language. It has also been extensively translated into several languages and has been thoroughly validated in these international adult and pediatric populations [34, 68–90]. The questionnaire consists of 22 items across 4 domains including function, pain, self-image, and mental health. Scoring is from 1 (worst outcome) to 5 (best outcome).

Defining "Value" in Spine Care

Emerging technology and an aging population have resulted in expanding surgical indications and an overall increase in healthcare costs associated with spine surgery. A study by Martin et al. analyzed spine-related healthcare expenditures from 1997 to 2005 and observed that total expenditures for patients with spine pathology increased 65% during this time period [91]. Similarly the number of patients who reported dysfunction related to neck or back problems increased 20.7% over this same time period. The complexities of delivering spine care and healthcare in general have become a dramatic problem, with healthcare spending growing at a rate greater than the nation's economic growth [92]. It is clear that these trends are applying significant pressure onto the already burdened healthcare system.

With this growing concerns regarding sustainability of our healthcare system, there has been a recent shift toward value-based care in spine surgery as expenditures for spine care are some of the highest of all pathologies. This presented as a mandate by the Affordable Care Act (ACA) to reduce expenditures through the pursuit of high-value care [93]. In an effort to obtain high-value care, the ACA authorized the Patient-Centered Outcomes Research Institute (PCORI) to invest in comparative effectiveness research which hoped to bring transparency to both physicians and patients regarding the comparative effectiveness of different procedures and interventions [93].

This methodology builds on the quality improvement shift that occurred though widespread implementation of PRO measures and expands the focus of care to not only provide the highest quality care but at the most efficient cost. This concept, referred to as value, or the quality divided by the cost, utilizes information gleamed from PRO tools and applies them to an economic model [94]. There has been increased utilization of these value models in spine care; however, accurate and precise modeling is still being developed [95]. In order to fully understand and interpret these models and how they can impact spine care, we must first understand how value in spine care is determined.

Defining the Value Model

As mentioned previously, value is defined as the quality of an intervention in relation to the cost of that intervention. One way that value can be modeled is through cost-effective analyses (CEAs). CEA defines the effectiveness or utility of an intervention compared to the cost. Defining quality can be difficult as we have seen previously in this chapter and can refer to clinician-centered data or PRO measures. Choosing the appropriate quality measure depends on the focus of the value model being analyzed. For instance, if taking a hospital or payer perspective, using clinician-centered data such as operating room time, length of hospital stay, or time to fusion may be more appropriate. However, as previously mentioned, given the shift to a more patient-centered focus of quality assessment, the use of PRO as a quality metric in value analysis is imperative. It is important that the quality metric chosen has several key characteristics including its numeric conversion for application in a value model, can be easily communicated among all key stakeholders, and has the ability to be compared across several disease states, allowing for standardization [94]. Two key metrics that meet these criteria and are widely used in value modeling are the utility score and the quality-adjusted life year (QALY), both of which will be covered in further detail.

Given the lack of transparency associated with spine care and healthcare costs in general, it can be quite challenging to define the cost portion of the value equation. There are currently two methods of which cost is determined, either the hospital/payer perspective or from the perspective of the society, which includes both direct costs of the procedure and the indirect costs from loss of productivity associated with a disease or post procedure state [94].

An additional concern with value analysis is determining the timeframe with which to model. Different interventions may require different time horizons from which to evaluate such as the comparison between a simple decompression and a more complex decompression with an associated fusion [94]. A powerful example of the effect of timeframe on value modeling can be seen in the 2- versus 4-year cost-effective data as presented in the Spine Patient Outcomes Research Trial (SPORT) study on degenerative spondylolisthesis. At a 2-year time horizon, Tosteson et al. demonstrated cost per QALY benefit of $115,600 for surgical treatment over nonoperative management [94, 96]. This 2-year time horizon factors in the high initial upfront costs are associated with fusion. However over the ensuing 2 years, as patients continue to heal and gain improvements in their quality of life, the cost per QALY gained from surgical intervention decreased to $64,300 in the 4-year follow-up study [94, 97, 98]. This case highlights the importance of understanding the natural history of disease and postsurgical states when appropriately modeling the timeframe of the economic model as this can have profound effects on the overall value of an intervention in spine care. Interventions that have lasting effects and produce continued improvements in health states can lead to increasing cost-effectiveness of an intervention, whereas those interventions with only temporizing effect, without lasting impact on health states, will have decreasing cost-effectiveness overtime [94].

Quality Measures and Utility Value

Quality can be defined based on clinician-centered measures or patient-centered metrics such as PRO metrics. Given the shift in focus of quality assessment to patient-centric models, using the PRO metrics in the value equation is ideal. However, not all PRO measures are equally suited for use in value assessment. It is important to utilize a PRO tool that allows numeric incorporation into the value equation and can also be compared across many different disease states to allow for appropriate standardization. One way to incorporate the PRO data into numeric value for use in CEA is by conversion into a health state utility (HSU) value. The HSU is a numeric assessment that reflects a patient's perspective on a particular health state. As previously mentioned it ranges from 0 (death) to 1.0 (ideal health). Calculating HSU values can be performed by direct or indirect means. The direct method, which is infrequently used, involves a standard gamble analysis which presents an individual with a theoretical choice between a certain health state and a gamble that can either improve or worsen the condition. The probabilities of obtaining the improved health state is then varied to the point in which the individual is indifferent between choosing the current health state and the gamble option. The HSU value is the probability at which the respondent is indifferent to the decision between the current health state and the gamble option [99, 100]. This method involves large focus groups and is both costly and time consuming.

The indirect method of calculating HSU is more commonly used in spine value modeling and involves conversion of PRO data to a numeric value. As mentioned not all PRO tools can be converted to HSU values. Most commonly used convertible metrics are the EQ-5D, SF-36 (and its associated sub-surveys the SF-6D and the SF-12), and most recently the NDI and NRS [30, 101–104].

Quality-Adjusted Life Year (QALY)

HSU values as obtained from PRO measures allow for value modeling from the patient's perspective and therefore allows for quality assessment of the economics of spine care to account for the true burden of disease (and intervention) on the patient. The use of HSU values is critical in calculating the QALY which is a measure of not only the quality of life but the duration of this benefit [105]. Dividing the QALY gained by an intervention by the cost of the intervention provides a unit of measure used to determine value. QALY is calculated by multiplying the HSU value associated with a given health state by the amount of time lived in that state, where a QALY of 1 indicates 1 year of life lived in perfect health. A QALY of 0.5 can represent a half a year lived in perfect health or 1 year lived in a debilitated state [105, 106]. Observing QALY changes over time can be used to compare the long-term effect of different treatment options on health states.

Cost Calculation in Spine Care

Cost calculation for spine care can be complex, with numerous perspectives to consider. Costs from the hospital perspective include the direct costs, those costs immediately associated with the provision of care. These costs include diagnostic tests, medications, outpatient visits, hospital admission, implants, supplies, physician fees, overhead, and disposable supplies. From the perspective of an insurer, the costs include the amount of money paid to the hospital for services and often include physician and surgeon fees involved in delivering care. Costs from the patient and societal perspective include all of these direct costs as well as the indirect costs such as caregiver fees and lost productivity secondary to time away from work. Lack of transparency and reimbursement differences across regions can complicate these calculations [94].

Assessing direct costs is typically performed through the use of publically available resources, such as Medicare and private payer payment data, or through cost to charge ratios. Some propose that the use of widely available Medicare data is a true reflection of the societal perspective of cost since Medicare payments to hospitals come in the form of monthly premiums collected from the patient pool. Similarly private payer payments can be derived from adjustments made from Medicare payment [94]. A less commonly used method to derive cost is through cost to charge ratios which convert hospital charges into cost estimate. Cost to charge ratios are different across hospital systems and are publically available through the work of the Healthcare Cost and Utilization Project [107].

Indirect costs, although more difficult to grasp given the many layers associated with patient care in the post-intervention period, is cited as the largest portion of the total cost of care in patients with low back pain [108]. This can be accounted for by the loss of productivity of the patient and caregivers who miss work to provide care for the patient and also the decreased productivity of patient initially upon returning to work. The most common way to calculate indirect cost is through the human capital approach which assumes that a patient's productivity is correlated to the patient's wages and benefits that would have been earned during the time in which the patient is unable to work [109]. Calculating indirect costs of caregivers missing work can be more challenging.

Cost-Effective Analysis (CEA): Putting Together the Value Equation

As mentioned previously CEA is the most common means of measuring value and quality from an economic perspective in spine care. It involves the comparison of two or more interventions in terms of outcome and cost per intervention [94]. It evaluates the cost necessary to produce a unit of benefit or as previously mentioned the cost per QALY ratio. With the recent push for more patient-centered quality assessments and the need to contain costs, the number of publications regarding cost-effectiveness has increased dramatically in the last several years [95]. In a systematic review published in 2014, Nwachukwu et al. observed that 70% of the identified CEA studies were published within the last 2 years of their study's publication date [95]. Given the rapid increase in studies, it is imperative to utilize guidelines to standardize this process. In 1996, the US panel on *Cost-Effectiveness in Health and Medicine* published recommendations for performing CEA research and identified four key recommendations: research should be performed from societal perspective, cost and health utility states should be discounted at the same rate for future time points, there should be consideration of use of utility measures, and there should be a need for incremental comparisons between two or more interventions [110].

These guidelines allow for patient-centered evaluation. The use of discounting accounts for the immediate high impact of time lost and money spent in the present versus the diminishing effect of time loss and money spent in the future. In addition using utility measures allows for comparison of health states across various disease states and therefore can weigh the economic and societal effects of spine interventions compared to other disease state interventions. Incremental accounting allows for comparison between two treatment arms and is imperative to determine which treatments are most effective for a given disease state [94]. This incremental cost-effectiveness ratio (ICER) is the crux of CEA and value analysis. It is measured by

$$\mathrm{ICER} = \mathrm{Cost}_{\mathrm{Tx1}} - \mathrm{Cost}_{\mathrm{Tx2}} / \mathrm{QALY}_{\mathrm{Tx1}} - \mathrm{QALY}_{\mathrm{Tx2}}$$

The ICER is a representation of the monetary value per QALY gained. However it is necessary to determine what this measure represents. It is also necessary to determine at what incremental cost per QALY is an intervention deemed cost-effective. In simple terms, an intervention that reduces cost and improves quality is always cost-effective. When discussing cost-effectiveness, it is necessary to consider the concept of willingness to pay. This concept helps guide cost-effectiveness when an intervention both increases health utility and also increases cost or decreases health utility while simultaneously decreasing cost. The willingness to pay threshold is the cost per QALY amount at which below interventions are considered cost-effective and above considered cost-ineffective. There is no consensus in the United States regarding what the willingness to pay threshold should be. It is currently set at $100,000/QALY based on analysis of health state preferences for renal dialysis set in the 1960s [111]. Economic modeling performed by Braithwaite et al. suggests that the current $100,000/QALY is outdated and will not keep up with societal trends [112]. The author's model suggests that the lower and upper limits of cost-effectiveness based on a current societal perspective are $183,000 and $264,000 per QALY, respectively.

It is clear that more work and refinement in the way clinicians' model value are needed. The work by Nwachukwu and colleagues identified several flaws in the current state of value modeling including a majority of studies that did not provide a comparator to the studied intervention [95]. Some studies that did utilize a comparison intervention did so only between surgical options and neglected the cost-benefit analysis of conservative or less invasive treatment options. In addition this report observed that a majority of studies modeled their CEA based on retrospective data and only utilized short follow-up of 2–5 years. This short duration of follow-up may not fully portray a lifetime of QALY gained or lost [94].

Further complicating these studies is the perspective taken from which CEAs are modeled. A robust example as described by Resnick et al. involves the CEA of anterior cervical discectomy and fusion (ACDF) with and without the use of a plate [93]. The original authors [113] concluded that as both procedures are cost-effective in terms of the cost per QALY, the ACDF intervention utilizing a plate would assume a higher overall cost related to the use of the implant ($1500) making ACDF without a plate the more cost-effective strategy. This rationale takes the perspective of the payer. However the authors also report that patients who underwent ACDF without a plate returned to work 3 weeks later than patients who underwent ACDF with a plate secondary to use of a hard cervical collar in the without plate cohort. Consider if a patient who has an ACDF without a plate typically earns at least $1500 or more during those 3 weeks off of work, then from a societal perspective, the ACDF with plate intervention may be more cost-effective [93]. Modeling value is a multifaceted process, and changes in perspectives and cost accounting can lead to drastically different results.

Conclusion

It is encouraging that a shift in the definition and assessment of quality in spine care is occurring in the United States. The early practice of using solely clinician-centered data only defines a small portion of the quality equation and has opportunity for improvement. The advent and widespread use of PRO measures aims to factor in the perspective of the patient. However the initial use of PRO has resulted in too many instruments created, many of which need validation and standardization in order to be applicable across populations. The consolidation of PRO use will only come as more studies use a select few tools and validate them across various disease states. The use of PRO metrics has spearheaded a new concept in spine quality assessment, the notion of value. The ideology of value and CEA allows both the physician and society to understand not only the burden of disease on the patient but also its associated costs. As best stated by Michael Porter in his *New England Journal of Medicine* article, "rigorous, disciplined measurement and improvement of value is the best way to drive system progress" [114].

The concept of value is not as simple to define as it may seem. Consideration of the many stakeholders' points of view, utilizing the appropriate time horizon, choosing appropriate cost accounting, and the need to compare against the numerous interventions (both operative and nonoperative), makes defining value difficult. CEA and value modeling are only in its infancy in spine care, and there is much improvement to be made. Given the significant cost burden on the healthcare system and the economy as a whole, it is up to all stakeholders to find ways to cut costs yet provide the highest quality of care. There is a great opportunity with the current state of healthcare to learn from the advances in quality assessment in the past and create value for spine patients in the future.

References

1. Deyo RA, Mirza SK, Martin BI, Kreuter W, Goodman DC, Jarvik JG. Trends, major medical complications, and charges associated with surgery for lumbar spinal stenosis in older adults. JAMA. 2010;303(13):1259–65.
2. Donabedian A. The quality of care: how can it be assessed? JAMA. 1988;260(12):1743–8.
3. Donabedian A. Evaluating the quality of medical care. 1966. Milbank Q. 2005;83(4):691–729.
4. Donabedian A. An introduction to quality assurance in health care, vol. 1. 1st ed. New York: Oxford University Press; 2003.
5. Teles AR, Khoshhal KI, Falavigna A. Why and how should we measure outcomes in spine surgery? J Taibah Univ Med Sci. 2016;11(2):91–7.
6. Weber C, Giannadakis C, Rao V, Jakola AS, et al. Is there an association between radiological severity of lumbar spinal stenosis and disability, pain, or surgical outcome: a multicenter observational study. Spine (Phila Pa 1976). 2016 Jan;41(2):E78–83.
7. Righesso O, Falavigna A, Avanzi O. Correlation between persistent neurological impairment and clinical outcome after microdiscectomy for treatment of lumbar disc herniation. Neurosurgery. 2012;70(2):390–6. discussion 396-7
8. Herkowitz HN, Kurz LT. Degenerative lumbar spondylolisthesis with spinal stenosis: a prospective study comparing decompression with decompression and intertransverse process arthrodesis. J Bone Joint Surg Am. 1991;73:802–8.
9. Lamberg TS, Remes VM, Helenius IJ, et al. Long-term clinical, functional and radiological outcome 21 years after posterior or posterolateral fusion in childhood and adolescence isthmic spondylolisthesis. Eur Spine J. 2005;14:639–44.
10. Haefeli M, Elfering A, Aebi M, Freeman BJ, Fritzell P, Guimaraes Consciencia J, et al. What comprises a good outcome in spinal surgery? A preliminary survey among spine surgeons of the SSE and European spine patients. Eur Spine J. 2008;17(1):104–16.
11. Zanoli G. Outcome assessment in lumbar spine surgery. Acta Orthop. 2005;76(suppl 318):2–4.
12. Guzman JZ, Cutler HS, Connolly J, Skovrlj B, Mroz TE, Riew KD, Cho SK. Patient-reported outcome instruments in spine surgery. Spine (Phila Pa 1976). 2016;41(5):429–37.
13. Bot SD, Terwee CB, van der Windt DA, Bouter LM, Dekker J, de Vet HC. Clinimetric evaluation of shoulder disability questionnaires: a systematic review of the literature. Ann Rheum Dis. 2004;63(4):335–41.

14. Mokkink LB, Terwee CB, Patrick DL, et al. The COSMIN study reached international consensus on taxonomy, terminology, and definitions of measurement properties for health related patient-reported outcomes. J Clin Epidemiol. 2010;63(7):737–45.
15. Terwee CB, Bot SD, de Boer MR, et al. Quality criteria were proposed for measurement properties of health status questionnaires. J Clin Epidemiol. 2007;60(1):34–42.
16. Lohr KN, Aaronson NK, Alonso J. Evaluating quality-of-life and health status instruments: development of scientific review criteria. Clin Ther. 1996;18(5):979–92.
17. Aaronson N, Alonso J, Burnam A, Lohr KN, et al. Assessing health status and quality-of-life instruments: attributes and review criteria. Qual Life Res. 2002;11(3):193–205.
18. McCormick JD, Werner BC, Shimer AL. Patient-reported outcome measures in spine surgery. J Am Acad Orthop Surg. 2013;21:99–107.
19. Copay AG, Glassman SD, Subach BR, Berven S, Schuler TC, Carreon LY. Minimum clinically important difference in lumbar spine surgery patients: a choice of methods using the Oswestry disability index, medical outcomes study questionnaire short form 36, and pain scales. Spine J. 2008;8(6):968–74.
20. Copay AG, Subach BR, Glassman SD, Polly DW Jr, Schuler TC. Understanding the minimum clinically important difference: a review of concepts and methods. Spine J. 2007;7(5):541–6.
21. Parker SL, Mendenhall SK, Shau DN, Adogwa O, et al. Minimum clinically important difference in pain, disability, and quality of life after neural decompression and fusion for same-level recurrent lumbar stenosis: understanding clinical versus statistical significance. J Neurosurg Spine. 2012;16(5):471–8.
22. Mattei TA. "Statistically significant" does not necessarily mean 'clinically different' on pain/quality of life scales: opportune remarks on clinical outcomes measures in cervical spondylotic myelopathy. Neurosurgery. 2012;71(2):E518–21.
23. Guilfoyle MR, Seeley H, Laing RJ. The short form 36 health survey in spine disease: validation against condition specific measures. Br J Neurosurg. 2009;23(4):401–5.
24. Haro H, Maekawa S, Hamada Y. Prospective analysis of clinical evaluation and self-assessment by patients after decompression surgery for degenerative lumbar canal stenosis. Spine J. 2008;8(2):380–4.
25. Ware JE Jr. SF-36 health survey update. Spine (Phila Pa 1976). 2000;25(24):3130–9.
26. Brazier J, Roberts J, Deverill M. The estimation of a preference-based measure of health from the SF-36. J Health Econ. 2002;21(2):271–92.
27. Cruz LN, Camey SA, Hoffmann JF, Rowen D, et al. Estimating the SF-6D value set for a population-based sample of Brazilians. Value Health. 2011;14(5 Suppl 1):S108–14.
28. The EuroQol Group. EuroQol: A new facility for the measurement of health-related quality of life. Health Policy. 1990;16(3):199–208.
29. Tosteson AN. Preference-based health outcome measures in low back pain. Spine (Phila Pa 1976). 2000;25(24):3161–6.
30. Solberg TK, Olsen JA, Ingebrigtsen T, Hofoss D, Nygaard OP. Health-related quality of life assessment by the EuroQol-5D can provide cost-utility data in the field of low-back surgery. Eur Spine J. 2005;14(10):1000–7.
31. Dolan P. Modeling valuations for EuroQol health states. Med Care. 1997;35(11):1095–108.
32. Braun J, McHugh N, Singh A, Wajdula JS, Sato R. Improvement in patient reported outcomes for patients with ankylosing spondylitis treated with etanercept 50 mg once-weekly and 25 mg twice-weekly. Rheumatology (Oxford). 2007;46(6):999–1004.
33. Papaioannou D, Brazier J, Parry G. How valid and responsive are generic health status measures, such as EQ-5D and SF- 36, in schizophrenia? A systematic review. Value Health. 2011;14(6):907–20.
34. Adobor RD, Rimeslåtten S, Keller A, Brox JI. Repeatability, reliability, and concurrent validity of the scoliosis research society-22 questionnaire and EuroQol in patients with adolescent idiopathic scoliosis. Spine (Phila Pa 1976). 2010;35(2):206–9.
35. Mueller B, Carreon LY, Glassman SD. Comparison of the EuroQOL-5D with the Oswestry disability index, back and leg pain scores in patients with degenerative lumbar spine pathology. Spine (Phila Pa 1976). 2013 Apr 20;38(9):757–61.

36. Wang P, Zhang J, Liao W, Zhao L, et al. Content comparison of questionnaires and scales used in low back pain based on the international classification of functioning, disability and health: a systematic review. Disabil Rehabil. 2012;34(14):1167–77.
37. Longo UG, Loppini M, Denaro L, Maffulli N, Denaro V. Rating scales for low back pain. Br Med Bull. 2010;94:81–144.
38. Gatchel RJ, Mayer TG. Psychological evaluation of the spine patient. J Am Acad Orthop Surg. 2008;16(2):107–12.
39. Ostelo RW, Deyo RA, Stratford P, et al. Interpreting change scores for pain and functional status in low back pain: towards international consensus regarding minimal important change. Spine (Phila Pa 1976). 2008;33(1):90–4.
40. Parker SL, Adogwa O, Paul AR, Anderson WN, Aaronson O, Cheng JS, McGirt MJ. Utility of minimum clinically important difference in assessing pain, disability, and health state after transforaminal lumbar interbody fusion for degenerative lumbar spondylolisthesis. J Neurosurg Spine. 2011;14(5):598–604.
41. Grotle M, Brox JI, Vøllestad NK. Concurrent comparison of responsiveness in pain and functional status measurements used for patients with low back pain. Spine (Phila Pa 1976). 2004;29(21):E492–501.
42. Childs JD, Piva SR, Fritz JM. Responsiveness of the numeric pain rating scale in patients with low back pain. Spine (Phila Pa 1976). 2005;30(11):1331–4.
43. DeVine J, Norvell DC, Ecker E, et al. Evaluating the correlation and responsiveness of patient-reported pain with function and quality-of-life outcomes after spine surgery. Spine (Phila Pa 1976). 2011;36(21 suppl):S69–74.
44. Fairbank JC, Couper J, Davies JB, O'Brien JP. The Oswestry low back pain disability questionnaire. Physiotherapy. 1980;66(8):271–3.
45. Fairbank JC, Pynsent PB. The Oswestry disability index. Spine (Phila Pa 1976). 2000;25(22):2940–52.
46. Fairbank JC. Use and abuse of Oswestry disability index. Spine (Phila Pa 1976). 2007;32(25):2787–9.
47. Hagg O, Fritzell P, Nordwall A, Swedish Lumbar Spine Study G. The clinical importance of changes in outcome scores after treatment for chronic low back pain. Eur Spine J. 2003;12(1):12e20.
48. Roland M, Fairbank J. The Roland-morris disability questionnaire and the Oswestry disability questionnaire. Spine (Phila Pa 1976). 2000;25(24):3115–24.
49. Fairbank JC. Why are there different versions of the Oswestry disability index? J Neurosurg Spine. 2014;20:83–6.
50. Vernon H, Mior S. The neck disability index: a study of reliability and validity. J Manip Physiol Ther. 1991;14(7):409–15.
51. MacDermid JC, Walton DM, Avery S, et al. Measurement properties of the neck disability index: a systematic review. J Orthop Sports Phys Ther. 2009;39(5):400–17.
52. Young IA, Cleland JA, Michener LA, Brown C. Reliability, construct validity, and responsiveness of the neck disability index, patient-specific functional scale, and numeric pain rating scale in patients with cervical radiculopathy. Am J Phys Med Rehabil. 2010;89(10):831–9.
53. Cleland JA, Fritz JM, Whitman JM, Palmer JA. The reliability and construct validity of the neck disability index and patient specific functional scale in patients with cervical radiculopathy. Spine (Phila Pa 1976). 2006;31(5):598–602.
54. Yonenobu K, Abumi K, Nagata K, Taketomi E, Ueyama K. Interobserver and intraobserver reliability of the Japanese orthopaedic association scoring system for evaluation of cervical compression myelopathy. Spine (Phila Pa 1976). 2001;26(17):1890–5.
55. Hirabayashi K, Miyakawa J, Satomi K, Maruyama T, Wakano K. Operative results and postoperative progression of ossification among patients with ossification of cervical posterior longitudinal ligament. Spine (Phila Pa 1976). 1981;6(4):354–64.
56. Kato S, Oshima Y, Oka H, et al. Comparison of the Japanese Orthopaedic Association (JOA) score and modified JOA (mJOA) score for the assessment of cervical myelopathy: a multicenter observational study. PLoS One. 2015;10:e0123022.

57. Kopjar B, Tetreault L, Kalsi-Ryan S, et al. Psychometric properties of the modified Japanese Orthopaedic Association scale in patients with cervical spondylotic myelopathy. Spine (Phila Pa 1976). 2015;40:E23–8.
58. Oshima K, Iwasaki M, Sakaura H, et al. Comparison of the Japanese orthopaedic association score and the Japanese orthopaedic association cervical myelopathy evaluation questionnaire scores: time-dependent changes in patients with cervical spondylotic myelopathy and posterior longitudinal ligament. Asian Spine J. 2015;9:47–53.
59. Faraj SSA, van Hooff ML, Holewijn RM, Polly DW Jr, Haanstra TM, de Kleuver M. Measuring outcomes in adult spinal deformity surgery: a systematic review to identify current strengths, weaknesses and gaps in patient-reported outcome measures. Eur Spine J. 2017;26(8):2084–93.
60. Asher MA, Lai SM, Burton D, Manna B. The reliability and concurrent validity of the SRS-22 patient questionnaire for idiopathic scoliosis. Spine. 2003;28(1):63–9.
61. Asher MA, Lai SM, Burton D, Manna B. Scoliosis Research Society-22 patient questionnaire: responsiveness to change associated with surgical treatment: preliminary results. Spine. 2003;28(1):70–3.
62. Asher MA, Lai SM, Burton DC. Further development and validation of the Scoliosis Research Society (SRS) outcomes instrument. Spine. 2000;25(18):2381–6.
63. Asher MA, Lai SM, Burton D, Manna B. Discrimination validity of the Scoliosis Research Society-22 patient questionnaire: relationship to idiopathic scoliosis curve pattern and curve size. Spine. 2003;28(1):74–8.
64. Asher MA, Lai SM, Glattes C, Burton DC, Alanay A, Bago J. Refinement of the SRS-22 health-related quality of life questionnaire function domain. Spine. 2006;31(5):593–7.
65. Lai SM, Asher MA, Burton D. Estimating SRS-22 quality of life measures with SF-36. Application in idiopathic scoliosis. Spine. 2006;31(4):473–8.
66. Monticone M, Nava C, Leggero V, Rocca B, Salvaderi S, Ferrante S, Ambrosini E. Measurement properties of translated versions of the Scoliosis Research Society-22 patient questionnaire, SRS-22: a systematic review. Qual Life Res. 2015 Aug;24(8):1981–98.
67. Berven S, Deviren V, Demir-Deviren S, et al. Studies in the modified Scoliosis Research Society Outcomes Instrument in adults: validation, reliability, and discriminatory capacity. Spine (Phila Pa 1976). 2003;28:2164–9.
68. Rosanova GC, Gabriel BS, Camarini PM, Gianini PE, Coehlo DM, Oliveira AS. Concurrent validity of the Brazilian version of SRS 22r with Br-SF-36. Rev Bras Fisioter. 2010;14(2):121–6.
69. Camarini PM, Rosanova GC, Gabriel BS, Gianini PE, Oliveira AS. The Brazilian version of the SRS-22r questionnaire for idiopathic scoliosis. Braz J Phys Ther. 2013;17(5):494–505.
70. Zhao L, Zhang Y, Sun X, Du Q, Shang L. The Scoliosis Research Society-22 Questionnaire adapted for adolescent idiopathic scoliosis patients in China: reliability and validity analysis. J Child Orthop. 2007;1(6):351–5.
71. Cheung K, Senkoylu A, Alanay A, Genc Y, Lau S, Luk KD. Reliability and concurrent validity of the adapted Chinese version of Scoliosis Research Society-22 (SRS-22) questionnaire. Spine. 2007;32(10):1141–5.
72. Li M, Wang CF, Gu SX, He SS, Zhu XD, Zhao YC, Zhang JT. Adapted simplified Chinese (mainland) version of Scoliosis Research Society-22 questionnaire. Spine. 2009;34(12):1321–4.
73. Qiu G, Qiu Y, Zhu Z, Liu Z, Song Y, Hai Y, et al. Re-evaluation of reliability and validity of simplified Chinese version of SRS-22 patient questionnaire: a multicenter study of 333 cases. Spine. 2011;36(8):E545–50.
74. Schlösser TP, Stadhouder A, Schimmel JJ, Lehr AM, van der Heijden GJ, Castelein RM. Reliability and validity of the adapted Dutch version of the revised Scoliosis Research Society 22-item questionnaire. Spine J. 2014 Aug 1;14(8):1663–72.
75. Beausejour M, Joncas J, Goulet L, Roy-Beaudry M, et al. Reliability and validity of adapted French Canadian version of Scoliosis Research Society outcomes questionnaire (SRS-22) in Quebec. Spine. 2009;34(6):623–8.

76. Lonjon G, Ilharreborde B, Odent T, Moreau S, Glorion C, Mazda K. Reliability and validity of the French-Canadian version of the Scoliosis Research Society 22 questionnaire in France. Spine. 2014;39(1):E26–34.
77. Niemeyer T, Schubert C, Halm HF, Herberts T, Leichtle C, Gesicki M. Validity and reliability of an adapted German version of Scoliosis Research Society-22 questionnaire. Spine. 2009;34(8):818–21.
78. Antonarakos PD, Katrinitsa L, Angelis L, Paganas A, Koen EM, Christodoulou EA, Christodoulou AG. Reliability and validity of the adapted Greek version of Scoliosis Research Society-22 (SRS-22) questionnaire. Scoliosis. 2009;4:14.
79. Potoupnis M, Papavasiliou K, Kenanidis E, Pellios S, Kapetanou A, Sayegh F, Kapetanos G. Reliability and concurrent validity of the adapted Greek version of the Scoliosis Research Society-22r questionnaire. A cross-sectional study performed on conservatively treated patients. Hippokratia. 2012;16(3):225–9.
80. Monticone M, Baiardi P, Calabrò D, Calabrò F, Foti C. Development of the Italian version of the revised Scoliosis Research Society-22 patient questionnaire, SRS-22r-I: cross-cultural adaptation, factor analysis, reliability, and validity. Spine. 2010;35(24):E1412–7.
81. Hashimoto H, Sase T, Arai Y, Maruyama T, Isobe K, Shouno Y. Validation of a Japanese version of the Scoliosis Research Society-22 patient questionnaire among idiopathic scoliosis patients in Japan. Spine. 2007;32(4):E141–6.
82. Lee JS, Lee DH, Suh KT, Kim JI, Lim JM, Goh TS. Validation of the Korean version of the Scoliosis Research Society-22 questionnaire. Eur Spine J. 2011;20(10):1751–6.
83. Mousavi SJ, Mobini B, Mehdian H, Akbarnia B, et al. Reliability and validity of the Persian version of the Scoliosis Research Society-22r questionnaire. Spine. 2010;35(7):784–9.
84. Glowacki M, Misterska E, Laurentowska M, Mankowski P. Polish adaptation of Scoliosis Research Society-22 questionnaire. Spine. 2009;34(10):1060–5.
85. Bago J, Climent JM, Ey A, Perez-Grueso FJ, Izquierdo E. The Spanish version of the SRS-22 patient questionnaire for idiopathic scoliosis: transcultural adaptation and reliability analysis. Spine. 2004;29(15):1676–80.
86. Climent JM, Bago J, Ey A, Perez-Grueso FJ, Izquierdo E. Validity of the Spanish version of the Scoliosis Research Society-22 patient questionnaire. Spine. 2005;30(6):705–9.
87. Danielsson AJ, Romberg K. Reliability and validity of the Swedish version of the Scoliosis Research Society-22 (SRS-22r) patient questionnaire for idiopathic scoliosis. Spine. 2013;38(21):1875–84.
88. Leelapattana P, Keorochana G, Johnson J, Wajanavisit W, Laohacharoensombat W. Reliability and validity of an adapted Thai version of the Scoliosis Research Society-22 questionnaire. J Child Orthop. 2011;5(1):35–40.
89. Sathira-Angkura V, Pithankuakul K, Sakulpipatana S, Piyaskulkaew C, Kunakornsawat S. Validity and reliability of an adapted Thai version of Scoliosis Research Society-22 questionnaire for adolescent idiopathic scoliosis. Spine. 2012;37(9):783–7.
90. Alanay A, Cil A, Berk H, Acaroglu RE, et al. Reliability and validity of adapted Turkish version of Scoliosis Research Society-22 (SRS-22) questionnaire. Spine. 2005;30(21):2464–8.
91. Martin BI, Deyo RA, Mirza SK, et al. Expenditures and health status among adults with back and neck problems. JAMA. 2008;299(6):656–64.
92. Holahan J, Blumberg LJ, McMorrow S, Zuckerman S, Waidmann T, Stockley K. Health Policy Center Occasional Paper. Washington, DC: The Urban Institute; 2011. Containing the growth of spending in the U.S. Health System.
93. Resnick DK, Tosteson AN, Groman RF, Ghogawala Z. Setting the equation: establishing value in spine care. Spine (Phila Pa 1976). 2014;39(22 Suppl 1):S43–50.
94. Rihn JA, Bradford CL, Phillips FM, Glassman SD, Albert TJ. Defining the value of spine care. J Am Acad Orthop Surg. 2013;21:419–26.
95. Nwachukwu BU, Schairer WW, Shifflett GD, Kellner DB, Sama AA. Cost-utility analyses in spine care: a qualitative and systematic review. Spine (Phila Pa 1976). 2015;40(1):31–40.
96. Tosteson AN, Lurie JD, Tosteson TD, et al. Surgical treatment of spinal stenosis with and without degenerative spondylolisthesis: cost-effectiveness after 2 years. Ann Intern Med. 2008;149(12):845–53.

97. Abdu WA, Lurie JD, Spratt KF, et al. Degenerative spondylolisthesis: does fusion method influence outcome? Four year results of the spine patient outcomes research trial. Spine (Phila Pa 1976). 2009;34(21):2351–60.
98. Tosteson AN, Tosteson TD, Lurie JD, et al. Comparative effectiveness evidence from the spine patient outcomes research trial: surgical versus nonoperative care for spinal stenosis, degenerative spondylolisthesis, and intervertebral disc herniation. Spine (Phila Pa 1976). 2011;36(24):2061–8.
99. Brazier J, Deverill M, Green C, Harper R, Booth A. A review of the use of health status measures in economic evaluation. Health Technol Assess. 1999;3(9):i–iv,1–164.
100. Qureshi S, Goz V, McAnany S, Cho SK, Hecht AC, Delamarter RB, Fehlings MG. Health state utility of patients with single-level cervical degenerative disc disease: comparison of anterior cervical discectomy and fusion with cervical disc arthroplasty. J Neurosurg Spine. 2014;20(5):475–9.
101. Bosch JL, van der Graaf Y, Hunink MG. Health-related quality of life after angioplasty and stent placement in patients with iliac artery occlusive disease: results of a randomized controlled clinical trial. Circulation. 1999;99:3155–60.
102. Bullens PH, van Loon CJ, de Waal Malefijt MC, Laan RF, Veth RP. Patient satisfaction after total knee arthroplasty: a comparison between subjective and objective outcome assessments. J Arthroplast. 2001;16:740–7.
103. Haentjens P, De Groote K, Annemans L. Prolonged enoxaparin therapy to prevent venous thromboembolism after primary hip or knee replacement. A cost-utility analysis. Arch Orthop Trauma Surg. 2004;124:507–17.
104. Carreon LY, Anderson PA, Glassman SD. Predicting SF-6D utility scores from the neck disability and numeric rating scales for neck and arm pain. Spine (Phila Pa 1976). 2011;36(6):490–4.
105. Sassi F. Calculating QALYs, comparing QALY and DALY calculations. Health Policy Plan. 2006;21(5):402–8.
106. Weinstein MC, Torrance G, McGuire A. QALYs: the basics. Value Health. 2009;12:S5–9.
107. Healthcare Cost and Utilization Project (HCUP). Cost-to-charge ratio files. Rockville: Agency for Healthcare Research and Quality. Available at: http://www.hcup-us.ahrq.gov/db/state/costtocharge.jsp. Accessed 9 May 2013.
108. Dagenais S, Caro J, Haldeman S. A systematic review of low back pain cost of illness studies in the United States and internationally. Spine J. 2008;8(1):8–20.
109. van den Hout WB. The value of productivity: human-capital versus friction-cost method. Ann Rheum Dis. 2010;69(suppl 1):i89–91.
110. Weinstein MC, Siegel JE, Gold MR, Kamlet MS, Russell LB. Recommendations of the panel on cost-effectiveness in health and medicine. JAMA. 1996;276(15):1253–8.
111. Hirth RA, Chernew ME, Miller E, Fendrick AM, Weissert WG. Willingness to pay for a quality-adjusted life year: in search of a standard. Med Decis Mak. 2000;20(3):332–42.
112. Braithwaite RS, Meltzer DO, King JT Jr, et al. What does the value of modern medicine say about the $50,000 per quality-adjusted life-year decision rule? Med Care. 2008;46:349–56.
113. Angevine PD, Zivin JG, McCormick PC. Cost-effectiveness of single-level anterior cervical discectomy and fusion for cervical spondylosis. Spine (Phila Pa 1976). 2005;30(17):1989–97.
114. Porter ME. What is value in health care? N Engl J Med. 2010;363(26):2477–81.

Part II

Methodology in Quality Assessment

4 Choice of Quality Metrics for Assessment of the Spine Patient

Taylor D. Ottesen, Kareem J. Kebaish, and Jonathan N. Grauer

Abbreviations

ACS-NSQIP	American College of Surgeons National Surgical Quality Improvement Program
AHRQ	Agency for Healthcare Research and Quality
APU	Annual payment update
CMS	Center for Medicare and Medicaid Services
DVT	Deep vein thrombosis
HCAHPS	Hospital Consumer Assessment of Healthcare Providers and Systems
EHR	Electronic health record
IVR	Interactive voice response
PCP	Primary care physician
PROM	Patient-reported outcome measures
VBP	Value-based purchasing program

The Importance and Role of Quality Metrics

In the United States, national healthcare expenditures reached over 3.2 billion dollars in 2015, an increase of 5.8% over the previous year [1]. The sustained rise in healthcare spending is expected to continue to rise and has led to increased examination of methods to reduce costs while maintaining or improving quality.

T. D. Ottesen · K. J. Kebaish · J. N. Grauer (✉)
Department of Orthopaedics and Rehabilitation, Yale University School of Medicine, New Haven, CT, USA
e-mail: jonathan.grauer@yale.edu

J. Ratliff et al. (eds.), *Quality Spine Care*,
https://doi.org/10.1007/978-3-319-97990-8_4

Unfortunately, despite the significant costs of healthcare in the United States, it has been estimated that less than 55% of patients receive the proper diagnosis and care [2]. As a result, healthcare is often fragmented in its delivery, overly complicated, and uncoordinated.

In an attempt to address some of these issues, quality metrics are being increasingly utilized to assess various types of healthcare data to evaluate performance from as granular as individual physicians and patients to entire healthcare systems. Evaluation of providers and policies against established quality standards establishes the performance of healthcare systems. The evaluation and adjustment based on these metrics are important to improve the care provided.

Quality metrics enable physicians, administrators, lawmakers, insurance entities, and governments to evaluate patient care and make necessary adjustments to give the highest quality of care to the patient. In addition, quality metrics help patients to make informed choices about their health and options for care.

Although the measurement of quality seeks to evaluate current healthcare models, their performance, and subsequent improvements in care quality itself has been hard to measure. A wide range of metrics have been developed in an effort to quantify quality. In general, these measures can be categorized into four major categories: (1) structural, (2) process, (3) outcome, or (4) patient experience [3]. Each system of metrics highlights a different aspect of care, all of which are important.

These metrics are particularly relevant in spine care with spinal issues being such a common reason for patients to seek medical attention and have mixed surgical outcomes for different surgical indications [4, 5]. Given the large assortment of tools to assess quality care, a basic knowledge of these tools and an understanding of their results are essential for today's spine surgeons [6]. This chapter seeks to delineate and explore quality metric techniques in spine care while recognizing that each system has pros and cons but bring important contributions to the evaluation of healthcare. It is through a balanced combination of these metrics that healthcare can ensure the highest level of care for patients.

Structural Measures

Every healthcare institution has a mix of initiatives and policies aimed at ensuring high-quality patient care – these are defined as structural measures. Structural measures, along with process and outcome measures, were first popularized in 1966 by Dr. Avedis Donabedian through an article published in *Milbank Quarterly* [7]. In its early form, structural measures focused on the quality of facilities and resources, administrative policies, and the qualification of providers [8]. Structural measures are useful in providing patients with information on how well-equipped health systems are for providing high-quality care.

An important distinction to note is that, unlike many other metrics, structural measures are not defined by outcomes but rather rely on the assumption that if an institution has the proper structures in place, then high-quality care will follow. There are a variety of different components that contribute to the structural measures utilized for spine patients, including the use of electronic health records (EHR), access to imaging, ratio of providers to patients, and available facilities and technology.

Though it has become a norm across virtually all healthcare providers, the use of EHR is a structural measure. There are many different EHR systems, each with their own advantages. Nonetheless, all systems share the goal of improving the coordination of care by making patient records accessible to all providers. Efficient access to records is especially valuable in spine patients, as these patients are likely to see a number of providers to manage their condition. For example, not all patients start by visiting a spine surgeon; some patients start by visiting a primary care physician (PCP). If the PCP does not find success with conservative treatment, they might refer them to a spine surgeon to evaluate their condition, as well as pain management specialist to help control the pain associated with their condition [9]. All three providers are capable of prescribing analgesics for pain relief, and having adequate records from the patients' previous visits is important for avoiding over-prescription of controlled drugs which could put patients at risk of serious complications such as addiction or overdose.

While in theory, EHR revolutionizes the synchrony of providers, in practice, this is not always the case. EHR has undeniably improved the documentation and communication within institutions; however, there is currently no centralized EHR system across different practices/institutions [10]. Unless a patient's provider utilizes the same system, a reliance on faxing records, sharing CDs of images, or having patients carry their documentation still exists. Some opponents of EHR have argued that it results in an increased burden on physicians, which could decrease the time spent with patients or result in higher rates of burnout among providers [11]. The example of EHR highlights one of the major shortcomings of structural measures. Institutions may be able to check off a long list of requirements but still fall short of high-quality care because of how a policy is executed.

Access to diagnostic images such as radiographs, computed tomography scans, and magnetic resonance imaging also plays a role in the coordination of quality care. Spine patients undergo many scans to evaluate the severity and progression of their condition. Patients might be seen by a number of different specialists, for second opinions and reevaluations, all of whom may need to review their scans. Ensuring that the scans are easily accessible to the providers can improve the quality of care by avoiding repetitive scans that subject the patient to unnecessary doses of radiation, with an additional benefit of reducing excess costs and use of resources.

Another structural measure is how well an institution is staffed at any given time. Some hospitals may mandate limits on the number of patients that can be seen by an attending physician. Such initiatives stem from the findings that a significant number of attending physician are seeing a higher volume of patients than what are considered to be "safe levels" and admit that this significantly impacts the quality of care they can provide [12].

The availability of facilities and resources is also a structural measure, indicating whether a hospital is equipped to provide high-quality care. This measure may be influenced by a number of different factors, such as the amount of radiographic equipment. This is especially important at trauma centers, as limited imaging equipment can lead to delays in critical diagnoses. Delays in the diagnoses of spinal injuries are associated with significantly worse prognosis [13–16]. The availability of intensive care unit beds can also influence this measure. Reduced availability of ICU beds is associated with worse outcomes and involuntary changes in patients' goals of care [17, 18]. When assessing these measures, not all hospitals should be compared to the same standard. Some hospitals have lower patient volumes or may be located in the same region as a larger hospital that is designated to receive difficult cases.

Structural measures are a useful metric and can provide spine patients with valuable insight and inform their decision of where to seek care for their condition. These examples are certainly not exhaustive, and every institution has countless structural measures to bolster the quality of care. The importance of structural measures is not in that they provide patients with any guarantees for their care but rather in that they inform them of whether an institution or provider has the capacity to provide a certain level of quality care. In addition, some structural measures are more relevant to certain patient populations and diagnoses. Ideally, there would be a direct relationship between the structural measures and the quality of care; however, this depends on how well initiatives or policies are executed.

Process Measures

In addition to structural and outcome measures, process measures became branded as one of the major methods by which to define quality through the early efforts of Dr. Avedis Donabedian [7]. Process measures focus strictly on the process by which care is administered irrespective of outcomes. These metrics evaluate how consistently a provider adheres to delineated guidelines of care with the belief that adherence to these guidelines will yield positive outcomes. Typically, these guidelines represent generally accepted procedures and treatments that improve the health of the patient and/or prevent future complications.

Process measures are objective in nature. In general, the metric gathers whether or not the provider or care team followed a guideline. Questions are often formatted in a yes or no format. For example, was prophylaxis for deep vein thrombosis (DVT) administered prior to surgery and were antibiotics administered prior to incision [19]? Others include whether the patient's medications were checked before prescribing any new medication, are providers regularly checking for cutaneous and soft tissue wounds on diabetic patients, and was smoking cessation counseling given?

One advantage of process measures is the ease of collection and interpretation. As a result, a large majority of quality metrics publically published for each hospital are made of up a combination of various process measures. The Centers for Medicare and Medicaid Services (CMS) maintains a central website named Hospital Compare that freely disseminates these numbers to the public. The publication of this information enables patients to make educated decisions about their medical care and establish expectations of what care they will receive both on a hospital-wide level and for a given condition. Additionally, dissemination of these metrics to the public keeps hospitals accountable and stimulates improvement on a hospital-wide level [20].

Process measures are particularly useful for physicians because it provides well-defined, clear tasks and action-based feedback to improve their delivery of quality care. Physicians can easily identify areas for improvement and make necessary adjustments in their routine without the limitations of subjective data found in outcome and patient-reported measures. On a hospital level, process measures enable reduction of inappropriate variation or deficits in the system. Administrators are easily able to identify areas of concern in care and redirect hospital policy and funds to reduce this variation. Problem areas may be as simple as a deficit in the number and availability of pressure-redistribution mattresses leading to increased pressure sore quantity and associated complications in the hospital. Regardless of the problem, careful monitoring of these metrics brings quick intervention and correction of deviations that could lead to decreased quality of care.

A potential drawback to process measures is that they do not always follow or predict quality outcomes. A benefit to this separation is that it reduces resistance for physicians and hospitals to take more difficult patients. When evaluated solely by outcomes, physicians can be hesitant or unwilling to operate on sick patients with challenging conditions. With process measures, as long as the physician strictly follows established guidelines, they will be in compliance with accepted standards and can strive for the best possible outcomes. Although several studies have shown positive correlations between hospital performance on CMS's Hospital Compare and outcomes [21, 22], other studies have shown little relationship between them [23].

Moreover, process measures frequently do not distinguish with granularity, the true quality of care that was given. Quality metrics that require smoking cessation advice treat all smoking cessation encounters the same without the opportunity to describe the depth of conversation or resources provided. The metric will be affirmative regardless of whether the physician mentioned cessation in passing or had a thorough conversation with acknowledgment of barriers to quitting and commitment to a cessation management plan.

Process measures are also absent or deficient in vital areas of care that have been shown to drive outcomes. Areas such as technology and coordination of care are largely underrepresented in process metrics. Inclusion of areas such as how treatment was coordinated and the inclusion of mental illness services as a part of the patient care team are needed for the future development of process measures.

Despite these disadvantages, process measures have become the status quo within quality metrics, while critics and supporters alike cite necessary improvements in the measures. Although process measures have been previously established based on research and observations, it is important to closely and regularly evaluate these measures to ensure they are truly tracking desired outcomes. Many measures have been shown to directly link to changes in quality of care; however, other process measures have been less successful. Recent studies have found that hospital performance has been very loosely tied to the CMS-defined sets of process measures and has shown no significant differences in mortality [21, 24] or readmission rates [25] between hospitals when evaluated based on these processed measures.

Additionally, as mentioned, metrics to measure coordination of care through discharge and beyond are largely missing. This represents an untapped area for improvement in the quality of care as care coordination, early primary care follow-up, and patient adherence to medication regimens have been associated with reduced readmission rates [25–32].

The data provided through process measures enables easy analysis of holes in quality of care and highlights straightforward methods to improve performance and ideally the resulting outcomes. The addition of some important expansion could enhance the value of process measures and further evidence-based delivery of quality care. The growth of publically reported measures, such as those found in Hospital Compare, to include complementary outcomes measures, could improve the patient experience and quality of care [25].

Objectively Assessed Outcome Measures

Since their creation along with structural and process measures, outcome measures have faced largely the same challenges. When first described by Dr. Donabedian, outcome measures assessed ranged from mortality rates to patient satisfaction. It was clear that certain outcomes were much easier to measure than others, and, eventually, this resulted in the division of this measure into objectively assessed outcome measures and patient-reported outcome measures. Objectively assessed outcome measures include variables such as infection rates, postsurgical mortality rates, and readmission rates. These measures can be quantified, are easily accessible, and are objective of the opinions of patients or providers.

As recently as 2009, mortality rates have been in the spotlight for assessing the quality of care; however, with advancements in technology and surgical mortality decreasing, there may be less room for improvement in this measure [33–35]. Thus, while maintaining focus on this measure, systems are turning attention more toward secondary measures such as reducing infection rates [36].

This change highlights an important consideration when using outcome measures; although the data on these measures may be readily available, measures must be carefully considered for their relevance and outcomes considered in relation to the influence of confounding factors. Nonetheless, measures that objectively undergo these considerations can be invaluable to providers in improving their techniques and practice. For institutions, they can inform choices in policies and initiatives and provide feedback for existing efforts.

Another great example of an outcome measure is readmission rate, as it is useful in highlighting some of the important considerations of how a measurement should be made and the potential confounders that can influence the measure. Readmission is particularly relevant to hospital administrators as hospitals assume responsibility for the incremental costs with the rise of bundle and pay-for-performance models. However, readmission can be difficult to define, for example, establishing timelines for a readmission as a result of surgery compared to a readmission as a result of poor health. The current standard, set by CMS, is to count a return to the hospital in the 30 days following the patients' discharge as a readmission resulting from surgery

[37]. Arguments can be made whether this too much or too little time and certainly each case is likely heavily dependent on the circumstances that lead to readmission and individual patient comorbidities.

With the current focus on outcomes, objectively assessed measures may seem to represent the gold standard in measuring the quality of care, but it is important to note that numerous factors can influence the outcomes of each patient. Every patient has a unique medical history and set of comorbidities that can increase their risk of complications and poorer outcomes compared to healthier patients. Some providers may have higher rates of adverse outcome as a result of their patient population, which is a factor they cannot control without limiting care to subpopulations with greater comorbidities or with challenging clinical presentations. One popular solution is the use of risk adjustment models, which have become well known for their use by Medicare and Medicaid to predict the cost of care based on characteristics of individual patients [38].

In addition to improved prediction of the cost of care, risk adjustment can also serve to inform the quality of care assessment for a particular provider or institution by adjusting for the difficulties in the patient populations they serve. Nonetheless, risk adjustment models are far from perfect and have undergone extensive evolution over the past two decades to better align with research findings, incentives, and matching healthcare resources to needs. Such evolution will continue in order to improve the utility of objectively assessed outcome measures and respond to advancements in treatment and patient care.

The caveats of mortality, infection, and readmission rates serve to highlight how even seemingly objective measures require careful consideration when they are used. Objectively assessed outcome measures are invaluable for quantifying the effects of different initiatives and providing patients with information on the performance of hospitals and providers. Providers can also make use of this outcome to inform them of how well their outcomes compare to their peers and use the results to guide improvements in care.

Registries

In order to study spine disorders and produce generalizable results for the whole population, data from multiple providers as well as national and international institutions can be used. Institutions can directly collaborate through multicenter studies; however, using registries can also be an efficient way to compile large datasets. The root of the modern-day medical registry can be traced back to 1967 when the Medical Birth Registry of Norway was created to track the incidence of congenital abnormalities and determine their causes [39]. Registries are collections of data on patients with specific diagnoses, pre-existing conditions, treatments, and other details related to their demographics and care. Many registries currently exist within the United States and internationally, consisting of data on surgical patients in general, as well as data specific to spine patients.

Each registry has its own unique characteristics based on its intended purpose and uses. For example, one of the goals of the Spine Registry, initiated by the North

American Spine Society, is to examine the natural history of spine disorders. This registry will fulfill this goal by collecting longitudinal data on patient outcomes and treatments. As another example, the American College of Surgeons National Surgical Quality Improvement Program (ACS-NSQIP) aims to reduce the rate of surgical complications by tabulating rates of surgical adverse events and establishing benchmarks to which these can be compared. This database used defined criteria for patient demographics, comorbidities, and perioperative outcomes to establish uniform reporting and allow for risk adjustment. Many other registries exist specifically for spine patients, and each of them varies in size and institutional participation and has their own methods and goals.

The utility of registries has become increasingly clear over the past decade. It is difficult for a single provider to study patients with unique circumstances and conditions. They may simply have too small of a sample to reach any statistically significant conclusion about treatment outcomes. Using registries can increase the power of such research to produce meaningful results. Registries provide additional utility in that they are less prone to the biases of single institutions, patient samples, or provider experience. For institutions, registries can provide a measure of their quality of care and guide policies for improvement. Registries can also provide feedback about the utility of structural or process measures.

While their development has certainly revolutionized medical research, registries are not without limitations. The most significant limitation of registries is that they lead to observational rather than experimentally comparisons. As such, it is important to exercise caution when drawing conclusions from such studies; the data can only be used to establish correlational relationships rather than causal relationships. Concerns about the quality of registry data have also been raised, particularly for orthopedic registries; many of these datasets do not contain disease-specific outcome measures [40] and may have variable data quality and completeness [41].

Despite the above-noted limitations, registries fill an important role in the larger picture of quality metrics, allowing for facile collaboration across different institutions. The collective data provides invaluable insight into treatment outcomes and understanding how to select the most appropriate plan of care for each patient. Providers can use the data to determine how to reduce these complications, while patients can use the data to determine which institutions have the most favorable outcomes for their conditions. Finally, under the pressure of insurance companies, institutions also make great use of registries for epidemiological purposes, as well as reduction of preventable complications such as infection.

Patient-Reported Outcomes Measures

The ultimate goal of using quality metrics is to ensure that patients receive the most appropriate care for their needs. As such, the patients' opinions about their quality of care are an important consideration and can serve as an indicator of how well their treatment course aligned with their goals of care. Patient-reported outcome measures (PROMs) are a quantification of patients' views on how well the treatment addressed their symptoms, enhanced their function, and fit their specific needs. This data is collected through surveys given to patient typically before and after surgery, which allows for comparison of both states and an understanding of the health gains from the procedure [42].

Using PROMs redefines what may be considered a successful treatment outcome by shifting the judgment from providers to patients, thus empowering patients in a number of different ways. Spine patients typically seek treatment for two primary reasons: (1) alleviation of pain and (2) restoration of functional status [43]. Reaching this understanding of the patients' goals may be as simple as interviewing or surveying them before treatment. For example, a patient might be asked, "Do you have difficulty tying your shoes?" The question would then be followed up with, "On a scale of 1–10 rate how important this is to you." The patient may then be asked a series of questions to assess their intensity of pain and how much it affects their desired daily function.

Through proper surveying and questioning, providers can gain a better understanding of what improvements are most important to the patient and what they prioritize. Previous research has utilized PROMs in assessing the success of different interventions in spine patients [44]. PROMs also provide institutions as well as prospective patients with valuable information about providers and can help guide practice and policies [45].

The use of PROMs does have a few setbacks; the most obvious of which is that despite the quantification of the data, asking for patient's opinions is a subjective measure and can be influenced by biases. These biases must be considered when determining how and when to collect data and how that data should be used. When using this data to judge a provider's effectiveness, it is necessary to account for the patients' experiences such as the occurrence of complications. Other challenges revolve around the difficulty of data collection. Distributing surveys can be costly and requires time and resources, and patient interest in completing such surveys can be limited. In addition to bias and cost, currently, there remains a deficit in uniform agreement on which PROMs to use. Some are general health oriented and some are more disease specific. Comparisons across systems that do not collect such measures or collect different measures can be difficult. Further, each of these measures can be influenced by many variables not related to the spine itself.

Tough and potentially subjective, PROMs are perhaps some of the most important quality metrics as the results are patient-derived. Their results highlight a key point that no matter how efficacious a treatment might be, a plan of care must align with the patients' goals in order to be effective. Providers can use this metric to understand how to better serve their patients and meet their goals of treatment. Institutions can utilize the results to assess their providers and inform policies for improving and optimizing quality of care. Some efforts are needed to improve the implantation of PROMs and increase institutional use and patient participation in these surveys. With an emphasis on high-value care, understanding how to continue making use of this metric and its role in insurance reimbursements will become an increasingly relevant question.

Patient-Reported Satisfaction

Another patient-reported metric that is being given increasing attention is patient-reported satisfaction. Studies have defined patient satisfaction to be "the degree to which a patient feels they have received high-quality health care," [41] and are evaluated in many specialties [46]. Patient-reported satisfaction gathers information directly from patients about many aspects of their clinical care. Surveys inquire about interpersonal aspects such as the ability of a physician or staff to communicate clearly and in an accessible vernacular as well as procedural aspects such as ease of making an appointment or obtaining timely test results. It should be noted that this is unique from other outcomes and process metrics, as satisfaction is a measurement that is entirely subjective [47].

In order to assess the experience of patients and their satisfaction with their experience, a variety of proprietary surveys have been created by private and government organizations. The industry leader has largely been Press Ganey Associates, Inc., which quickly became one of the leading health consultant agencies for patient experience after its inception in 1985 [48]. Branded as the expert in patient satisfaction, they have developed many tools that gather both general information and information unique to each patient [49].

Other companies have also tried to assess the patient experience through metrics such as the patient expectation survey developed by Arbor Associates [49]. Additionally, the Patient Satisfaction and Loyalty Measurement System by the Jackson Organization, Research Consultants Inc. has added to the available techniques by assessing patient loyalty as a result of satisfaction [49]. Still others, such as the Health Plan Effectiveness Data and Information Set, were developed to further evaluate patient's experience with the healthcare system [48, 50].

As healthcare has become more and more of a service industry, hospitals have utilized these commercial surveys to understand the patient experience. However, the copious number of measurement options makes patient satisfaction a difficult metric to standardize. In an effort to create continuity and standardization across hospital systems, CMS and the Agency for Healthcare Research and Quality (AHRQ) created the Hospital Consumer Assessment of Healthcare Providers and Systems (HCAHPS) survey [48]. The current HCAHPS survey consists of 32 questions and focuses on aspects of the clinical experience such as communication of doctors and nurses to the patient, how well a patient's pain was controlled, the cleanliness of the facilities, and whether they would recommend the hospital to their friends and family.

Following pilot programs, the HCAHPS survey was approved for use on a national scale in 2005 [51], and over the next 3 years, the program was refined and expanded. During this time, individual hospital results began to be public, so patients could make informed decisions about their healthcare [52]. Access by the public to these scores acted as an incentive for hospitals to evaluate their staff and facilities to address deficiencies that could lower their HCAHPS survey scores.

The incentive for hospitals to increase the quality of care through the HCAHPS patient satisfaction metric was further solidified in 2008 when government reimbursements to hospitals began to be tied to survey results [38]. Acute care institutions were mandated to use and report HCAHPS in all their facilities in order to receive their annual payment update (APU) and hospitals who did not report these and other quality metric measures would be penalized 2% of their APU [52]. Hospitals were further motivated by additional rewards for hospitals with higher HCAHPS scores under the value-based purchasing program (VBP) [53].

CMS compliance requirements have evolved since 2008, but, currently, a minimum of 300 HCAHPS surveys must be completed by a random sampling of eligible patients over a 12-month reporting period [54]. These surveys can be completed via telephone, mail, mixed telephone and mail, or active interactive voice response (IVR) which allows patients to take the survey on the phone with live access to an operator [48, 52, 54].

Although HCAHPS has become a major model to evaluate quality, opinions are mixed on its effectiveness. Many non-orthopedic studies have presented positive correlations between HCAHPS responses and outcomes, some even referring to satisfaction as "the ultimate endpoint to the health-care pathway" [46, 55]. For example, higher HCAPS scores have been shown to correlate with decreased heart failure readmissions [56], increased observed-to-expected survival rates [57], and 30-day readmission and perioperative mortality rates [58]. Spine surgery-specific studies found a positive correlation between the amount of time that was spent with a patient and a patient's postoperative pain score [59]. Additionally, shorter hospital stays were associated with patients who responded "always" when asked "how often was your pain well controlled," and increased scores on "how often did the hospital staff do everything they could to help you with your pain" were associated with a decrease in operation time and pain scores [60].

In contrast to the aforementioned studies, critics believe satisfaction to only be a measure of service regardless of more important outcomes [47]. Some critics argue that a patient's satisfaction is determined to a greater degree based on "concierge" services provided by the hospital rather than the actual quality of the care received [48, 58, 61]. For the spine patient, perhaps the most difficult and important part of their care is done under anesthesia making it impossible for the patient to truly evaluate the full range of their care. Patients are then left with their morning breakfast selection and cleanliness of the facility to determine their satisfaction with their care. Some studies have conversely showed decreased or no correlation between satisfaction scores and outcomes such as in lumbar surgery [62]. Patients who developed nosocomial infections showed no difference in HCAHPS scores than their non-infected counterparts [63], and two orthopedic studies were unable to establish a connection between satisfaction scores and received surgical care [62, 63].

For both positive and negative results, it is important to consider confounding factors inherent to HCAHPS data. For example, one study found that patients who responded to the survey via telephone or IVR were much more likely to give higher scores than those who took the survey via mail [64]. Moreover, demographic patient factors can have an effect on survey responses [62, 64–66]. Factors such as age, sex, economic status, education, and religious beliefs can influence a response [55, 67].

In one study, males, African Americans, those of lower economic status, and those with a shorter length of stay were found to have higher HCAHPS scores [68]. Variation in preadmission medications was also shown to be associated with satisfaction scores [60].

Unfortunately, when metrics become quantifiable and compensation becomes tied to these numbers, there can be unforeseen results. Some studies have suggested that in an effort to increase scores, physicians have satisfied patients' requests for treatments that are unnecessary or contraindicated in that patient population [69]. This can be damaging to both patients and the healthcare system by leading to antibiotic-resistant bacteria, overexposure to radiation, overmedication, and medication abuse [48]. Regardless of specialty, it can be agreed that care that is unsafe or ineffective is low quality irrespective of the declared satisfaction by the patient.

Patient satisfaction is an important part of healthcare, and it will continue to play an important role in the delivery of US healthcare. Although both patient satisfaction and PROMs are extremely subjective measures of quality, they are important to the patient experience. Patients and physicians need to work together to achieve health for their patients. Although there are limitations to these quality measures, additional research and reporting will influence future healthcare access and reimbursement strategies.

Enactment of Quality Measures

Such a variety of quality measures serves to highlight the vast number of methods for measuring quality and abundance of opinions on what measures can best reflect the quality of patient care. There is certainly no standard across institutions, which gives hospitals the liberty to choose their own set of quality measures.

Currently, standardizing quality metrics across a group of institutions would be challenging. Difficulties would arise in the collection of these metrics in a manner that is consistent and useful across all institutions. Perhaps electronic medical records could be used, as systems such as Cerner, McKesson, and Epic have spread across the country.

Nonetheless, if the collection issues are resolved, the next issue would be the debates over which metrics should be used. Registries attempt to bypass these obstacles, providing standardized data from multiple institutions. Nonetheless, as outlined previously, registries are not without fault, and problems with compliance and accuracy are known. Further, there is no evidence to show that completely aligning quality metrics across institutions would yield to the larger goal of optimizing quality of care.

Currently, many institutions are focusing on optimizing their own existing quality metrics while contributing and following more centralized standards. This process can be both through internal evaluation and comparison with other institutions. Outcome measures are useful indicators of the quality of care because they can be used to assess the efficacy of other measures and inform how initiatives are best executed by comparing different institutions without standardizing metrics. An internal evaluation would be useful in dictating what measures should be used across different specialties and patient populations. Structural measures can be useful across an entire institution, whereas specific process measures may be useful for some specialties but serve little utility for others. There must be a balance between the metrics used to assess a particular specialty and the metrics used across the entire institution. Each specialty has its own unique set of procedures and thus should have their own unique set of metrics to rate them. Furthermore, quality measures should not be mutually exclusive within a specialty. For example, pairing structural measures with other quality metrics such as outcome measures that directly assess the effects of these policies are necessary to ensure that sufficient evidence exists for these structural initiatives.

Conclusion

If one thing is certain about quality metrics, it is that the constant changes in health insurance policy have put pressure on hospitals to improve their measures and align them with the expectations of insurers. Ideally, these expectations would realistically translate to higher quality of care rather than simply fulfilling checklists or compromising care to inflate patient satisfaction measures. Every measure has its own unique advantages and brings light to different aspects of care. However, no measure alone can sufficiently provide a full scope of the quality of care an institution provides. Hospitals and insurers should find utility in every measure and have an open line of communication to coordinate how they use these measures. Breaking down such barriers would result in a significant improvement in the usage of quality metrics, which would be advantageous to all players. Patients would benefit from higher-quality care, insurers would have better control of reimbursement costs, and hospitals would be able to continue generating stable and consistent growth.

References

1. US National Health Expenditure Data, NHE Fact Sheet Centers for Disease Control and Prevention, National Center for Health Statistics [updated June 2017]. Available from: https://www.cms.gov/research-statistics-data-and-systems/statistics-trends-and-reports/nationalhealthexpenddata/nhe-fact-sheet.html.
2. McGlynn EA, Asch SM, Adams J, Keesey J, Hicks J, DeCristofaro A, et al. The quality of health care delivered to adults in the United States. N Engl J Med. 2003;348(26):2635–45.
3. Morris C, Bailey K. Measuring health care quality: an overview of quality measures. Washington, DC: Families USA; 2014.
4. Hart LG, Deyo RA, Cherkin DC. Physician office visits for low back pain. Frequency, clinical evaluation, and treatment patterns from a U.S. national survey. Spine. 1995;20(1):11–9.
5. Andersson GB. Epidemiological features of chronic low-back pain. Lancet (London, England). 1999;354(9178):581–5.
6. Teles AR, Khoshhal KI, Falavigna A. Why and how should we measure outcomes in spine surgery? J Taibah Univ Sci. 2016;11(2):91–7.
7. Best M, Neuhauser D. Avedis Donabedian: father of quality assurance and poet. Qual Saf Health Care. 2004;13(6):472–3.

8. Donabedian A. Evaluating the quality of medical care. Milbank; Memorial Fund Quaterly. 1965.
9. Atlas SJ, Deyo RA. Evaluating and managing acute low back pain in the primary care setting. J Gen Intern Med. 2001;16(2):120–31.
10. Alpert JS. The electronic medical record in 2016: advantages and disadvantages. Digit Med. 2016;2(2):48.
11. Shanafelt TD, Dyrbye LN, Sinsky C, Hasan O, Satele D, Sloan J, et al., editors. Relationship between clerical burden and characteristics of the electronic environment with physician burnout and professional satisfaction. Mayo Clin Proc. 2016.: Elsevier;91:836–48.
12. Michtalik HJ, Yeh H-C, Pronovost PJ, Brotman DJ. Impact of attending physician workload on patient care: a survey of hospitalists. JAMA Intern Med. 2013;173(5):375–7.
13. Anderson S, Biros MH, Reardon RF. Delayed diagnosis of thoracolumbar fractures in multiple-trauma patients. Acad Emerg Med. 1996;3(9):832–9.
14. Platzer P, Hauswirth N, Jaindl M, Chatwani S, Vecsei V, Gaebler C. Delayed or missed diagnosis of cervical spine injuries. J Trauma Acute Care Surg. 2006;61(1):150–5.
15. Davis DP, Wold RM, Patel RJ, Tran AJ, Tokhi RN, Chan TC, et al. The clinical presentation and impact of diagnostic delays on emergency department patients with spinal epidural abscess. J Emerg Med. 2004;26(3):285–91.
16. Davis JW, Phreaner DL, Hoyt DB, Mackersie RC. The etiology of missed cervical spine injuries. J Trauma Acute Care Surg. 1993;34(3):342–6.
17. Tran BT. Reduced Icu bed availability is associated with worse outcomes on the general wards. Crit Care Alert. 2014;22(6):41–2.
18. Stelfox HT, Hemmelgarn BR, Bagshaw SM, Gao S, Doig CJ, Nijssen-Jordan C, et al. Intensive care unit bed availability and outcomes for hospitalized patients with sudden clinical deterioration. Arch Intern Med. 2012;172(6):467–74.
19. Shekelle PG, Wachter RM, Pronovost PJ, Schoelles K, McDonald KM, Dy SM, et al. Making health care safer II: an updated critical analysis of the evidence for patient safety practices. Evid Rep Technol Assess (Full Rep). 2013;211:1–945.
20. Fung CH, Lim YW, Mattke S, Damberg C, Shekelle PG. Systematic review: the evidence that publishing patient care performance data improves quality of care. Ann Intern Med. 2008;148(2):111–23.
21. Werner RM, Bradlow ET. Relationship between Medicare's hospital compare performance measures and mortality rates. JAMA. 2006;296(22):2694–702.
22. Lilford RJ, Brown CA, Nicholl J. Use of process measures to monitor the quality of clinical practice. Br Med J. 2007;335(7621):648–50.
23. Fonarow GC, Abraham WT, Albert NM, Stough WG, Gheorghiade M, Greenberg BH, et al. Association between performance measures and clinical outcomes for patients hospitalized with heart failure. JAMA. 2007;297(1):61–70.
24. Jha AK, Orav EJ, Li Z, Epstein AM. The inverse relationship between mortality rates and performance in the hospital quality alliance measures. Health Aff. 2007;26(4):1104–10.
25. Stefan MS, Pekow PS, Nsa W, Priya A, Miller LE, Bratzler DW, et al. Hospital performance measures and 30-day readmission rates. J Gen Intern Med. 2013;28(3):377–85.
26. Shepperd S, Parkes J, McClaren J, Phillips C. Discharge planning from hospital to home. Cochrane Database Syst Rev. 2004;1:Cd000313.
27. van Walraven C, Seth R, Austin PC, Laupacis A. Effect of discharge summary availability during post-discharge visits on hospital readmission. J Gen Intern Med. 2002;17(3):186–92.
28. Jack BW, Chetty VK, Anthony D, Greenwald JL, Sanchez GM, Johnson AE, et al. A reengineered hospital discharge program to decrease rehospitalization: a randomized trial. Ann Intern Med. 2009;150(3):178–87.
29. Parrish MM, O'Malley K, Adams RI, Adams SR, Coleman EA. Implementation of the care transitions intervention: sustainability and lessons learned. Prof Case Manag. 2009;14(6):282–93. quiz 94-5
30. Parry C, Min SJ, Chugh A, Chalmers S, Coleman EA. Further application of the care transitions intervention: results of a randomized controlled trial conducted in a fee-for-service setting. Home Health Care Serv Q. 2009;28(2–3):84–99.

31. Coleman EA, Smith JD, Frank JC, Min SJ, Parry C, Kramer AM. Preparing patients and caregivers to participate in care delivered across settings: the care transitions intervention. J Am Geriatr Soc. 2004;52(11):1817–25.
32. Daly BJ, Douglas SL, Kelley CG, O'Toole E, Montenegro H. Trial of a disease management program to reduce hospital readmissions of the chronically critically ill. Chest. 2005;128(2):507–17.
33. Control CfD, Prevention. QuickStats: death rate from complications of medical and surgical care among adults aged >45 years, by age group–United States, 1999–2009. MMWR Morb Mortal Wkly Rep. 2012;61(37):750.
34. Roche J, Wenn RT, Sahota O, Moran CG. Effect of comorbidities and postoperative complications on mortality after hip fracture in elderly people: prospective observational cohort study. BMJ. 2005;331(7529):1374.
35. Goodkin DA, Bragg-Gresham JL, Koenig KG, Wolfe RA, Akiba T, Andreucci VE, et al. Association of comorbid conditions and mortality in hemodialysis patients in Europe, Japan, and the United States: the Dialysis Outcomes and Practice Patterns Study (DOPPS). J Am Soc Nephrol. 2003;14(12):3270–7.
36. Control CfD, Prevention. QuickStats: rates of Clostridium difficile infection among hospitalized patients aged ≥65 years, by age group – National Hospital Discharge Survey, United States, 1996–2009. MMWR Morb Mortal Wkly Rep. 2011;60(34):1171.
37. Horwitz L, Partovian C, Lin Z, Herrin J, Grady J, Conover M, et al. Hospital-wide all-cause 30-day risk-standardized readmission measure: Final technical report. 2013. Accessed at https://www.qualitynet.org/dcs/ContentServer?cid=1219069855273&pagename=QnetPublic%2FPage%2FQnetTier3&c=Page.
38. Pope GC, Kautter J, Ellis RP, Ash AS, Ayanian JZ, Iezzoni LI, et al. Risk adjustment of Medicare capitation payments using the CMS-HCC model. Health Care Financ Rev. 2004;25(4):119.
39. Irgens L. The origin of registry-based medical research and care. Acta Neurol Scand. 2012;126(s195):4–6.
40. Barrie J, Marsh D. Quality of data in the Manchester orthopaedic database. BMJ. 1992;304(6820):159–62.
41. Arts DG, De Keizer NF, Scheffer G-J. Defining and improving data quality in medical registries: a literature review, case study, and generic framework. J Am Med Inform Assoc. 2002;9(6):600–11.
42. Neil W. Wagle M, MBA. Implementing Patient-Reported Outcome Measures (PROMs) NEJM Catalyst: NEJM Catalyst; 2017. Available from: https://catalyst.nejm.org/implementing-proms-patient-reported-outcome-measures/.
43. Carey TS, Garrett JM, Jackman AM. Beyond the good prognosis: examination of an inception cohort of patients with chronic low back pain. Spine. 2000;25(1):115.
44. Weinstein JN, Lurie JD, Tosteson TD, Skinner JS, Hanscom B, Tosteson AN, et al. Surgical vs nonoperative treatment for lumbar disk herniation: the Spine Patient Outcomes Research Trial (SPORT) observational cohort. JAMA. 2006;296(20):2451–9.
45. Black N. Patient reported outcome measures could help transform healthcare. Br Med J. 2013;346:f167.
46. Korolija D, Wood-Dauphinee S, Pointner R. Patient-reported outcomes. How important are they? Surg Endosc. 2007;21(4):503–7.
47. Godil SS, Parker SL, Zuckerman SL, Mendenhall SK, Devin CJ, Asher AL, et al. Determining the quality and effectiveness of surgical spine care: patient satisfaction is not a valid proxy. Spine J. 2013;13(9):1006–12.
48. Malpani R, Hilibrand AS, Grauer JN. Evolution and use of Hospital Consumer Assessment of Healthcare Providers and Systems (HCAHPS) surveys and their application for spinal surgery patients. Contemporary Spine Surgery (Accepted). 2017.
49. Urden LD. Patient satisfaction measurement: current issues and implications. Outcomes Manag. 2002;6(3):125–31.
50. Assurance NCfQ. Medicare special needs plans performance results: HEDIS 2014. 2014.
51. Tevis SE, Kennedy GD, Kent KC. Is there a relationship between patient satisfaction and favorable surgical outcomes? Adv Surg. 2015;49:221–33.

52. Giordano LA, Elliott MN, Goldstein E, Lehrman WG, Spencer PA. Development, implementation, and public reporting of the HCAHPS survey. Med Care Res Rev. 2010;67(1):27–37.
53. Services DoHaHSCfMaM. Hospital value-based purchasing. Medicare Learning Network. 2015.
54. Services DoHaHSCfMaM. CAHPS® Hospital Survey (HCAHPS) Quality Assurance Guidelines Version 12.0. 2017.
55. Chow A, Mayer EK, Darzi AW, Athanasiou T. Patient-reported outcome measures: the importance of patient satisfaction in surgery. Surgery. 2009;146(3):435–43.
56. Dy SM, Chan KS, Chang HY, Zhang A, Zhu J, Mylod D. Patient perspectives of care and process and outcome quality measures for heart failure admissions in US hospitals: how are they related in the era of public reporting? Int J Qual Health Care. 2016;28(4):522–8.
57. Srinivas R, Chavin KD, Baliga PK, Srinivas T, Taber DJ. Association between patient satisfaction and outcomes in kidney transplant. Am J Med Qual. 2015;30(2):180–5.
58. Tsai TC, Orav EJ, Jha AK. Patient satisfaction and quality of surgical care in US hospitals. Ann Surg. 2015;261(1):2–8.
59. Etier BE Jr, Orr SP, Antonetti J, Thomas SB, Theiss SM. Factors impacting Press Ganey patient satisfaction scores in orthopedic surgery spine clinic. Spine J. 2016;16(11):1285–9.
60. Maher DP, Wong W, Woo P, Padilla C, Zhang X, Shamloo B, et al. Perioperative factors associated with HCAHPS responses of 2,758 surgical patients. Pain Med. 2015;16(4):791–801.
61. Joseph B, Azim A, O'Keeffe T, Ibraheem K, Kulvatunyou N, Tang A, et al. American College of Surgeons level I trauma centers outcomes do not correlate with patients' perception of hospital experience. J Trauma Acute Care Surg. 2017;82(4):722–7.
62. Levin JM, Winkelman RD, Smith GA, Tanenbaum J, Benzel EC, Mroz TE, et al. The association between the Hospital Consumer Assessment of Healthcare Providers and Systems (HCAHPS) survey and real-world clinical outcomes in lumbar spine surgery. Spine J. 2017;17:1586.
63. Day MS, Hutzler LH, Karia R, Vangsness K, Setia N, Bosco JA 3rd. Hospital-acquired conditions after orthopedic surgery do not affect patient satisfaction scores. J Healthc Qual. 2014;36(6):33–40.
64. Elliott MN, Zaslavsky AM, Goldstein E, Lehrman W, Hambarsoomians K, Beckett MK, et al. Effects of survey mode, patient mix, and nonresponse on CAHPS hospital survey scores. Health Serv Res. 2009;44(2 Pt 1):501–18.
65. Levin JM, Winkelman RD, Smith GA, Tanenbaum JE, Benzel EC, Mroz TE, et al. Impact of preoperative depression on hospital consumer assessment of healthcare providers and systems survey results in a lumbar fusion population. Spine. 2017;42(9):675–81.
66. Fenton JJ, Jerant AF, Bertakis KD, Franks P. The cost of satisfaction: a national study of patient satisfaction, health care utilization, expenditures, and mortality. Arch Intern Med. 2012;172(5):405–11.
67. Carr-Hill R, Sheldon T. Rationality and the use of formulae in the allocation of resources to health care. J Public Health Med. 1992;14(2):117–26.
68. Peres-da-Silva A, Kleeman LT, Wellman SS, Green CL, Attarian DE, Bolognesi MP, et al. What factors drive inpatient satisfaction after knee arthroplasty? J Arthroplast. 2017;32(6):1769–72.
69. Zusman EE. HCAHPS replaces Press Ganey Survey as quality measure for patient hospital experience. Neurosurgery. 2012;71(2):N21–4.

Patient-Reported Outcomes

5

Melissa R. Dunbar and Zoher Ghogawala

The importance of the patient perspective in US healthcare is broadly recognized. There is a growing realization that patient experience, satisfaction, and outcome are essential to improving overall quality in spine care. While process measures and 30-day complications data have helped focus attention on improving quality in medicine, there are unique aspects to spinal care that demand the monitoring of long-term patient-reported outcomes.

The most important aspect of spinal care is restoration of function and productivity and reduction of pain. Patients are the best source to provide that feedback. There is a need for practical validated patient-reported outcomes tools in our quest to optimize outcomes within spine care.

Characteristics of Patient-Reported Outcomes Tools

Patient-reported outcome (PRO) measures should have three characteristics. They should be reliable, valid, and responsive [1–3]. Reliability refers to reproducibility. There is interobserver (degree to which different observers obtain similar results) reliability and intraobserver (degree to which the same observer gets the same result on repeated testing) reliability. There is also the concept of test-retest reliability, which examines how well an instrument performs when tested between two separate time points.

M. R. Dunbar
Department of Neurosurgery, Lahey Hospital & Medical Center, Burlington, MA, USA

Z. Ghogawala (✉)
Department of Neurosurgery, Lahey Hospital & Medical Center, Burlington, MA, USA

Department of Neurosurgery, Tufts University School of Medicine, Boston, MA, USA
e-mail: Zoher.Ghogawala@Lahey.org

J. Ratliff et al. (eds.), *Quality Spine Care*,
https://doi.org/10.1007/978-3-319-97990-8_5

Typically, the reliability of a PRO is assessed with a kappa (κ) statistic, which measures agreement between observers. An outcomes tool is considered to be highly reliable if $\kappa > 0.8$, is moderately reliable if κ statistic falls between 0.6 and 0.8, and is not reliable if κ is below 0.6 [4]. There is also assessment of how an individual test domain performs in relation to the overall composite result [5]. This is measured using the Cronbach α, which assesses whether individual domains of an outcomes tool correlate with the final composite score [6, 7].

Validity represents to what extent the measure actually assesses the measure of interest. For example, the Oswestry Disability Index (ODI) is widely used because it has been validated as being an accurate measure of disability from spinal disorders [8]. Typically, newer measures are judged to be accurate and valid when they correlate with previously validated and widely used instruments like the ODI.

Similarly, responsiveness is assessed by correlating performance to a previously validated tool such as ODI or SF-36 [9]. Recently, the Scoliosis Research Society-22 (SRS-22) instrument has been validated to be more responsive than ODI for detecting improvement in patients treated surgically for adult spinal deformity [10, 11].

Disease-Specific Versus General Health-Related Quality of Life

A PRO may focus upon assessment of a specific disease's impact on a patient or may focus upon general health-related quality of life. Instruments like ODI have been validated and used for the assessment of treatments for low back pain. Instruments like the SF-36 or SF-12 survey examine overall health-related quality of life. The distinction is vital in understanding applicability of PROs to specific clinical and research questions.

For example, two recently published RCTs on the benefit of lumbar fusion in patients with lumbar spondylolisthesis reached different conclusions [12]. While there are multiple differences between the trials in terms of study population and design, one used ODI as the primary outcome measure and concluded that there was no advantage to adding a fusion to a decompression when treating patients with lumbar spondylolisthesis [13], while the other trial used SF-36 as the primary outcome measure and reached the opposite conclusion [14]. The SF-36, and more recently the SF-12, have been demonstrated as being reliable, valid, and responsive for assessing patients with both cervical and lumbar spinal disorders [15].

Minimum Clinical Important Difference

When assessing a response to treatment, it is important to know whether the change in a validated PRO is clinically meaningful or not. Copay and colleagues have rigorously examined a large group of patients with spinal disorders to calculate the minimal clinically important difference (MCID) for commonly used PROs. They reported MCID for ODI as 12.8 points and MCID for SF-36 physical component summary (PCS) at 4.9 points [16]. Researchers often use MCID values to calculate sample size for clinical trials by asking how many patients would be required to detect a meaningful clinical difference between two study populations when comparing the effectiveness to two or more treatments [17].

Cost-Utility Analysis

Cost-utility analysis is a specific type of cost-effectiveness evaluation that permits the direct comparison of cost and outcome for different treatments. The outcome for these analyses requires the assessment of preference-based health-related quality of life such as the EQ-5D (EuroQol group) [18]. Preference-based health-related quality of life is reported as a score between 0 (death) and 1 (perfect health). The score is then multiplied by time (years) to generate quality-adjusted life years (QALYs) so that cost can be compared in terms of cost/QALYs gained by one treatment versus another. The validated PRO, SF-36, can be converted to QALYs by transforming 11 questions from SF-36 into the preference-based SF-6D [19].

PROMIS

One of the challenges with the collection of PROs in registry quality efforts is the burden placed on patients. Completion of validated PROs is often time-consuming, and many registries have suboptimal completion rates over time. In addition, many validated PROs require licenses and considerable expense for healthcare researchers to use on a routine basis.

The NIH-funded Patient-Reported Outcomes Measurement Information System (PROMIS®) has been developed and validated recently by multiple groups for both cervical and lumbar spinal disorders [20, 21]. There is no fee associated with or license required for the use of PROMIS® for noncommercial use. PROMIS® assesses a breadth of domains and allows for a great range of responses which enables the measures to be responsive both for those in the healthy, general population as well as those suffering from chronic conditions.

PROMIS® employs computer-adaptive testing (CAT) technology that reduces the number of questions that each patient must complete based on answers to previous questions. One recent study found that PROMIS®-physical function took 1.1 min for patients to complete as opposed to 4 min for completing SF-12 [20].

Anxiety/Depression

Multiple groups have found that PROs are affected by anxiety and depression. These two common mental disorders complicate the ability to compare outcomes of different spinal treatments. In the past, it has been difficult to account for anxiety and depression other than to acknowledge their overall negative impact upon PRO results. With the development of PROMIS® anxiety and depression domains, it has been possible to learn more about the impact of these conditions in evaluating treatment for spinal disorders. For example, a recent study found that PROMIS® depression scores >50 were associated with worse PROMIS® physical function and ODI disability scores before and after lumbar decompression surgery; however, depressed patients had greater improvement in PROMIS® physical function after surgery despite having lower absolute scores postoperatively compared with non-depressed patients [22].

Summary

The importance of measuring PROs for assessing quality efforts in spine care has been established. A given PROs must be reliable, valid, and responsive. In addition, PROs are useful for cost-utility analyses. National and international registry efforts have underscored the need for PROs to be free of cost and simple to complete for patients. Recent developments in CAT have increased the feasibility of including PROs in everyday spinal practice.

References

1. Deyo RA, Andersson G, Bombardier C, et al. Outcome measures for studying patients with low back pain. Spine. 1994;19:2032S–6S.
2. Deyo RA, Diehr P, Patrick DL. Reproducibility and responsiveness of health status measures. Statistics and strategies for evaluation. Control Clin Trials. 1991;12:142S–58S.
3. Kopec JA, Esdaile JM. Functional disability scales for back pain. Spine. 1995;20:1943–9.
4. Hadley MN, Walters BC, Grabb PA, et al. Guidelines for the management of acute cervical spine and spinal cord injuries. Clin Neurosurg. 2002;49:407–98.
5. Karanicolas PJ, Bhandari M, Kreder H, et al. Evaluating agreement: conducting a reliability study. J Bone Joint Surg Am. 2009;91(Suppl 3):99–106.
6. Cronbach LJ, Meehl PE. Construct validity in psychological tests. Psychol Bull. 1955;52:281–302.
7. Cronbach LJ. Test reliability; its meaning and determination. Psychometrika. 1947;12:1–16.
8. Fairbank JC, Couper J, Davies JB, O'Brien JP. The Oswestry low back pain disability questionnaire. Physiotherapy. 1980;66:271–3.
9. Guilfoyle MR, Seeley H, Laing RJ. The short form 36 health survey in spine disease – validation against condition-specific measures. Br J Neurosurg. 2009;23:401–5.
10. Ghogawala Z, Resnick DK, Watters WC 3rd, et al. Guideline update for the performance of fusion procedures for degenerative disease of the lumbar spine. Part 2: assessment of functional outcome following lumbar fusion. J Neurosurg Spine. 2014;21:7–13.
11. Bridwell KH, Berven S, Glassman S, et al. Is the SRS-22 instrument responsive to change in adult scoliosis patients having primary spinal deformity surgery? Spine. 2007;32:2220–5.
12. Ghogawala Z, Resnick DK, Glassman SD, Dziura J, Shaffrey CI, Mummaneni PV. Randomized controlled trials for degenerative lumbar spondylolisthesis: which patients benefit from lumbar fusion? J Neurosurg Spine. 2017;26:260–6.
13. Forsth P, Olafsson G, Carlsson T, et al. A randomized, controlled trial of fusion surgery for lumbar spinal stenosis. N Engl J Med. 2016;374:1413–23.
14. Ghogawala Z, Dziura J, Butler WE, et al. Laminectomy plus fusion versus laminectomy alone for lumbar spondylolisthesis. N Engl J Med. 2016;374:1424–34.

15. Lee CE, Browell LM, Jones DL. Measuring health in patients with cervical and lumbosacral spinal disorders: is the 12-item short-form health survey a valid alternative for the 36-item short-form health survey? Arch Phys Med Rehabil. 2008;89:829–33.
16. Copay AG, Glassman SD, Subach BR, Berven S, Schuler TC, Carreon LY. Minimum clinically important difference in lumbar spine surgery patients: a choice of methods using the Oswestry disability index, medical outcomes study questionnaire short form 36, and pain scales. Spine J. 2008;8:968–74.
17. Ghogawala Z, Resnick DK, Glassman SD, Dziura J, Shaffrey CI, Mummaneni PV. Achieving optimal outcome for degenerative lumbar spondylolisthesis: randomized controlled trial results. Neurosurgery. 2017;64:40–4.
18. Rabin R, de Charro F. EQ-5D: a measure of health status from the EuroQol group. Ann Med. 2001;33:337–43.
19. Brazier J, Roberts J, Deverill M. The estimation of a preference-based measure of health from the SF-36. J Health Econ. 2002;21:271–92.
20. Boody BS, Bhatt S, Mazmudar AS, Hsu WK, Rothrock NE, Patel AA. Validation of Patient-Reported Outcomes Measurement Information System (PROMIS) computerized adaptive tests in cervical spine surgery. J Neurosurg Spine. 2018;28:268–79.
21. Sharma M, Ugiliweneza B, Beswick J, Boakye M. Concurrent validity and comparative responsiveness of PROMIS – SF versus legacy measures in the cervical and lumbar spine population: longitudinal analysis from baseline to post surgery. World Neurosurg. 2018;115:e664.
22. Merrill RK, Zebala LP, Peters C, Qureshi SA, McAnany SJ. Impact of depression on patient-reported outcome measures after lumbar spine decompression. Spine. 2018;43:434–9.

Registries in Spine Care in the United States

6

Owoicho Adogwa, Joseph Cheng, and John E. O'Toole

Introduction

Spinal disorders are extremely common, debilitating, and costly to patients, payers, and society as a whole [1]. The increasing frequency of spinal-related interventions along with increasing cost has triggered a paradigm shift to the delivery of value-based spine care [2]. The goal of this shift is the expected convergence of the interests of patients, payers, politicians, and clinicians. Value in healthcare is expressed as patient-centered outcomes (*effectiveness of care*) divided by related cost of care. Integral to the value equation is the ability to track patient outcomes longitudinally over time. Health registries, when designed properly, have the potential to provide the necessary statistical power and real-world setting required for true value measurement in both individuals and populations. In this chapter, we provide a summary of spinal registries in the United States.

The United States spends more on health care than any other industrialized country in the world [3–5]. Healthcare, as a proportion of the gross domestic product has increased faster than any other sector [3–5]. The increase in healthcare expenditure is driven by a multitude of factors including increasing use of emerging technologies, broader indications for interventions, and an increased demand from an aging population interested in more aggressive interventions to improve the quality of their life [6]. This increase in healthcare spending is particularly relevant to spine.

In 2010, healthcare expenditures related to spine problems were estimated to be US$100 billion. This represents an over 300% increase from 1995 [3, 5, 6]. A disproportionate amount of these expenditures are attributable to the use of

O. Adogwa (✉) · J. E. O'Toole
Rush University Medical Center, Chicago, IL, USA

J. Cheng
Department of Neurosurgery, University of Cincinnati College of Medicine, Cincinnati, OH, USA

J. Ratliff et al. (eds.), *Quality Spine Care*,
https://doi.org/10.1007/978-3-319-97990-8_6

nonsurgical treatment strategies for management of spinal pain. These costs can be funneled into three categories – treatment cost (surgical/nonsurgical), employer cost, and employee cost due to lost wages and adverse effects on quality of life. A study of Medicare patients found that the rate of surgery for spinal stenosis alone rose 20-fold over the past decade [7]. More recently, the Agency for Healthcare Research and Quality reported that spinal fusions were the most expensive surgical procedure performed in the United States, with annual expenditure approaching $200 billion [8]. Despite this increase in healthcare resource utilization and costs, there was no corresponding improvement in patient-related outcomes over the same time period. In fact, the Institute Of Medicine estimates that up to 30% of diagnostic and therapeutic spine interventions are unnecessary or ineffective [9]. Also worrisome, is the marked variation in the use of spinal surgery between regions in the United States. Given these circumstances, efforts to improve healthcare quality and control costs remain at the forefront of current reform initiatives in the United States.

Healthcare Costs Conundrum

Providers in the US healthcare system embrace some of the most technologically available treatments anywhere [7, 10, 11]. These new and often more expensive technologies, at times, offer little or no incremental benefit. This is particularly relevant for spine care, a field with growing use of osteobiologics and new, novel devices to treat a growing number of patients. The expected benefits or advantage of these treatment regiments over existing technologies have not been clearly defined. In the healthcare quality/cost conundrum, attempts to maximize quality alone could potentially exacerbate the problem since there is no upper limit to the demand for additional health benefits irrespective of the cost [8, 9, 12]. In a healthcare economy with finite resources, the benefits of care must be considered along with the cost of delivering care; and measuring value (*patient-centered outcomes/cost*) appears to be the most comprehensive way to account for healthcare quality and cost [13, 14].

Over the past 50 years, there have been several attempts to reform the healthcare system. Most recently, there has been a paradigm shift away from the traditional fee-for-service model toward the development of a value-based model. In the traditional fee-for-service model, reimbursement was independent of outcomes, with minimal attention (if any) given to cost [12]. A value-based model, with the dual emphasis on improving quality and controlling cost, has several advantages: (1) focusing on cost alone without considering the quality component is shortsighted and likely ignores the ultimate goal of medicine, which is to deliver better health to patients and society, and (2) focusing solely on cost usually results in cost shifting rather than cost savings and creates a perverse incentive structure to increase volume in profitable service lines in response to a decrease in reimbursements and the potential unintentional consequence of not treating riskier, more costly patients [8, 9]. Ultimately, patients want a better health status and not more healthcare, and the current healthcare crisis demands reform initiatives that consider both quality and cost.

When evaluating spinal conditions, it is important to appreciate that spine disorders are a heterogeneous group of conditions often with a lack of diagnostic clarity. Thus, in both surgical and nonsurgical spinal interventions, there are wide variations in practice. Grouping these patients together into a single category (or a few broad categories) for the purpose of assessing treatments, as has been commonly done with large administrative databases, fails to provide useful or meaningful data. For instance, while the majority of patients with back pain require no intervention, back pain secondary to instability and spinal deformity respond well to spinal arthrodesis; therefore this treatment modality should be considered of significant *value* in these subsets of patients. Hence, when contemplating value with different treatment strategies, these diagnostic nuances are more important than lumping patients together in nonmeaningful clinical categories.

Transition to Value-Based Healthcare

Value is defined as the quality of the intervention divided by the cost of the intervention measured longitudinally over time. While appearing straightforward, both cost and quality are quite challenging to measure. Quality of care is a multidimensional construct and can be defined in many ways – i.e., doing the right thing, at the right time, in the right way, for the right patient, and having the best possible results [2, 3, 15–17]. Following this definition, several measures can be used to assess quality of care including safety measures, process measures, or patient-reported outcomes metrics. Outcome measures can be disease-specific or apply to the patient's general health. The goals of measuring outcomes of surgical or medical interventions should be (1) to capture those outcomes that are most important to the patient (*patient-centered metrics*) and (2) to use outcome measures that can be effectively communicated among various stakeholders and allow for comparison across disease states.

There is ongoing debate as to the utility of process measures in the value equation. Process measures are specific steps in a process that lead either positively or negatively to a particular outcome. These measures are usually recorded at point of contact and are easy to recall for research purposes. Examples of process measures pertinent to patients undergoing spinal surgery may include operative time, estimated blood loss, duration of surgery, administration of preoperative antibiotics, as well as length of hospital stay. These measures are often evidence-based best practices manifested from a health system's efforts at quality improvement. They are less burdensome to collect and form the basis for the current physician quality reporting initiatives required by the government. The question remains, however, whether or not process measures accurately reflect the quality of care delivered. Does decreased average operative time or timely administration of antibiotics translates to the improved overall quality of care delivered to an individual patient? Many would argue that these measures do not address the parameters that are most important to patients and therefore should not be included in the value analysis [8, 9, 14, 15, 18].

Patient-centered measures for elective spine care focus on those dimensions most reflective of the patient's preferences and values. These measures can be disease specific or capture the patient's general health state. The most commonly utilized health-related quality of life measures include the Oswestry Disability Index (ODI) [19], Neck Disability Index (NDI), the Short Form 36 (SF-36) general health survey [20], Numeric Rating Pain Scale (NRS) [21], Patient Satisfaction Index [22], and EuroQol (EQ-5D) [23]. Measures may also include items such as return to work or return to favorite activity. The individual outcome measures will be discussed in more detail later in this chapter.

Cost of the medical or surgical intervention is the denominator of the value equation. Assessing cost accurately can be equally daunting in healthcare. Costs can be divided into direct and indirect costs incurred during the episode of care. Direct costs are those that are related to the patient's initial treatment or management of any subsequent complication. For similar treatments, these costs may vary across payers, regions, and states. Due to this aforementioned variation, direct costs are usually estimated based on a standardized payment amount, for instance, the Medicare national payment amount [23]. As one might imagine, this approach may over- or underestimate the direct cost of providing treatment. Indirect costs should also be accounted for and can include domains such as lost productivity or lost income of a secondary caregiver; it can be calculated based on a standard human capital approach. Indirect costs can vary considerably depending on the patient population (young patient versus elderly patient), and this variation can significantly affect the calculated value of any surgical intervention.

The final and least discussed component of the value equation is time. It is important to consider the durability of any treatment intervention in the value equation. For instance, if the desired outcome following spinal arthrodesis lasts only 12 months with a subsequent decline in outcomes and a need for further treatments, this intervention may have good short-term but not long-term value. Irrespective of the treatment rendered, the long-term clinical outcome of a medical or surgical intervention may deteriorate over time leading to increased cost or the decrease in value over time [7, 11–13, 18, 24]. Given this, when assessing the value of both surgical and nonsurgical care, emphasis should be placed on long-term follow-up to determine the durability of that intervention.

Value in Spine Care: *Useful Outcome Measures*

Value in spine care is measured by comparing outcomes delivered against cost of delivering those outcomes. In a patient-centered care model, both measurable and observable health outcomes are evaluated, along with the patient's perception of healthcare quality. Integral to the determination of effectiveness of healthcare delivery is the acquisition of reliable and valid outcomes data [2, 15–17, 20]. Below we describe the most commonly utilized health-related quality of life measures for the study of spinal disorders.

The Oswestry Disability Index (ODI) is a disease-specific validated questionnaire that was first published in 1980 [19]. It is a valid, reliable, and responsive outcomes questionnaire and considered by many researchers as the gold standard for assessing the degree of functional disability and estimating the quality of life in a person with low back pain. It is a self-administered questionnaire that contains ten subdomains including pain intensity, ability to care for oneself, ability to walk, ability to sit, ability to stand, social life, sleep quality, travel ability, sexual function, as well as lifting ability. The questionnaire is easy to administer and score, with scores ranging from 0 to 100. Higher scores equate to more severe functional disability.

The Neck Disability Index (NDI) is a modification of the Oswestry Disability Index. It is a valid, reliable outcomes instrument with good responsiveness and a high test-retest reliability [7, 19]. It is a self-administered, condition-specific questionnaire with ten subdomains including pain, personal care, lifting, reading, headaches, concentration, driving, sleeping, work and recreation. Each section is scored on a 0–5 rating scale, where 0 means "No Pain" and 5 means "Worst Imaginable Pain." It can be scored as a raw score, with a maximum score of 50, or expressed as a percentage.

The Numeric Rating Pain Scale is a unidimensional measure of pain that has been widely used in diverse patient populations to capture treatment effectiveness. It is a simple, reliable, and validated measure widely used due to its simplicity and adaptability to a broad range of spinal conditions. The scores range from 0 to 10, with high scores indicating greater pain intensity [22].

SF-36 is a validated widely used general health measure consisting of eight subdomains including physical pain and bodily function [23]. It is generally divided into two main groups; the physical and mental component scores. It has been shown to be valid and reliable for patients undergoing non-operative and operative treatments of the lumbar spinal disorders. The SF-36 questionnaire does not include a preference-weighting system and does not yield a single summary score that allows for a straightforward means of quality-adjusted life years (QALYs) [21].

SF-12 is an abbreviated version of the SF-36 consisting of a subset of 12 items selected from the original SF-36 and is less burdensome for the patient and administrator. It has been shown to be valid, reliable, and responsive for patients with cervical and lumbar disorders. Unlike SF-36, the SF-12, cannot be reliably broken down into eight domains of health and but rather is reported as physical and mental component scores [11, 22, 23, 25]. SF-36 and SF-12 can be converted to SF-6D for use as a health utility measure, particularly in cost-effectiveness studies.

The EuroQol-5D is a general measure of health initially developed by a group of European investigators for comparative effectiveness and cost effectiveness research across disease states. The EQ-5D is a preference-based measure of general health that assesses 5 dimensions of health-related quality of life [26]: morbidity, self-care, daily activities, pain and discomfort. Each dimension is scored on a scale of 1–3, with 1 indicating no problems, 2 indicating some problems, and 3 indicating extreme problems. Using a combination of these dimensions, a total of 243 possible health states exist. EQ-5D has been shown to be valid, reliable, and responsive when compared to other disease-specific measures.

Quality-adjusted life year (QALY) is a generic measure of disease burden, accounting for both the quantity and quality of life lived [2, 8, 9, 16]. It is typically utilized in economic evaluations to assess the value for money of medical or surgical interventions. It is commonly used in cost-effectiveness analysis, expressed as costs divided by the QALYs gained from the treatment of a specific disease state. Perfect health for 1 year is assigned a QALY value of 1. If an individual's health is below this maximum, then QALYs are accrued at a rate of less than 1 per year. Death is associated with 0 QALYs. The utility score used to calculate QALY has been determined from numerous existing health-related measures, including EQ-5D and SF-6D. The QALYs of a certain treatment is calculated by multiplying the utility value of that treatment by the duration of the treatment effect [20, 23, 26].

The Rationale for a Spine Registry

The growing utilization of spinal surgery underscores the need for valid and reliable data to define the value delivered by these procedures. Numerous stakeholders are motivated to improve spine care – particularly providers, patients, and payers – and each has an interest in properly defining the value of spinal surgery [12]. To date, most of the data on hospital safety, perioperative complications, resource utilization, as well as outcomes after spinal surgery vary widely in the literature and are obtained from retrospective reviews or a limited number of tightly controlled studies. Furthermore, there is a paucity of data on expected benchmarks of acceptable morbidity and treatment effectiveness.

Purely based on study design, randomized trials have been the standard-bearer for high-quality medical evidence, and observational methods like prospective and retrospective cohort studies are thought to provide lower-quality evidence [2, 17]. This view, however, ignores the obvious limitations of randomized controlled trials – which at times can be difficult to conduct, inappropriate or inadequate to the question at hand, as well as prohibitively costly and time-consuming. The false conflict between advocates of randomized controlled trials in all situations and proponents of observational studies needs to be replaced with a mutual understanding of the complementary roles of the two approaches. While the narrow inclusion/exclusion criteria of randomized controlled trials ensure internal validity and data quality and thereby a high level of evidence, these restrictions limit external validity and therefore the ability to generalize the conclusions of the studies [25]. Prospective registries provide a lower level of evidence but are cost-effective and easily scaled and have a higher feasibility of being closer to "real-world" clinical situations. Well-organized registries with data of high validity and representativeness can produce level I prognostic evidence and level II evidence on the effectiveness of care.

Summary of Existing Spine Registries in the United States

Over the past 2 decades, there has been increased multi-stakeholder interest in developing prospective registries to assess the value of spine surgery. These registries are designed to be easily scaled, to document care in real-world clinical settings, and to address some of the inaccuracies often contained in administrative claims databases. Presented below is a summary of available prospective clinical spine registries. Administrative databases and non-spine databases were excluded from this review.

Detailed information was obtained on 12 existing prospective spinal registries. The majority of registries prospectively collected patient information and continued to accumulate data as of December 2017. Most of the registries had start dates after 2001, with registry populations ranging from 1000 to over 50,000 unique patients. Follow-up periods ranged from 1 to 2 years, with 2-year follow-up rates estimated to be between 50% and 80%. Universally, longer follow-up times consistently produced lower follow-up rates. The majority of the registries collected process variables as well as patient-reported outcome measures and required data extractors to input patient information. Relevant outcome measures included pain scores, Oswestry Disability Index, EuroQol-5D, SF-12/36, or return to baseline activity. Two registries collected data on healthcare resource utilization, and one registry collected data on direct and indirect cost. Details of US registries are presented in Tables 6.1, 6.2, and 6.3.

Table 6.1 Spine registries in the United States

Registry name	Registry sponsor	Setting	Year started	Design	Anatomical location	Conditions evaluated	Method of data collection
QOD	NPA, AANS	Multi-institutional	2012	Prospective	Cervical, thoracic, lumbar	Lumbar stenosis, spondylolisthesis, degenerative disc disease, cervical myelopathy, radiculopathy	Data extractors, clinical interviewers
SMISS	SMISS	Multi-institutional	2011	Prospective	Thoracic, lumbar	Focused on minimally invasive treatment of degenerative lumbar stenosis, spondylolisthesis, degenerative scoliosis	NR
AO (non-fusion)	AO Spine Foundation	Multi-institutional	NR	Prospective	Cervical, thoracic, lumbar	Cervical myelopathy, degenerative lumbar stenosis, degenerative spondylolisthesis, degenerative scoliosis	NR
KP	Kaiser Permanente	Multi-institutional, California	2009	Prospective	Cervical, thoracic, lumbar	Focused on spinal implants: pedicle screws, rods, arthroplasty	Electronically collected from referring physicians
SSD	AO Spine Foundation	International	NR	Prospective	Cervical, thoracic, lumbar	Focused on patients with scoliosis	Electronically collected from referring physicians
SOD	Setting Scoliosis Straight Foundation, Harms Study Group	Multi-institutional	2008	Prospective	Thoracic, lumbar	Adolescent patients between ages 10 years and 21 years with diagnosis of idiopathic scoliosis	Data extractors, clinical interviewers
TBI	TBI	Institutional	2015	Prospective	Cervical, thoracic, lumbar	Cervical myelopathy, degenerative lumbar stenosis, degenerative spondylolisthesis, degenerative scoliosis	Data extractors, clinical interviewers, electronically collected directly from patients

NSN	National Spine Network	Multi-institutional	1994	Prospective	NR	NR	NR
Chest wall and spine deformity	Children's Spine Foundation	Multi-institutional	2005	Prospective	Thoracic, lumbar	Focused on children with chest wall and spine deformities	Data extractors, clinical interviewers
VSR	Vanderbilt University Medical Center	Institutional	2010	Prospective	Cervical, thoracic, lumbar	All patients undergoing elective spine surgery at Vanderbilt Spine Center	Data extractors, clinical interviewers
ATSD	NR	Multi-institutional	2010	Prospective	Thoracic, lumbar	Focused on adult patients with spinal deformity	Data extractors, clinical interviewers
NASS	NASS	Multi-institutional	2016	Prospective	Lumbar	Focused on patients with degenerative stenosis, spondylolisthesis, scoliosis, disc herniation, radiculopathy	Electronically collected directly from patients

QOD Quality Outcomes Database, *SMISS* Society for Minimally Invasive Spine Surgery, *KP* Kaiser Permanente Spine Implant Registry, *SSD* Scoliosoft Scoliosis Database, *SOD* Scoliosis Outcomes Database, *TBI* Texas Back Institute, *NSN* National Spine Network, *VSR* Vanderbilt Spine Registry, *ATSD* adult thoracolumbar spinal deformity database, *NASS* North American Spine Society Database, *NPA* Neuropoint Alliance, *AANS* American Association of Neurological Surgery, *NR* not reported or could not be identified

Table 6.2 Detailed registry information

		Outcomes assessments				
Registry name	Demographic data collected	Functional status	Pain	Quality of life	Other	PROMs assessment intervals
QOD	Age, gender, race, weight, BMI, smoking history, depression, symptoms, occupation, diagnosis, surgical levels, baseline disability	ODI, NDI	NRS	SF-36, EQ-5D	Return to work, complications, readmissions	Before surgery, 3-months, 12 months
SMISS	Age, gender, race, weight, BMI, smoking history, primary diagnosis, depression, surgical levels	ODI	NRS	NR	Complications, readmissions, radiographic parameters	Before surgery, 1-year, 2-year
AO (non-fusion)	Age, gender, race, weight, BMI, smoking history, primary diagnosis, surgical levels	NR	NR	NR	Complications, readmissions	NR
KP	Age, gender, race, weight, BMI, smoking history, primary diagnosis, surgical levels, implant used	NR	NR	NR	Post-operative complications, readmissions	NR
SSD	Age, gender, race, weight, BMI, smoking history, primary diagnosis, surgical levels, operative characteristics	NR	NR	NR	Radiographic outcomes	NR
SOD/HSG	Patients between ages 10 and 21, gender, race, weight, BMI, history of idiopathic scoliosis, surgical levels, operative characteristics	SRS-22, SRS-24	NRS	NR	Radiographic outcomes, level of activity, patient satisfaction	Baseline, 2-years
TBI	Age, gender, race, weight, BMI, smoking history, primary diagnosis, surgical levels, operative characteristics	ODI, NDI	NRS	SF-36, EQ-5D	Return to work, complications, readmissions	Before surgery, 3-months, 12 months. 24-months
NSN	Age, gender, race, weight, BMI, smoking history, primary diagnosis, surgical levels, operative characteristics	NR	NR	NR	NR	NR
Chest wall and spine deformity	Patients between ages 10 and 21, gender, race, weight, BMI, primary diagnosis, surgical levels, operative characteristics	SRS-22, SRS-24	NRS	NR	Radiographic outcomes, level of activity, patient satisfaction	Baseline, 2-years

VSR	Age, gender, race, weight, BMI, smoking history, depression, symptoms, occupation, diagnosis, surgical levels, baseline disability	ODI, NDI	NRS	SF-36, EQ-5D	ZUNG depression questionnaire, return to work, complications, readmissions	Before surgery, 3-months, 12 months, 24-months
ATSD	Age, gender, race, weight, BMI, smoking history, primary diagnosis, surgical levels, operative characteristics	NR	NR	NR	Radiographic outcomes	NR
NASS	Age, gender, race, weight, BMI, smoking history, depression, symptoms, occupation, diagnosis, surgical levels, baseline disability	ODI	NRS	EQ-5D	Complications, readmissions	Before surgery, 3-months, 12-months, 24-months

QOD Quality Outcomes Database, *SMISS* Society for Minimally Invasive Spine Surgery, *KP* Kaiser Permanente Spine Implant Registry, *SSD* Scoliosoft Scoliosis Database, *SOD* Scoliosis Outcomes Database, *TBI* Texas Back Institute, *NSN* National Spine Network, *VSR* Vanderbilt Spine Registry, *ATSD* adult thoracolumbar spinal deformity database, *NASS* North American Spine Society Database, *NPA* Neuropoint Alliance, *AANS* American Association of Neurological Surgery, *NR* not reported or could not be identified, *ODI* Oswestry Disability Index, *NRS* numeric rating scale, *EQ-5D* EuroQol-5D, *SF-36/12* Short Form-36/12, *ZUNG* Zung depression questionnaire, *PROMs* patient-reported outcome measures

Table 6.3 Outcomes reported and data quality assurance

Registry name	Outcomes reported	Process for monitoring data quality	Website
QOD	NRS, EQ-5D, ODI, NDI, return to work, complication rates, readmission	Site audits by independent auditors, internal weekly audits, quarterly compliance reports	http://www.neuropoint.org/NPA%20N2QOD.aspx
SMISS	Age, gender, race, weight, BMI, smoking history, primary diagnosis, depression, surgical levels	NR	NR
AO (non-fusion)	NR	Internal audits	NR
KP	Age, gender, race, weight, BMI, smoking history, primary diagnosis, surgical levels, implant used	Internal audits	https://national-implantregistries.kaiserpermanente.org/
SSD	Radiographical outcomes before and after surgery	NR	https://aospine.aofoundation.org/Structure/pages
SOD/HSG	Radiographical outcomes before and after surgery	Internal audits	NR
TBI	NR	Internal audits	NR
NSN	NR	NR	http://www.nationalspinenetwork.org/
Chest wall and spine deformity	NR	Individual sites conduct internal audits	NR
VSR	NRS, ODI, NDI, SF-12, EQ-5D, ZUNG	Internal audits	https://my.vanderbilt.edu/spineoutcomeslab/
ATSD	Age, gender, race, weight, BMI, smoking history, primary diagnosis, surgical levels, operative characteristics	Individual sites conduct internal audits	NR
NASS	Age, gender, race, weight, BMI, smoking history, depression, symptoms, occupation, diagnosis, surgical levels, baseline disability	Individual sites conduct internal audits	https://www.spine.org/ResearchClinicalCare/Research/SpineRegistry

QOD Quality Outcomes Database, *SMISS* Society for Minimally Invasive Spine Surgery, *KP* Kaiser Permanente Spine Implant Registry, *SSD* Scoliosoft Scoliosis Database, *SOD* Scoliosis Outcomes Database, *TBI* Texas Back Institute, *NSN* National Spine Network, *VSR* Vanderbilt Spine Registry, *ATSD* adult thoracolumbar spinal deformity database, *NASS* North American Spine Society Database, *NPA* Neuropoint Alliance, *AANS* American Association of Neurological Surgery, *NR* not reported or could not be identified, *ODI* Oswestry Disability Index, *NRS* numeric rating scale, *EQ-5D* EuroQol-5D, *SF-36/12* Short Form-36/12, *ZUNG* Zung depression questionnaire

Conclusion

Prospective, longitudinal, patient-reported outcomes registries are useful tools that facilitate the measurement of treatment durability, safety, cost-effectiveness, and healthcare value. Disease-specific registries are superior to administrative claims databases and provide valuable insights to treatment effectiveness and form the basis for patient-centered value-based reform efforts. More spine-focused registries are needed to power current reform initiatives.

References

1. Skovrlj B, Gologorsky Y, Haque R, Fessler RG, Qureshi SA. Complications, outcomes, and need for fusion after minimally invasive posterior cervical foraminotomy and microdiscectomy. Spine J. 2014;14(10):2405–11.
2. Roder C, Muller U, Aebi M. The rationale for a spine registry. Eur Spine J. 2006;15(Suppl 1):S52–6.
3. Good CR, Auerbach JD, O'Leary PT, Schuler TC. Adult spine deformity. Curr Rev Musculoskelet Med. 2011;4(4):159–67.
4. Li G, Passias P, Kozanek M, et al. Adult scoliosis in patients over sixty-five years of age: outcomes of operative versus nonoperative treatment at a minimum two-year follow-up. Spine (Phila Pa 1976). 2009;34(20):2165–70.
5. Uddin OM, Haque R, Sugrue PA, et al. Cost minimization in treatment of adult degenerative scoliosis. J Neurosurg Spine. 2015;23(6):798–806.
6. Bridwell KH, Glassman S, Horton W, et al. Does treatment (nonoperative and operative) improve the two-year quality of life in patients with adult symptomatic lumbar scoliosis: a prospective multicenter evidence-based medicine study. Spine (Phila Pa 1976). 2009;34(20):2171–8.
7. Fairbank J. Spinal disorders, quality-based healthcare and spinal registers. Acta Orthop. 2015;86(5):521–2.
8. Rihn JA, Berven S, Allen T, et al. Defining value in spine care. Am J Med Qual. 2009;24(6 Suppl):4S–14S.
9. Resnick DK, Tosteson AN, Groman RF, Ghogawala Z. Setting the equation: establishing value in spine care. Spine (Phila Pa 1976). 2014;39(22 Suppl 1):S43–50.
10. Agrawal BM, Brooks NP, Resnick DK. Wisconsin spine outcome study-pilot: preliminary data. Neurosurg Focus. 2012;33(1):E15.
11. Chang V, Schwalb JM, Nerenz DR, et al. The Michigan spine surgery improvement collaborative: a statewide collaborative quality initiative. Neurosurg Focus. 2015;39(6):E7.
12. McGirt MJ, Parker SL, Asher AL, Norvell D, Sherry N, Devin CJ. Role of prospective registries in defining the value and effectiveness of spine care. Spine (Phila Pa 1976). 2014;39(22 Suppl 1):S117–28.
13. Niederlander CS, Kriza C, Kolominsky-Rabas P. Quality criteria for medical device registries: best practice approaches for improving patient safety – a systematic review of international experiences. Expert Rev Med Devices. 2017;14(1):49–64.
14. Paxton EW, Kiley ML, Love R, Barber TC, Funahashi TT, Inacio MC. Kaiser Permanente implant registries benefit patient safety, quality improvement, cost-effectiveness. Jt Comm J Qual Patient Saf. 2013;39(6):246–52.
15. Roder C, Chavanne A, Mannion AF, Grob D, Aebi M. SSE Spine Tango – content, workflow, set-up. www.eurospine.org-SpineTango. Eur Spine J. 2005;14(10):920–924.
16. Roder C, El-Kerdi A, Grob D, Aebi M. A European spine registry. Eur Spine J. 2002;11(4):303–7.
17. van Hooff ML, Jacobs WC, Willems PC, et al. Evidence and practice in spine registries. Acta Orthop. 2015;86(5):534–44.

18. Cheng JS, Lee MJ, Massicotte E, et al. Clinical guidelines and payer policies on fusion for the treatment of chronic low back pain. Spine (Phila Pa 1976). 2011;36(21 Suppl):S144–63.
19. Fairbank JC. Oswestry disability index. J Neurosurg Spine. 2014;20(2):239–41.
20. Glassman SD, Bridwell KH, Shaffrey CI, et al. Health-related quality of life scores underestimate the impact of major complications in lumbar degenerative scoliosis surgery. Spine Deform. 2018;6(1):67–71.
21. Asher AL, Kerezoudis P, Mummaneni PV, et al. Defining the minimum clinically important difference for grade I degenerative lumbar spondylolisthesis: insights from the quality outcomes database. Neurosurg Focus. 2018;44(1):E2.
22. Adogwa O, Owens R, Karikari I, et al. Revision lumbar surgery in elderly patients with symptomatic pseudarthrosis, adjacent-segment disease, or same-level recurrent stenosis. Part 2. A cost-effectiveness analysis: clinical article. J Neurosurg Spine. 2013;18(2):147–53.
23. Adogwa O, Parker SL, Davis BJ, et al. Cost-effectiveness of transforaminal lumbar interbody fusion for grade I degenerative spondylolisthesis. J Neurosurg Spine. 2011;15(2):138–43.
24. Ohnmeiss DD. The fate of prospective spine studies registered on www.ClinicalTrials.gov. Spine J. 2015;15(3):487–491.
25. Asher AL, Speroff T, Dittus RS, et al. The National Neurosurgery Quality and Outcomes Database (N2QOD): a collaborative North American outcomes registry to advance value-based spine care. Spine (Phila Pa 1976). 2014;39(22 Suppl 1):S106–16.
26. Lamu AN, Gamst-Klaussen T, Olsen JA. Preference weighting of health state values: what difference does it make, and why? Value Health. 2017;20(3):451–7.

Registries in Spine Care: UK and Europe 7

Bernhard Meyer, Ehab Shiban, and Sandro M. Krieg

Introduction

Beginning in the mid-1990s, registries were set up throughout medicine in order to potentially gain more comprehensive data on the care provided [1]. While the Swedish Spine Registry was the first structured spine registry on a larger scale, Spine Tango was the first international registry [2, 3]. We have thus gained a lot of experience with this kind of data acquisition for almost two decades. Now it is time to analyze and evaluate what we have gained in a systemic fashion in order to optimize this modality for future use.

While randomized controlled trials (RCTs) provide level I evidence but have the disadvantage that they need to focus on well-defined subgroups, registries, in contrast, have the potential advantage to gather datasets from the complete population suffering from a specific disease, receiving a specific device/procedure, etc.

Since they involve the interest of many stakeholders, such as healthcare providers, payors, professional/scientific societies, etc., many interests collide resulting in compromises. For instance, healthcare providers and payors want to get a good estimate of quality measures across hospitals, while governmental data protection legislation might hamper this approach despite interests in improving healthcare costs by better data.

B. Meyer (✉) · E. Shiban · S. M. Krieg
Department of Neurosurgery, Universitätsklinikum rechts der Isar der Technischen Universität München, Munich, Germany
e-mail: Bernhard.Meyer@tum.de

J. Ratliff et al. (eds.), *Quality Spine Care*,
https://doi.org/10.1007/978-3-319-97990-8_7

Most importantly, however, registries rely on the quality and completeness of data entered into their databases. Data quality, however, is usually very low if data entries do not undergo any monitoring as required by good clinical practice (GCP) guidelines or if national specifics require anonymized data entries making it impossible to obtain any relevant follow-up or reoperation data.

This chapter therefore provides an overview on the current major registries in spinal care in the UK and Europe, by demonstrating their design and specifics, as well as outlining the strengths and weaknesses of registries and the medical, socioeconomic, and scientific value.

Overview on Current Spine Registries in Europe

We performed a search for currently ongoing spine registries via Medline, Google, clinicaltrials.gov, and inquiries to societies. We mainly included spine registries with focus on scientific, socioeconomic, and healthcare provider perspectives, which are used and acknowledged by national scientific societies or governmental organizations. For the purpose of this chapter, we did not consider registries of scientific organizations and/or universities/hospitals, focusing on one specific spinal disease or one scientific question. Table 7.1 provides an overview on major spine registries in Europe, as well as their focus and particularities.

Registry Design and Monitoring

Limitations and Pitfalls

Although there are registries on conservative treatment of spinal disease, most currently used registries focus on surgical treatment [5]. The basic motivation for a registry is either for quality assurance or scientific questions. If we want to investigate and better understand differences of treatment modalities or their cost-effectiveness in a real-world setting, registries should ideally not be reduced to one disease or treatment option despite the necessity for very comprehensive data acquisition. To compensate for that, the data need to be more general in order to make them more comparable across different treatment options which reduce the data accuracy and precision. "Granularity" is the term experts use when talking about standardized description of patient particularities. The finer the granularity, the better the distinction between patients, which comes at the price of an unrealistically high number of items per patient. More focused registries allow for disease-based data entries with a lesser number of items and the same precision per patient. Overall, we can define four types of registries:

- General data collection: one group of disease, such as spine disease
- Disease-focused data collection: e.g., degenerative spine disorders

Table 7.1 Overview on current European spine registries, including UK

Registry name	Location	Setting[a]	Since	Location spine	Outcomes lumbar spine: Functional status	Outcomes lumbar spine: Pain	Outcomes lumbar spine: Quality of life	PROMS[b] assessments	ICHOM-LBP[c] PROMS criteria	Benchmark[d]	Scientific publications/ EBM[e] level
Swespine	Sweden	N	1998	L; C; D; T; I; M	ODI	VAS B&L	SF36; EQ5D	B; P; 12; 24; O; 5y	Yes	Average and individual centers	Yes, 37
NORspine	Norway	N	2006	L; D	ODI	NPRS B&L	EQ5D	B; P; 3; 12	No	Average	Yes, 21
Danespine	Denmark	N	2009	L; C; D; T; I; M	ODI	VAS and B&L	EQ5D; SF36	B; P; 3; 6; 12; 24; 5y; 10y	No	Average	Yes, 5
Dutch Spine Surgery Registry	The Netherlands	N	2014	L; D; C; T; I; M	ODI	NRPS B&L	EQ5D SF36	B; P; 2/6; 12; 24	Yes	Average and individual centers	No
British Spine Registry	UK	N	2012	L; C; D; T; I; M	ODI	VAS and B&L	EQ5D	B; 3; 12; 24; O, 5y	No	Average and individual centers	No
Spanish National Health Service	Spain	N	2002	L; C	RMDQ	NRPS B&L	Not meas.	B; P; 3; O, each 3 mo	No	Only own data	Yes, 9
SWISSspine	Switzerland	N	2005	L; C; D; T; I; M	RMDQ	NASS; NRPS B&L	EQ5D	B; P; 3; 6; 12; 24; O,	No	Average	Yes, 14

(continued)

Table 7.1 (continued)

Registry name	Location	Setting[a]	Since	Location spine	Outcomes lumbar spine: Functional status	Outcomes lumbar spine: Pain	Outcomes lumbar spine: Quality of life	PROMS[b] assessments	ICHOM-LBP[c] PROMS criteria	Benchmark[d]	Scientific publications/ EBM[e] level
Spine Tango	33 departments worldwide	M	2002	L; C; D; T; I; M	ODI; COMI	COMI: NPRS B&L	EQ5D	B; P; 6w; 3; 12; 24	Yes	Average	Yes, 62
Spine Society of Germany	Germany, Austria	M	2016	L; C; D; T; I; M	ODI; COMI	COMI: NPRS B&L	EQ5D	B; P; 6w; 3; 12; 24	Yes	Average	No

This table serves as an overview on current European spine registries focusing on the general question of the registry (general spine registry vs. specific questions), focus (socioeconomic, healthcare provider perspective, etc.), monitoring of the registry entries, etc.
Modified & updated from Van Hooff et al. [4]
[a]Settings: *N* national, *M* multicenter, *I* institutional
[b]*PROMS* patient-reported outcome measures (PROMs)
[c]*ICHOM-LBP* the International Consortium for Health Outcomes Measurement- Low Back Pain
[d]Benchmark Benchmarking is performed against the average value of participating institutions in ten registries
[e]*EBM* evidence-based medicine
Locations: *L* lumbar spine, *C* cervical spine, *D* deformity, *T* trauma, *I* infection, *M* metastases, *O* others
Functional status: *ODI* Oswestry Disability Index, *RMDQ* Roland and Morris Disability Questionnaire, *COMI* Core Outcome Measures Index
Pain: *B&L* back and leg, *VAS* visual analog scale, *NPRS* numeric pain rating scale
Quality of life: *SR22r* Scoliosis Research Society 22 questions, *EQ5D* EuroQol 5 dominions (including EuroQol VAS)
PROMS at: *B* baseline, *P* perioperative, *6w* 6 weeks, *1* 1 months, *3* 3 months, *6* 6 months, *12* 12 months

- Symptom-oriented data collection: e.g., back pain as a symptom of various diseases requiring different diagnostics and treatment
- Treatment-oriented data collection: focused only on surgical vs. medical vs. ablative treatment

All European registries taken into account for this chapter fall into the first ambitious category. As mentioned above, the reliability and usefulness of the results are inherently dependent on the quality and completeness of data entries in the first place. RCTs undergo regular monitoring visits to ensure accurate data entry, but registries usually do not, at least none of those listed in Table 7.1.

Results from RCTs are also independent from the country and healthcare system since the inclusion criteria, follow-up, and reimbursement are managed by a sponsor to create a controlled study environment. This is not the case in registries. Indication, patient selection, and patient specifics, including follow-up, etc., depend on the healthcare system. Thus, registry data in a stricter sense are only valid in the respective country or system.

Also highly dependent on the environment is the possibility to follow-up patients. While some countries with national healthcare systems assign one lifetime number to each citizen allowing for lifelong follow-up over decades even when treated in different hospitals, other countries, such as Germany, usually do only allow anonymized rather than pseudonymized data entry, making it impossible to follow up patients after discharge. Without changes in data protection legislation, it is impossible to gather reliable data beyond the time between admission and the day of discharge.

In their first report, the organizers of Spine Tango reported their experience when implementing their registry in 25 centers in 9 countries. They stated "To cope with administrative issues and the legal requirements of data anonymization, national Spine Tango modules are inevitable" [1]. This means that even when using anonymized patient data, as Spine Tango does, national data protection laws as well as local institutional specifics will prohibit meaningful follow-up.

One approach, used by the recently implemented North American spine registry is that the "N2QOD is designated for quality improvement rather than research enterprise and therefore allows collection of protected health information (PHI) data without the need for written informed consent" [6]. Nonetheless, this prospectively collected data is analyzed post hoc for scientific questions. Waiving written informed consent is, however, not an option in most European countries. Moreover, the requirements of electronic data storage systems also vary widely across the world.

As mentioned, registries potentially have some advantages over RCTs, but they are also more prone to bias and confounders. In order to reduce these biases and confounders, several measures are required.

As outlined in this chapter, the requirement of obtaining informed consent will cause severe selection bias, as participation rates were shown to drop dramatically from 96% to 34% after informed consent was made mandatory in the Acute Coronary Syndrome Registry [7].

Moreover, without monitoring, the danger of selective reporting/entry is obvious either by omitting whole groups of high-risk patients or liberal interpretation of what constitutes a complication. Both things are known to happen if no rigorous guidelines for reporting are established and ultimately controlled. To our knowledge this is not the case for any European Spine Registry.

In order to account for the actual variances between centers concerning outcomes, multivariate analyses could be able to adjust for covariates [8]. But multivariate analyses can only handle known covariates or biases. If these are unknown or not recorded by the registry, there is no possibility to clear the registry data from these influences potentially leading to wrong or biased results.

The Vanderbilt group analyzed and compared clinical outcome and patient satisfaction data in study using SF-12, ODI, NRS, EQ-5D, and NDI as patient-related outcome measures (PROMs), surgical morbidity for defining quality, and reduction in disability and QoL to measure effectiveness of care. Yet, despite considerable multivariate analysis, they were not able to find any correlation between clinical outcome and patient satisfaction data telling us that surrogate markers may not be a valid tool to be used in spine registries or any other study type due to the vast amount of covariables [9].

Scientific Output of Spine Registries and Impact on Quality

Effects on the quality of healthcare through registries have been reported. The Swedish Hip Registry, for instance, led to reduced revision rates and potential clinical problems during the early course [10, 11]. The same is true for catheter-related bloodstream infection on ICUs, a study which was done by a collaborative registry of five US ICUs [12]. Yet, this only means that just by standardized and comprehensive external analysis of outcome data, the care already improves considerably. This phenomenon was also described for the Swedish spine registry by demonstrating that patient-related outcome measures, such as length of inpatient stay, improve over time due to the presence of the register [3, 4].

There is one major review available by Van Hoof and colleagues analyzing the actual impact of spine registries on the quality of spine care and outcomes. They reported that they could not find any impact of spine registries on the quality of spine care and outcomes [4]. Yet, they argue that articles originating from spine registries were at least able to provide moderate evidence for treatment options or risk factors.

From the Swedish spine registry originated data showing that elderly patients with lumbar spinal stenosis might benefit from limited surgery by decompression alone rather than fusion procedures, which then led to a RCT confirming the same result with level I evidence for outcome, complications, and costs [13, 14].

According to us this constitutes the only valid way to use unmonitored and thus biased registry data in a scientific context. This however is not the case for the majority of other studies in Table 7.2. Only in exceptional cases the limitations of the results are acknowledged in an appropriate manner. Considerable loss to follow-up, selective reporting of unmonitored and uncontrolled data, and inappropriate comparison of treatment modalities are only some of the limitations inherent to the published results. Despite being sometimes labeled as level 2 evidence, in our opinion this holds true for almost none of the publications. Despite huge efforts, the actual scientific output is also somewhat low (Table 7.2). A lot of scientific articles have been published just analyzing the registry data. However, most of them are more or less of descriptive nature reporting various risk factors or factors predicting favorable or unfavorable outcome. Moreover, in many instances single center data are extracted from the registry not representing the whole cohort (Table 7.1).

The Swedish spine registry has a high output of articles with data based on the complete registry dataset providing an adequate level of evidence (Table 7.2). The same is true for NORspine and SWISSspine. This is in contrast to Spine Tango, having the highest number of publications (n = 62), which are to a larger extent based on single center series.

Discussion

According to us, registries should serve primarily quality management purposes and then limited and specific scientific ones. For both purposes, however, complete datasets of high quality with a minimum follow-up of 12 months are equally important.

As outlined above for most European spine registries this is not yet the case. Being at a decisive moment of substantial changes in healthcare, such as outcome-centered reimbursement, changes in medical device legislation etc., it is necessary to adapt current registries to these requirements.

Data restriction to key short- and long-term parameters is one prerequisite, especially with ambitious general registries striving for the complete spectrum of spinal diseases. It may however prove better to convert to disease-specific data collection.

If not, the amount of items should not exceed a clinically relevant number since this hampers completeness and integrity of the datasets. On the other hand, the acquired data need to have a certain granularity in order to capture all particularities of the respective patient and to be able to differentiate two similar but different patients by the data entries. It was shown that more items, such as health-related, psychological, social, and biomedical indicators, potentially impact the clinical results of interventions for disorders of the lumbar spine [4, 15]. Thus, at least the International Consortium for Health Outcomes Measurement (ICHOM) agreed on a minimum set of data [4, 16].

Patient-related factors, such as age, gender, previous medical history, comorbidities, previous spine surgeries, and previous spine implants, are quite straightforward. PROMs have to be adapted very much to the disease and should preferably be easy to measure. For low back pain, for instance, the ICHOM published recommendations that PROMs shall be used to measure interventional outcomes [16]. These are the EuroQol 5 dimensions (EQ5D), the Oswestry Disability Index (ODI), and

Table 7.2 Scientific output of current European spine registries including the UK

Registry	Type of data	#	Title	Journal, year	EBM level
Swespine	*Registry data*	1	Reliability of the prospective data collection protocol of the Swedish Spine Register. Test-retest analysis of 119 patients	Acta Orthop 2006	**3**
		2	Dural lesions in lumbar disc herniation surgery: incidence, risk factors, and outcome	Eur Spine J 2010	**2**
		3	Smokers show less improvement than nonsmokers 2 years after surgery for lumbar spinal stenosis: a study of 4555 patients from the Swedish spine register	Spine 2011	**2**
		4	Cost effectiveness of disc prosthesis versus lumbar fusion in patients with chronic low back pain: randomized controlled trial with 2-year follow-up	Eur Spine J. 2011	**1**
		5	Cost-effectiveness of balloon kyphoplasty (BKP) vs. standard medical treatment in patients with osteoporotic vertebral compression fracture – a Swedish multicenter RCT with 2-year follow up	Spine 2011	**1**
		6	Adverse events in spine surgery in Sweden: a comparison of patient claims data and national quality register (Swespine) data	Acta Orthop. 2011	3
		7	Dural lesions in decompression for lumbar spinal stenosis: incidence, risk factors and effect on outcome	Eur Spine J. 2012	2
		8	Prognostic factors in lumbar spinal stenosis surgery – A prospective study of imaging and patient related factors in 109 patients operated on by decompression	Acta Orthop. 2012	2
		9	Instrumentation in lumbar fusion improves back pain but not quality of life 2 years after surgery. A study of 1310 patients with degenerative disc disease from the Swedish Spine Register SWESPINE	Acta Orthop. 2013	2
		10	Dural lesions in decompression for lumbar spinal stenosis: incidence, risk factors and effect on outcome	Acta Orthop. 2013	2
		11	Does fusion improve the outcome after decompressive surgery for lumbar spinal stenosis?: a two-year follow-up study involving 5390 patients	Bone Joint J. 2013	2
		12	Obesity is associated with inferior results after surgery for lumbar spinal stenosis: a study of 2633 patients from the Swedish Spine Register	Spine 2013	2
		13	The impact of pain on function and health related quality of life in lumbar spinal stenosis: a register study of 14.821 patients	Spine 2013	2

		14	Pre- and postoperative quality of life in patients treated for scoliosis	Acta Orthop.	3
		15	Obese patients report modest weight loss after surgery for lumbar spinal stenosis: a study from the Swedish spine register	Spine (Phila Pa 1976). 2014	3
		16	Recurrent Versus Primary Lumbar Disc Herniation Surgery: Patient-reported Outcomes in the Swedish Spine Register Swespine	Clin Orthop Relat Res. 2015	3
		17	Preoperative pain pattern predicts surgical outcome more than type of surgery in patients with central spinal stenosis without concomitant spondylolisthesis: a register study of 9051 patients	Spine 2014	3
		18	Outcome of surgical treatment of lumbar disc herniation in young individuals	Bone Joint J. 2015	3
		19	Clinical outcomes after treatment with disc prostheses in three lumbar segments compared to one- or two segments	Int J Spine Surg. 2015	3
		20	Lumbar disc herniation surgery in children: outcome and gender differences	Eur Spine J. 2016	3
		21	Gender differences in patients scheduled for lumbar disc herniation surgery: a National Register Study including 15,631 operations	Eur Spine J. 2016	2
		22	Inferior Outcome of Lumbar Disc Surgery in Women Due to Inferior Preoperative Status: a Prospective Study in 11,237 Patients	Spine (Phila Pa 1976). 2016	2
		23	Similar result after non-elective and elective surgery for lumbar disc herniation: an observational study based on the SweSpine register	Eur Spine J. 2016	3
		24	Gender differences in the surgical treatment of lumbar disc herniation in elderly	Eur Spine J. 2016	3
		25	The outcome of lumbar disc herniation surgery is worse in old adults than in young adults	Acta Orthop. 2016	2
		26	The value of patient global assessment in lumbar spine surgery: an evaluation based on more than 90,000 patients	Eur Spine J. 2017	2
		27	Surgical treatment of lumbar disc herniation in different ages – evaluation of 11,237 patients	Spine J. 2017	2
		28	Women do not fare worse than men after lumbar fusion surgery: two-year follow-up results from 4780 prospectively collected patients in the Swedish National Spine Register with lumbar degenerative disc disease and chronic low back pain	Spine J. 2017	2

(continued)

Table 7.2 (continued)

Registry	Type of data	#	Title	Journal, year	EBM level
	Philosophy and background	29	The Swedish national register for lumbar spine surgery	Acta Orthop Scand 2001	5
		30	The role of national registration	Acta Orthop Scand 2002	5
		31	A practical approach to spine registers in Europe. The Swedish experience	Eur Spine J 2006	5
		32	Swedish Society of Spinal Surgeons. The Swedish Spine Register: development, design and utility	Eur Spine J 2009	5
		33	The national quality registries: long and complicated way if the medical profession doesn't see the advantages	Läkartidn 2011	5
	Single center analysis	34	X-Stop versus decompressive surgery for lumbar neurogenic intermittent claudication – a randomized controlled trial with 2 years follow-up	Spine 2013	1
		35	Gender differences in lumbar disc herniation surgery	Acta Orthop 2008	3
		36	SF-36 scores in degenerative lumbar spine disorders: analysis of prospective data from 451 patients	Acta Orthop 2006	3
		37	Health-related quality of life in patients before and after surgery for a herniated lumbar disc	J Bone Joint Surg 2005	3
NORspine	*Registry data*	1	Can we define success criteria for lumbar disc surgery?: estimates for a substantial amount of improvement in core outcome measures	Acta Orthop. 2013	2
		2	Minimally invasive decompression versus open laminectomy for central stenosis of the lumbar spine: pragmatic comparative effectiveness study	BMJ. 2015	2
		3	Public and private health service in Norway: a comparison of patient characteristics and surgery criteria for patients with nerve root affections due to discus herniation	Eur Spine J. 2014	2
		4	Comparative effectiveness of microdecompression and laminectomy for central lumbar spinal stenosis: study protocol for an observational study	BMJ Open. 2014	2
		5	The Risk of Getting Worse: predictors of Deterioration After Decompressive Surgery for Lumbar Spinal Stenosis: a Multicenter Observational Study	World Neurosurg. 2015	2

		6	Does Obesity Affect Outcomes After Decompressive Surgery for Lumbar Spinal Stenosis? A Multicenter, Observational, Registry-Based Study	World Neurosurg. 2015	2
		7	Does daily tobacco smoking affect outcomes after microdecompression for degenerative central lumbar spinal stenosis? – A multicenter observational registry-based study	Acta Neurochir (Wien). 2015	2
		8	Surgery for Lumbar Spinal Stenosis in Individuals Aged 80 and Older: a Multicenter Observational Study	J Am Geriatr Soc. 2016	2
		9	Is There an Association Between Radiological Severity of Lumbar Spinal Stenosis and Disability, Pain, or Surgical Outcome?: A Multicenter Observational Study	Spine (Phila Pa 1976). 2016	2
		10	Does surgical technique influence clinical outcome after lumbar spinal stenosis decompression? A comparative effectiveness study from the Norwegian Registry for Spine Surgery	Eur Spine J. 2017	2
		11	The effectiveness of decompression alone compared with additional fusion for lumbar spinal stenosis with degenerative spondylolisthesis: a pragmatic comparative non-inferiority observational study from the Norwegian Registry for Spine Surgery	Eur Spine J. 2017	3
		12	Surgery for lumbar spinal stenosis in patients with rheumatoid arthritis: a multicenter observational study	Eur J Rheumatol. 2016	2
		13	Risk factors for surgical site infections among 1772 patients operated on for lumbar disc herniation: a multicentre observational registry-based study	Acta Neurochir (Wien). 2017	2
		14	Variation in selection criteria and approaches to surgery for Lumbar Spinal Stenosis among patients treated in Boston and Norway	Clin Neurol Neurosurg. 2017	3
		15	Lumbar microdiscectomy for sciatica in adolescents: a multicentre observational registry-based study	Acta Neurochir (Wien). 2017	2
		16	Total disc replacement versus multidisciplinary rehabilitation in patients with chronic low back pain and degenerative discs: 8-year follow-up of a randomized controlled multicenter trial	Spine J. 2017	1

(continued)

Table 7.2 (continued)

Registry	Type of data	#	Title	Journal, year	EBM level
		17	Criteria for failure and worsening after surgery for lumbar disc herniation: a multicenter observational study based on data from the Norwegian Registry for Spine Surgery	Eur Spine J. 2017	2
		18	Lumbar Microdiscectomy in Obese Patients: A Multicenter Observational Study	World Neurosurg. 2017	2
		19	Surgery for Herniated Lumbar Disc in Daily Tobacco Smokers: A Multicenter Observational Study	World Neurosurg. 2018	2
	Philosophy and background	20	Open discectomy vs microdiscectomy for lumbar disc herniation – a protocol for a pragmatic comparative effectiveness study	F1000Res. 2016	5
	Single center analysis	21	Microsurgical decompression for central lumbar spinal stenosis: a single-center observational study	Acta Neurochir (Wien). 2015	3
Danespine	*Registry data*	1	Patient are satisfied 1 year after decompression surgery for lumbar spinal stenosis	Dan Med J. 2016	3
		2	Predictors of Hospital Readmission and Surgical Site Infection in the United States, Denmark, and Japan: Is Risk Stratification a Universal Language?	Spine (Phila Pa 1976) 2017	2
	Philosophy and background	3	Implementation of the Danish national database Danespine for spinal surgery	Ugeskr Laeger. 2014	5
	Single center analysis	4	Patient-reported outcome measures unbiased by loss of follow-up. Single-center study based on DaneSpine, the Danish spine surgery registry	Eur Spine J. 2016	3
		5	Return to work after lumbar disc surgery is related to the length of preoperative sick leave	Dan Med J. 2017	3
SWISSspine	*Registry data*	1	Superior outcomes of decompression with an interlaminar dynamic device versus decompression alone in patients with lumbar spinal stenosis and back pain: a cross registry study	Eur Spine J. 2015	3
		2	Viscoelastic Disc Arthroplasty Provides Superior Back and Leg Pain Relief in Patients with Lumbar Disc Degeneration Compared to Anterior Lumbar Interbody Fusion	Int J Spine Surg. 2015	3
		3	Five-year results of lumbar disc prostheses in the SWISSspine registry	Eur Spine J. 2014	3

		4	Real-life results of balloon kyphoplasty for vertebral compression fractures from the SWISSspine registry	Spine J. 2014	3
		5	Incidence and risk factors for early adjacent vertebral fractures after balloon kyphoplasty for osteoporotic fractures: analysis of the SWISSspine registry	Eur Spine J. 2014	3
		6	Cement volume is the most important modifiable predictor for pain relief in BKP: results from SWISSspine, a nationwide registry	Eur Spine J. 2013	3
		7	Five-year results of cervical disc prostheses in the SWISSspine registry	Eur Spine J. 2013	3
		8	Comparative effectiveness research across two spine registries	Eur Spine J. 2012	2
		9	Influence of preoperative leg pain and radiculopathy on outcomes in mono-segmental lumbar total disc replacement: results from a nationwide registry	Eur Spine J. 2012	3
		10	Influence of preoperative nucleus pulposus status and radiculopathy on outcomes in mono-segmental lumbar total disc replacement: results from a nationwide registry	BMC Musculoskelet Disord. 2011	3
		11	Benchmarking in the SWISSspine registry: results of 52 Dynardi lumbar total disc replacements compared with the data pool of 431 other lumbar disc prostheses	Eur Spine J. 2010 Dec	3
		12	SWISSspine: the case of a governmentally required HTA-registry for total disc arthroplasty: results of cervical disc prostheses	Spine (Phila Pa 1976). 2010	3
		13	SWISSspine – a nationwide health technology assessment registry for balloon kyphoplasty: methodology and first results	Spine (Phila Pa 1976). 2010	3
		14	SWISSspine: a nationwide registry for health technology assessment of lumbar disc prostheses	Eur Spine J. 2009	3
Spine Tango	*Registry data*	1	Incidental durotomy in decompression for lumbar spinal stenosis: incidence, risk factors and effect on outcomes in the Spine Tango registry	Eur Spine J. 2017	3
		2	The Oswestry Disability Index, confirmatory factor analysis in a sample of 35,263 verifies a one-factor structure but practicality issues remain	Eur Spine J. 2017	2
		3	Is the duration of pre-operative conservative treatment associated with the clinical outcome following surgical decompression for lumbar spinal stenosis? A study based on the Spine Tango Registry	Eur Spine J. 2017	2

(continued)

Table 7.2 (continued)

Registry	Type of data	#	Title	Journal, year	EBM level
		4	Predictors of improvement in quality of life and pain relief in lumbar spinal stenosis relative to patient age: a study based on the Spine Tango registry	Eur Spine J. 2017	3
		5	A novel use of the Spine Tango registry to evaluate selection bias in patient recruitment into clinical studies: an analysis of patients participating in the Lumbar Spinal Stenosis Outcome Study (LSOS)	Eur Spine J. 2017	3
		6	Predictors of improvement in quality of life and pain relief in lumbar spinal stenosis relative to patient age: a study based on the Spine Tango registry	Eur Spine J. 2017	3
		7	Determination of the Oswestry Disability Index score equivalent to a “satisfactory symptom state” in patients undergoing surgery for degenerative disorders of the lumbar spine – a Spine Tango registry-based study	Spine J. 2016	2
		8	Influence of previous surgery on patient-rated outcome after surgery for degenerative disorders of the lumbar spine	Eur Spine J. 2016	3
		9	Total disc arthroplasty versus anterior cervical interbody fusion: use of the Spine Tango registry to supplement the evidence from randomized control trials	Spine J. 2016	3
		10	Superior outcomes of decompression with an interlaminar dynamic device versus decompression alone in patients with lumbar spinal stenosis and back pain: a cross-registry study	Eur Spine J. 2015	3
		11	Viscoelastic Disc Arthroplasty Provides Superior Back and Leg Pain Relief in Patients with Lumbar Disc Degeneration Compared to Anterior Lumbar Interbody Fusion	Int J Spine Surg. 2015	3
		12	Patient outcomes after laminotomy, hemilaminectomy, laminectomy and laminectomy with instrumented fusion for spinal canal stenosis: a propensity score-based study from the Spine Tango registry	Eur Spine J. 2015	2
		13	Do surgeon credentials affect the rate of incidental durotomy during spine surgery	Eur Spine J. 2014	2
		14	The influence of comorbidity on the risks and benefits of spine surgery for degenerative lumbar disorders	Eur Spine J. 2014	2
		15	Comparative effectiveness research across two spine registries	Eur Spine J. 2012	2

		16	Reliability and validity of the cross-culturally adapted French version of the Core Outcome Measures Index (COMI) in patients with low back pain	Eur Spine J. 2012	2
		17	Reliability and validity of the cross-culturally adapted Italian version of the Core Outcome Measures Index. Eur Spine J	Eur Spine J. 2012	2
		18	Predictors of surgical, general and follow-up complications in lumbar spinal stenosis relative to patient age as emerged from the Spine Tango Registry	Eur Spine J. 2012	2
		19	Development of a documentation instrument for the conservative treatment of spinal disorders in the International Spine Registry, Spine Tango	Eur Spine J. 2011	2
		20	Ratings of global outcome at the first postoperative assessment after spinal surgery: how often do the surgeon and patient agree? Eur Spine J. 2009	Eur Spine J. 2009	2
		21	Microdiscectomy compared with standard discectomy: an old problem revisited with new outcome measures within the framework of a spine surgical registry	Eur Spine J. 2009	2
		22	The international spine registry SPINE TANGO: status quo and first results Eur Spine J. 2008	Eur Spine J. 2008	3
	Philosophy and background	23	A European spine registry	Eur Spine J. 2002	5
		24	SSE Spine Tango: a European Spine Registry promoted by the Spine Society of Europe (SSE)	Eur Spine J. 2004	5
		25	Does it take two to tango?	Eur Spine J. 2005	5
		26	SE Spine Tango – content, workflow, setup. www.eurospine.org – Spine Tango	Eur Spine J. 2005	5
		27	The rationale for a spine registry	Eur Spine J. 2006	5
		28	Benchmarking with Spine Tango: potentials and pitfalls	Eur Spine J. 2009	5
		29	How to Tango: a manual for implementing Spine Tango	Eur Spine J. 2009	5
	Single center analysis	30	Comparison of peri-operative and 12-month lifestyle outcomes in minimally invasive transforaminal lumbar interbody fusion versus conventional lumbar fusion	Br J Neurosurg. 2017	4
		31	Quality of Life and Functional Outcome after Microsurgical Decompression in Lumbar Spinal Stenosis: a Register Study	Z Orthop Unfall. 2017	4

(continued)

Table 7.2 (continued)

Registry	Type of data	#	Title	Journal, year	EBM level
		32	Spine Tango in Turkish: development of a Local Registry System	Turk Neurosurg. 2017	4
		33	Non-operative treatment of lumbar spinal stenosis	Technol Heal Care. 2016	4
		34	What level of pain are patients happy to live with after surgery for lumbar degenerative disorders?	Spine J. 2016	4
		35	Patient-reported outcome of surgical treatment for lumbar spinal epidural lipomatosis	Spine J. 2016	4
		36	Dynamic posterior stabilization for degenerative lumbar spine disease: a large consecutive case series with long-term follow-up by additional postal survey	Eur Spine J. 2016	4
		37	Adult degenerative scoliosis: comparison of patient-rated outcome after three different surgical treatments	Eur Spine J. 2016	4
		38	Patient-Rated Outcomes of Lumbar Fusion in Patients With Degenerative Disease of the Lumbar Spine: Does Age Matter?	Spine (Phila Pa 1976). 2016	4
		39	Spine Tango registry data collection in a conservative spinal service: a feasibility study	Eur Spine J. 2016	3
		40	Influence of gender on patient-oriented outcomes in spine surgery	Eur Spine J. 2016	4
		41	Assessment of outcome in patients undergoing surgery for intradural spinal tumor using the multidimensional patient-rated Core Outcome Measures Index and the modified McCormick Scale	Neurosurg Focus. 2015	4
		42	The influence of cervical plate fixation with either autologous bone or cage insertion on radiographic and patient-rated outcomes after two-level anterior cervical discectomy and fusion	Eur Spine J. 2015	4
		43	Lumbar facet joint effusion on MRI as a sign of unstable degenerative spondylolisthesis: should it influence the treatment decision?	J Spinal Disord Tech. 2015	4
		44	Spinal fracture reduction with a minimal-invasive transpedicular Schanz Screw system: clinical and radiological one-year follow-up	Injury. 2015	4
		45	Could less be more when assessing patient-rated outcome in spinal stenosis?	Spine (Phila Pa 1976). 2015	3

		46	A novel translaminar crossover approach for pathologies in the lumbar hidden zone	J Clin Neurosci Off J Neurosurg Soc Australas. 2015	4
		47	Applications of the ultrasonic bone cutter in spinal surgery – our preliminary experience	Br J Neurosurg. 2014	4
		48	Back pain in patients with degenerative spine disease and intradural spinal tumor: what to treat? when to treat?	Eur Spine J. 2014	4
		49	A comparative effectiveness study of patient-rated and radiographic outcome after 2 types of decompression with fusion for spondylotic myelopathy: anterior cervical discectomy versus corpectomy	Neurosurg Focus. 2013	3
		50	The assessment of complications after spine surgery: time for a paradigm shift?	Spine J. 2013	3
		51	Cross-cultural adaptation and validation of the Polish version of the core outcome measures index for low back pain	Eur Spine J. 2013	3
		52	Hospital for joint diseases participates in international spine registry Spine Tango after successful pilot study	Bull NYU Hosp Jt Dis. 2012	3
		53	A prospective, cohort study comparing translaminar screw fixation with transforaminal lumbar interbody fusion and pedicle screw fixation for fusion of the degenerative lumbar spine	J Bone Jt Surg (Br). 2009	3
		54	An observational study of patient-rated outcome after atlantoaxial fusion in patients with rheumatoid arthritis and osteoarthritis	Clin Orthop Relat Res. 2011	3
		55	The patient's perspective on complications after spine surgery	Eur Spine J. 2009	3
		56	A comparison of outcomes of cervical disc arthroplasty and fusion in everyday clinical practice: surgical and methodological aspects	Eur Spine J. 2010	3
		57	Development of a documentation instrument for the conservative treatment of spinal disorders in the International Spine Registry, Spine Tango	Eur Spine J. 2011	3
		58	The outcome of decompression surgery for lumbar herniated disc is influenced by the level of concomitant preoperative low back pain	Eur Spine J. 2011	3
		59	The influence of preoperative back pain on the outcome of lumbar decompression surgery	Spine (Phila Pa 1976).	3

(continued)

Table 7.2 (continued)

Registry	Type of data	#	Title	Journal, year	EBM level
		60	Ratings of global outcome at the first postoperative assessment after spinal surgery: how often do the surgeon and patient agree?	Eur Spine J. 2009	3
		61	Spinal surgery in the elderly: does age have an influence on the complication rate?	Orthopade. 2008	3
		62	Outcome assessment in low back pain: how low can you go?	Eur Spine J. 2005	3
Spanish National Health Service	*Registry data*	1	Predicting outcomes of neuroreflexotherapy in patients with subacute or chronic neck or low back pain	Spine J. 2014	2
		2	Predicting the evolution of low back pain patients in routine clinical practice: results from a registry within the Spanish National Health Service	Spine J. 2012	2
		3	Prevalence and factors associated with low back pain and pelvic girdle pain during pregnancy: a multicenter study conducted in the Spanish National Health Service	Spine (Phila Pa 1976). 2012	3
		4	The prognostic value of catastrophizing for predicting the clinical evolution of low back pain patients: a study in routine clinical practice within the Spanish National Health Service	Spine J. 2012	2
		5	The correlation between pain, catastrophizing, and disability in subacute and chronic low back pain: a study in the routine clinical practice of the Spanish National Health Service	Spine (Phila Pa 1976). 2011	2
		6	Minimal clinically important change for pain intensity and disability in patients with nonspecific low back pain. Spine	(Phila Pa 1976). 2007	2
		7	Fear avoidance beliefs influence duration of sick leave in Spanish low back pain patients	Spine (Phila Pa 1976). 2007	2
		8	Prognostic factors for neuroreflexotherapy in the treatment of subacute and chronic neck and back pain: a study of predictors of clinical outcome in routine practice of the Spanish National Health Service	Spine (Phila Pa 1976). 2007	2
		9	The influence of fear avoidance beliefs on disability and quality of life is sparse in Spanish low back pain patients	Spine (Phila Pa 1976). 2005	2

In this table, the scientific output of peer-reviewed publication from registry data is illustrated

the numeric pain rating scale (NPRS) for leg and back pain separately. The European registries outlined in Table 7.1 mainly use at least these three measures.

Most registries suffer from severe bias due to low granularity and missing long-term follow-up [4]. By reviewing the literature, PROMs are considered to be representative up to 1 year after surgery at least, meaning that this should be the minimum follow-up period for a spine registry [17, 18]. One study investigated the correlation in outcome data between 3 months and 12 months after surgery and did not find any proper correlation therefore proving that any spine study should have at least a 12-month follow-up period [19].

While the focus of patient satisfaction and effectiveness are more on long-term data, the quality of surgical care has short- and long-term implications. Short-term measurements are an important marker for surgical care, such as 30-day readmission rates, intraoperative complications, infection rates, and surgical and medical complications during the inpatient stay. Yet, although being considered important markers for surgical quality, these items do not correlate with the actual (long-term) treatment outcome [19–23].

It is further crucial to allow for proper risk adjustment by the data entries in order to not penalize surgeons who provide treatment to high-risk patients or diseases, which are more prone to complications than others.

Yet, for scientific purposes, follow-up data remain crucial and problematic. It is known that any loss of follow-up larger than 20% of the enrolled cases leads to bias [24]. In the above-cited study by McGirt et al., a follow-up rate in spine registries was found to be between 22% and 79% [25]. Consequently, even the study with the best follow-up rate was worse than minimally recommended rate. Accordingly, when analyzing and publishing registry data, a thorough analysis of non-responders and their baseline characteristics is required in order to rule out potential bias. Another important analysis issue is how to deal with these incomplete datasets. If they are completely discarded, there is a high risk of underestimating variability. It is therefore crucial to analyze if data are randomly missing or if there is a correlation between present and lacking data. Thus, although we should strive for complete datasets after all, missing data should not be discarded since it may cause bias of unknown direction and extent [26–28]. However, information on how these aspects were dealt with is not provided in the published articles in Table 7.2. We are therefore very skeptical with regard to the validity of most published series, which actually might prove to be counterproductive. Conclusions should be very careful, and a presumed trend should always be confirmed by a proper study design before taken as valid.

The Vanderbilt group also investigated 13 existing international spine surgery registries. The further conclusion of their work is meaningful: "Prospective, longitudinal, patient-reported outcomes registries are powerful tools that allow measurement of cost, safety, effectiveness, and health care value across clinically meaningful episodes of care. Registries entirely based on claims or billing data, safety measures alone, process measures, or other proxies of outcome offer valuable insights, but do not provide comprehensive data to drive patient-centered value-based reform." [25]. The same was shown by the Dutch group of Van Hooff et al. who searched 4273 references of registry data. After thoroughly analyzing the methodology of 34 registries, they found that 17 were at a high risk to be biased and therefore concluded that they "… found a lack of evidence that registries have had an impact on the quality of spine care, regardless of whether the intervention was non-surgical and/or surgical." As a result of their analysis, this group published a list of recommendations which need to be considered for a proper registry design [4].

Conclusion

In our opinion, it is time that major European spine registries undergo several adjustments – to different extent for respective registries – in order to fulfill the requirements for reliable quality assurance and benchmarking as well as for valid gain of knowledge and scientific progress. As they stand now, inherent biases endanger these goals and with high probability conclusions drawn from the actual data are flawed, skewed, or wrong.

Changes to be implemented include, but are not restricted to:

- Completeness of data by automated extraction and reduction of items
- High-quality data by strict definition of key parameters and mandatory monitoring
- Sufficient financing to achieve this

Unfortunately to date there is still a high reluctance to implement these changes for various reasons.

Conflict of Interest SK is consultant for Brainlab AG (Munich, Germany) and Nexstim Plc (Helsinki, Finland). BM is consultant for Ulrich Medical (Ulm, Germany), Medtronic (Dublin, Ireland), Relievant Medsystems Inc. (Redwood City, USA), DePuy Synthes (West Chester, USA), and Brainlab AG (Munich, Germany). ES is consultant for Nevro Corp. (Redwood City, USA) and receiving research grants from Icotec (Altstaetten, Switzerland) and Inomed (Emmendingen, Germany).

References

1. Melloh M, Staub L, Aghayev E, Zweig T, Barz T, Theis JC, et al. The international spine registry SPINE TANGO: status quo and first results. Eur Spine J. 2008;17(9):1201–9.
2. Fritzell P, Stromqvist B, Hagg O. A practical approach to spine registers in Europe: the Swedish experience. Eur Spine J. 2006;15(Suppl 1):S57–63.
3. Stromqvist B, Fritzell P, Hagg O, Jonsson B, Sanden B, Swedish Society of Spinal Surgeons. Swespine: the Swedish spine register : the 2012 report. Eur Spine J. 2013;22(4):953–74.
4. van Hooff ML, Jacobs WC, Willems PC, Wouters MW, de Kleuver M, Peul WC, et al. Evidence and practice in spine registries. Acta Orthop. 2015;86(5):534–44.
5. Kessler JT, Melloh M, Zweig T, Aghayev E, Roder C. Development of a documentation instrument for the conservative treatment of spinal disorders in the international spine registry, Spine Tango. Eur Spine J. 2011;20(3):369–79.

6. McGirt MJ, Speroff T, Dittus RS, Harrell FE Jr, Asher AL. The National Neurosurgery Quality and Outcomes Database (N2QOD): general overview and pilot-year project description. Neurosurg Focus. 2013;34(1):E6.
7. Armstrong D, Kline-Rogers E, Jani SM, Goldman EB, Fang J, Mukherjee D, et al. Potential impact of the HIPAA privacy rule on data collection in a registry of patients with acute coronary syndrome. Arch Intern Med. 2005;165(10):1125–9.
8. Wood AM, White IR, Thompson SG. Are missing outcome data adequately handled? A review of published randomized controlled trials in major medical journals. Clin Trials. 2004;1(4):368–76.
9. Godil SS, Parker SL, Zuckerman SL, Mendenhall SK, Devin CJ, Asher AL, et al. Determining the quality and effectiveness of surgical spine care: patient satisfaction is not a valid proxy. Spine J. 2013;13(9):1006–12.
10. Hailer NP, Weiss RJ, Stark A, Karrholm J. The risk of revision due to dislocation after total hip arthroplasty depends on surgical approach, femoral head size, sex, and primary diagnosis. An analysis of 78,098 operations in the Swedish Hip Arthroplasty Register. Acta Orthop. 2012;83(5):442–8.
11. Karrholm J. The Swedish Hip Arthroplasty Register (http://www.shpr.se). Acta Orthop 2010;81(1):3–4.
12. Pronovost P, Needham D, Berenholtz S, Sinopoli D, Chu H, Cosgrove S, et al. An intervention to decrease catheter-related bloodstream infections in the ICU. N Engl J Med. 2006;355(26):2725–32.
13. Forsth P, Michaelsson K, Sanden B. Does fusion improve the outcome after decompressive surgery for lumbar spinal stenosis?: a two-year follow-up study involving 5390 patients. Bone Joint J. 2013;95-B(7):960–5.
14. Forsth P, Olafsson G, Carlsson T, Frost A, Borgstrom F, Fritzell P, et al. A randomized, controlled trial of fusion surgery for lumbar spinal stenosis. N Engl J Med. 2016;374(15):1413–23.
15. van Hooff ML, van Loon J, van Limbeek J, de Kleuver M. The Nijmegen decision tool for chronic low back pain. Development of a clinical decision tool for secondary or tertiary spine care specialists. PLoS One. 2014;9(8):e104226.
16. Clement RC, Welander A, Stowell C, Cha TD, Chen JL, Davies M, et al. A proposed set of metrics for standardized outcome reporting in the management of low back pain. Acta Orthop. 2015;86(5):523–33.
17. Weinstein JN, Lurie JD, Tosteson TD, Zhao W, Blood EA, Tosteson AN, et al. Surgical compared with nonoperative treatment for lumbar degenerative spondylolisthesis. Four-year results in the Spine Patient Outcomes Research Trial (SPORT) randomized and observational cohorts. J Bone Joint Surg Am. 2009;91(6):1295–304.
18. Mannion AF, Brox JI, Fairbank JC. Comparison of spinal fusion and nonoperative treatment in patients with chronic low back pain: long-term follow-up of three randomized controlled trials. Spine J. 2013;13(11):1438–48.
19. Parker SL, Asher AL, Godil SS, Devin CJ, McGirt MJ. Patient-reported outcomes 3 months after spine surgery: is it an accurate predictor of 12-month outcome in real-world registry platforms? Neurosurg Focus. 2015;39(6):E17.
20. Chotai S, Parker SL, Sivaganesan A, Sielatycki JA, Asher AL, McGirt MJ, et al. Effect of complications within 90 days on patient-reported outcomes 3 months and 12 months following elective surgery for lumbar degenerative disease. Neurosurg Focus. 2015;39(6):E8.
21. Guerin P, El Fegoun AB, Obeid I, Gille O, Lelong L, Luc S, et al. Incidental durotomy during spine surgery: incidence, management and complications. A retrospective review. Injury. 2012;43(4):397–401.
22. Desai A, Ball PA, Bekelis K, Lurie J, Mirza SK, Tosteson TD, et al. SPORT: Does incidental durotomy affect longterm outcomes in cases of spinal stenosis? Neurosurgery. 2015;76(Suppl 1):S57–63. discussion S
23. Desai A, Ball PA, Bekelis K, Lurie JD, Mirza SK, Tosteson TD, et al. Outcomes after incidental durotomy during first-time lumbar discectomy. J Neurosurg Spine. 2011;14(5):647–53.

24. Schulz KF, Grimes DA. Sample size slippages in randomised trials: exclusions and the lost and wayward. Lancet. 2002;359(9308):781–5.
25. McGirt MJ, Parker SL, Asher AL, Norvell D, Sherry N, Devin CJ. Role of prospective registries in defining the value and effectiveness of spine care. Spine (Phila Pa 1976). 2014;39(22 Suppl 1):S117–28.
26. Biering K, Hjollund NH, Frydenberg M. Using multiple imputation to deal with missing data and attrition in longitudinal studies with repeated measures of patient-reported outcomes. Clin Epidemiol. 2015;7:91–106.
27. Schmidt CO, Raspe H, Pfingsten M, Hasenbring M, Basler HD, Eich W, et al. Does attrition bias longitudinal population-based studies on back pain? Eur J Pain. 2011;15(1):84–91.
28. Twisk J, de Vente W. Attrition in longitudinal studies. How to deal with missing data. J Clin Epidemiol. 2002;55(4):329–37.

Concepts of Risk Stratification in Measurement and Delivery of Quality

8

Tejbir Singh Pannu, Virginie Lafage, and Frank J. Schwab

Abbreviations

ABS	Activity-based costing
ACS NSQIP	American College of Surgeons National Surgical Quality Improvement Program
ASA	American Society of Anesthesiologists score
CCI	Charlson comorbidity index
CCR	Capacity cost rate
CDVC	Care delivery value chain
CSHA	Canadian Study of Health and Aging
EBL	Estimated blood loss
HCUP	Healthcare Cost and Utilization Project
HRQoLs	Health-related quality of life
ICD-10-CM	International Classification of Diseases, Tenth Revision, Clinical Modification diagnosis code
LOS	Length of stay
MCID	Minimal clinically important difference
mFI	Modified frailty index
N2QOD	National Neurosurgery Quality and Outcomes Database
NDI	Neck disability index
NRS	Numeric rating scale
ODI	Oswestry Disability Index
QALY	Quality adjusted life years

T. S. Pannu · V. Lafage (✉) · F. J. Schwab
Hospital for Special Surgery, New York, NY, USA
e-mail: lafagev@hss.edu

J. Ratliff et al. (eds.), *Quality Spine Care*,
https://doi.org/10.1007/978-3-319-97990-8_8

RAM	RAND appropriateness method
SCIP	Surgical Care Improvement Project
SPORT	Spine Patient Outcomes Research Trial
SSI	Surgical site infections
TDABC	Time-driven activity-based costing
VAS	Visual analog scale

Introduction

The importance of quality is gaining increased attention from governments, payers, and employers [1]. Interest stems from the high regional variability of clinical outcomes in patients with pathology of similar kind and severity. Poor quality of care is known to translate into increased cost of medical care [2].

Among the many specialties, spine care has captured substantial attention in the last decade due to prevalence of back conditions, high variability in cost and care, as well as perceived disparities in the quality of care across different areas and increasing cost and frequency of spine surgeries. There has been a 15-fold increase in complex fusion procedures in the Medicare population from 2002 to 2007 [3]. The question has arisen if the rising number of spinal procedures is actually improving the quality of life for the population of back pain sufferers.

There has been interest to shift toward value-based healthcare delivery systems [2]. Such systems consider quality and cost together as the determinants of the value in healthcare. The goal of this system is to provide the best quality of care at the lowest possible cost.

If quality is a new metric for physicians, then hospitals and healthcare systems need to be assessed and to be tracked over time to assess success. In addition, quality is anticipated to show variation between physicians [2]. For example, more experienced surgeons expectedly have a better quality start point; whereas, surgeons at the beginning of their careers are expected to show more improvement in quality over a span of time.

In regard to spine care, it will be necessary for providers and networks to relativize quality. The delivery of the best quality in spine care will depend on factors that affect the likelihood of reaching a desired outcome or performance. These factors may be related to the primary pathology, (e.g., severity of the disease) or independent of the primary pathology (e.g., presence of comorbidities).

Measuring and Delivering Quality

Measuring Quality

Measuring the quality of an intervention is a complex task, and numerous methods and tools have been described in the literature [3]; these include:

1. *Process of Care Measures Associated with an Intervention*:
   This tool is mainly used by hospitals and payers. These measures include perioperative data such as length of stay at the hospital (LOS); rate of complications; rate of readmissions; and adherence to the Surgical Care Improvement Project (SCIP) measures that are used to grade physicians and hospitals, but are not patient-centered.
2. *Patient-Reported Health-Related Quality-of-Life (HRQoLs) Measurement Questionnaires*:
   These measures are patient-centered and best for measuring the quality of an intervention. The most common can be categorized as *general health* (such as the 36-Item Short-Form Health Survey [SF-36] or the SF-12), or *disease-specific* (such as the Oswestry Disability Index [ODI], neck disability index [NDI], or Roland-Morris Disability Questionnaire).
3. *Pain scales*: Visual analog scales (VAS), numeric rating scales (NRS).
4. *Safety of an intervention.*
5. *Patient satisfaction*: This measure has been used with increased frequency in healthcare.

As it is easy to collect, it has often been used as a proxy for quality. It represents a patient's subjective perception of the care received. However, it has recently been proven to not be a valid measure of overall quality or effectiveness [4].

Calculating Quality

When the aforementioned measures are not available, quality can be calculated by dividing the value by the cost (*quality = value/cost*). The different methods for cost and value calculation are described hereafter.

Calculating the Cost Using Cost Accounting Tools [5]

Conventional Methods

Standard full costing, variance analysis, and bottom-line management constitute the conventional methods used for cost accounting. The standard full-cost-per-service unit is the basic parameter used to compute the total cost. There are three stages of cost allocation. Stage I represents direct costs to cost objects, stage II involves allocating and reallocating cost objects, and stage III includes indirect costs. The major drawback of these methods is that they require a large number of employees, which is burdensome.

Activity-Based Costing (ABC)

This method considers "activities" as the fundamental cost objects and uses the costs of these activities as building blocks for compiling the costs of other cost objects. The allocation bases used are called cost drivers, which include any factor which increases the cost of the activity. In healthcare, patients are unique products themselves. The first step in ABC is to identify all activities that are required in the treatment of the patient. Then, the costs are accumulated for each activity that consume resources and added to get the total cost. The standard treatment protocol can be utilized to account for services provided to a patient with a specific diagnosis. This method has been proven to be more useful than the conventional one, but given that most cost drivers are required for this method, there is a need for robust and expensive resources in data collection and measurement.

Time-Driven Activity-Based Costing (TDABC): Kaplan and Anderson, 2004 [6]

This is the most recent cost accounting tool. This modified version of ABC aimed to improve the balance between validity in costing and the resources used and prioritizes accuracy over precision (i.e., "approximately right rather than precisely wrong"). TDABC demands fewer resources by requiring only two key parameters: capacity cost rate (CCR) and the time required to perform activities. The CCR is the cost of capacity-supplying resources divided by the practical capacity of those resources. For calculating CCR, theoretical capacity is defined as the total number of days each resource or employee was available for work each year excluding holidays and sick leave. The cost of each resource used should be collected. CCR can be calculated by dividing the cost of a resource by its practical capacity over a given time period. Calculation of resource-level CCRs than the entire resource pool allows more thorough analysis and accurate results. When planning a TDABC analysis, availability of funding should be considered when selecting the level of the CCR.

In situations of resource constraints in healthcare, it might be useful to begin with a low-cost, crude process-level CCR, followed by refining the analysis to resource pools, and then to individual resources. For assessing CCR to the total cost, multiply the CCR of each resource by its duration of use (time component) in each activity, and sum the cost of each activity to obtain the cost of a process. The cost of each process is summed to generate the cost of a complete cycle of care for patients with a given medical condition. With the exception of defining the medical condition and the entire care delivery value chain (CDVC), all steps are mandatory for any TDABC analysis. Cost assignment through CCRs was described as more simple than ABC allocation methods, and CCRs together with contextual observations generated more accurate cost estimates, which suggests that TDABC is more able to address complexity in healthcare. The application of the TDABC methodology to healthcare follows a seven-step process as illustrated in Table 8.1.

Table 8.1 Seven steps of time-driven activity-based costing (TDABC) for healthcare organizations

Step 1	Select the medical disease
Step 2	Define the care delivery value chain
Step 3	Develop process maps that include each activity in patient care delivery
Step 4	Obtain time estimates for each activity and resources used
Step 5	Estimate the cost of supplying patient care resources (direct and indirect)
Step 6	Estimate the capacity of each resource and calculate CCR
Step 7	Calculate the total cost

Data from: Kaplan and Anderson [6]
CCR capacity cost rate

Defining the Cost Using Common Parameters

Direct Costs [3]

These represent the costs directly attributable to the hospital care of the patient. These include diagnostic work-up, drugs, outpatient visits, admission to the hospital, surgical and anesthesia fees, physical therapy, resource products (e.g., implants and blood products), disposable products (e.g., syringes, drapes, and electrocautery devices), staff, and utilities. Ideally, the direct costs should be derived from the hospital cost data. However, it is difficult to acquire detailed and accurate hospital data due to a lack of transparency caused by concerns over confidential data. Additionally, these data vary with respect to the area and vendor. Due to these shortcomings, the Medicare payment data and private payer payment data or cost to charge ratios are used to obtain direct costs. Direct costs estimated from the payment data represent the cost of an intervention from a societal perspective albeit payment by society to the Medicare and private insurer in form of monthly premiums. Thus, Medicare allowable payments for each component of the treatment are utilized to estimate the cost. Adjustment of Medicare payment rate on basis of percentage can be used to get private payer payment rates.

The cost-to-charge ratios are the coefficients which convert hospital charges for each component of care into the cost estimate for that care. Since these ratios vary from hospital to hospital, a database developed by the Healthcare Cost and Utilization Project (HCUP) is available which has ratios for each hospital. All the resources to calculate the direct costs are publicly available.

Indirect Costs [3]

Indirect costs represent those costs that are not directly related to the hospital care. Indirect costs are incurred due to productivity loss at a patient's workplace. This includes missed time from work or homemaking, missed time from work for an unpaid caretaker, and underperformance due to residual disability. Evidence shows that these costs account for the majority of total cost.

Two methods commonly used to estimate the indirect costs are as follows:

1. Human capital method: This is often the method of choice. In this method, indirect costs are calculated by multiplying the patient's time off work by the sum of the patient's wages and benefits for the period. It works under the assumption that productivity at work equates to the sum of wages and benefits of the patient.
2. Friction method: Friction period is defined as the time taken by an employer to replace the patient off work. This is multiplied by the wages and benefits to get the indirect costs. This method is highly useful for patients on permanent disability or for those who are out of work for an extended period of time.

Societal Perspective

From a societal point of view, both direct costs of care and the indirect costs related to the loss of workplace productivity should be summed to obtain the cost of an intervention [3].

Importance of Time in Measurement of Cost

Long-term follow-up is imperative in spine care. An adequate time horizon is necessary to assess the quality, cost, and value of an intervention. An intervention may be considered expensive upfront but might prove to be cost-effective on long-term follow-up. For example: 2- and 4-year Spine Patient Outcomes Research Trial (SPORT) on patients treated for degenerative spondylolisthesis showed the importance of adequate follow-up [7]. At 2-year follow-up, the surgical management added significant health benefits over non-operative treatment (cost/QALY, $115,600/QALY). At 4-year follow-up, operative treatment was found to be durable and to give lasting benefit while decreasing the cost to $64,300/QALY. The 4-year outcome was twice as cost-effective compared to calculations at 2-year outcome. Evaluation of quality and value of an intervention requires an adequate follow-up period.

Defining the Value

The definition of value depends upon the perspective as follows:

Patient Centric

Patient-centered value is an ideal definition and is highly recommended. The value depends on whether or not the set of patient needs were achieved. Value for an individual patient depends upon several factors:

- Access to appropriate care: depends on the equipment and facilities at the hospital (tertiary care versus secondary medical care).
- Highest level of medical care: describes patients who want relief from a disease regardless of costs.
- Specific outcome in treatment received: is based on what matters most to the patient. For example, in a spinal deformity case, the patient wants their physician to focus on pain rather than spinal curvature.

In this definition, the value should integrate all services, determined by a patient's medical condition and interconnected set of medical issues [2]. For example, in case of an integrative care for conditions such as adult spinal deformity, degenerative disc disease, spinal stenosis, and lumbar radiculopathy, the value should be determined for everything included in this care, outlining the concept of integrated accountable care.

Societal

From a societal perspective, value is related to the cost of surgery and productivity loss after surgery. This includes missed time from work, any persistent disability, or underperformance [3].

Employer

From the perspective of the hospital and physician, value depends only on the expenditure of all the resources used in an intervention. This includes patient visits, diagnostics, medications, and operative cost [3]. In this case, the value tends to vary depending on a set of thinking:

- Cost containment at a preset limit or growth over time: is encouraged at many hospitals. Value, cost, and quality all go hand in hand. Whereas, a more severe procedure might lead to better quality of outcome, but it will also raise the cost. In this sense, a cap on cost of an intervention may impact its value.
- Long-term view of improvement in outcomes, rather than weeks or months: is important in an effort to improve value. Some physicians have started to focus on long-term (2Y, 4Y, 10Y) quality of clinical outcome. The SPORT trial showed that the spine procedure increases in value if there are durable and good quality clinical outcomes [8].
- Prepayment versus fee for service scenario: impacts the value of care. Prepayment for a procedure can result in more freedom for risk for the physician. This makes the quality of the outcome and, therefore, the value more variable.

Risk Stratification

Definition

Risk stratification is defined as the identification of the parameters that are likely to influence a measured or desired outcome in a negative fashion. For any given patient or treatment, risk stratification can vary depending upon the specific outcome or performance measured. For example, for cost of care, the pathology and its complexity are critical risk factors, while for patient satisfaction, the incremental improvement and minimizing disability are key, and risks could be poor psychological profile such as depression or failed past treatment.

Concept: Patient and Procedural Factors

The concept of risk stratification is based on recognizing the potential factors which impact the quality of life achieved after an intervention. The patient's profile is an important factor which determines the quality of clinical outcome achieved in each patient. Demographic characteristics (age, gender, BMI) [9], diagnosis (disc disease, deformity, spondylolisthesis, tumor, or infection) [10], and comorbidities [11] (diabetes mellitus, coronary artery disease, renal disease, psychiatric illness, lung disease, etc.) are chief constituents of the patient's profile. With respect to an individual patient, the concept of risk stratification emphasizes the need to analyze preoperative risk factors for predicting postoperative complications and poor quality of life.

In addition, procedural risk factors also affect the clinical outcomes. These include the choice of the procedure and other surgical variables like approach, OR time, American Society of Anesthesiologists score (ASA), estimated blood loss (EBL), blood transfusion, intraoperative monitoring issues, adverse event during surgery, etc. [7, 12, 13].

As the evidence of the value of assessing these risk factors is growing, this concept is increasingly applied in clinical practice to tailor the surgical approach, resort to protective measures, and adjust expectations of quality of life after surgery.

Importance

Risk stratification empowers an informed choice for patients and assesses feasibility of the procedure in regard to likely success. Risk calculation and stratification reveal the natural history and can potentially predict the postoperative clinical quality of outcome. Variability in surgical approach and the constellation and expertise of clinical teams to the same spinal pathology is common. Hence, the predictive risk factors also vary regionally, as well as globally. Risk stratification is a beginning to assess factors (often modifiable) that must be considered to reduce this variability and improve the quality of spine care. Focusing on the value, cost, and quality of interventions, we are treading toward an epoch of accountability in healthcare [14].

Risk Modeling: Building Risk Stratification Approaches in Value and Cost

Defining Endpoints for Building Models

For some time, complications and poor outcomes have alarmed the spine community, and consequently there have been efforts to develop risk stratification models, which can be applied to predict quality of life after surgery. The definition of the endpoint is the most important component of a model. Depending on the type of endpoint, its incidence, magnitude, and impact, the quality and value of an intervention may be perceived differently. Statistically, the endpoints in a model represent the outcome or dependent variables. The goal of these models is to predict these outcome variables with the predictor or independent variables, which encompass the risk factors identified in the patient profile. Learning from past and other disciplines, the chief endpoints in spine care to evaluate quality and value are as follows: complications, length of stay (LOS), discharge disposition, readmission, reoperation, cost of hospitalization, 30- or 90-day procedure cost, and return to work.

Statistical Methods to Build Risk Models

Predictive analytics can provide information valuable to patients, especially when discussing the risks of surgery during clinical work-up. From a statistical point of view, several methodologies have been reported in the literature.

Logistic Regression

Currently, there are only a few predictive models in the field of spine surgery. Logistic regression is the most common statistical tool used in order to get odds ratios for developing the outcome of interest [15–18]. The output of logistic regression includes relative risk (RR) and confidence interval (CI). Translation of these odds ratio into gross probability is more understandable to patients. Strengths of methodology are prospective cohort and multicentric involvement and interpretation of results in the form of gross probability. Limitations of methodology are loss to follow-up, no validation, and assumptions used.

Modern Predictive Analytics in Spine (2004–2016)

Recently, modern predictive analytics have been used which provide accurate and patient-specific predictive models as compared to the traditional ones. The role of advanced predictive analytics is growing as the data available gets larger. Over the years, studies have shifted methodology-wise to focus on the development of one or multiple decision trees and to perform their analysis with novel tools. Spratt et al. (2004) were the first group to use modern predictive analysis [19]. They used the chi-square automatic interaction detection (CHAID) decision tree analysis to predict successful outcome following decompression for lumbar stenosis. Their model correctly classified 90.1% of successful outcomes with a positive predictive value of 85.7% and a negative predictive value of 100%. A few years later, Daubs et al. (2007) used an ensemble of 50 decision trees, rather than one, in order to evaluate predictors of psychological distress in patients presenting for evaluation of a spinal disorder [20]. Usage of an ensemble of 50 decision trees was a novel method and increased the predictability of the model, which was 92% accurate, 92% sensitive, and 95% specific in predicting a patient's level of psychological distress using 6 variables for 188 patients. More recently, Azimi et al. (2015) used a novel methodology to build a risk model [21]. An artificial neural network was developed to predict 2-year surgical satisfaction in 168 patients with lumbar spinal canal stenosis undergoing surgery and compared to traditional logistic regression. Artificial neural network was found to be more accurate than logistic regression.

Recently, Scheer et al. (2016) developed an innovative predictive model using an ensemble of decision trees to predict surgical complications in 557 patients [22]. The decision tree algorithm used five different bootstrapped models. This was followed by "internal validation" with 70:30 data split for training and testing the model, respectively. Final overall predictions were integrated and chosen by voting with random selection for tied votes. Overall accuracy and the area under a receiver operator characteristic curve (AUC) were calculated as well as predictor importance. The overall model accuracy was 87.6% correct with an AUC of 0.89 indicating a very good model fit.

An ensemble of many tree models leads to combined predictions from each of those trees, making the model more accurate. Decision trees are recommended as these incorporate both continuous and categorical variables, handle hundreds of variables, and are feasible even with missing data. Data split used by Scheer et al. for training and testing of the predictive model increased the generalizability of the model.

Expert Panels

Delphi/Modified Delphi Approach [23, 24]

The Delphi method involves systematic, iterative surveys that integrate qualitative and quantitative feedback to achieve consensus on responses or statements presented to expert panelists. Its principle is that the group opinion is more reliable than an individual opinion. The Delphi technique provides a systematic process for obtaining consensus opinion on issues that have not yet been investigated in clinical trials. The process can be used to achieve consensus for best practice in spine surgery, especially in patient selection and preoperative planning. As we wait for more evidence in support of risk stratification, this technique can be utilized to develop consensus on preoperative risk factors, likely to result in poor outcome in a particular patient. Statements can be designed for the preoperative patient characteristics and comorbidities which impact the quality and value of an intervention. According to recommendations for multidisciplinary panels, a panel can range from 7 to 15 individuals and should constitute spine surgeons, anesthesiologists, and registered nurses and may also include neurosurgeons or rheumatologists depending on the pathology. This panel composition reflects the perspectives of experts across different specialties on a patient's condition and ensures proportionate effect of stakeholders on the treatment decision. Sometimes, the experts are chosen from multiple medical centers to ensure geographic representation. The panelists need to have a requisite amount of experience in the surgery under discussion. The topic of analysis should be defined properly (e.g., posterior spinal fusion with interbody fusion and with discharge within 2 days). All best practice statements in the Delphi survey would pertain to the objective. This technique has three rounds in most of the cases. The consensus should be predetermined at a set percentage (i.e., for statements with answers, "agree" or "disagree").

- 1st Round: involves statements which are generated by conducting a structured review of the literature and available guidelines on the surgery in other disciplines. Grouping of statements can be done in line with the perioperative pathway for outpatient surgery.
- 2nd Round: includes structured questionnaires which are developed from the first round statements and sent to the panel members for feedback using an electronic survey tool. Each panelist is required to rate their level of agreement with each statement on a five-point Likert scale (1 (strongly disagree) to 5 (strongly agree)).

- 3rd Round: if required, it is used to rate updated or new items generated from the second round. Each panelist is provided information on their individual ratings, as well as full panel ratings from the original statements, and is asked to rerate the updated statements. Final frequency analysis from this round determines consensus levels for each statement, and panelists are given statements that achieved and did not achieve consensus.

RAND Appropriateness Method (RAM) [25]

RAM is another expert opinion method. When applied for spinal surgery, this methodology can be applied to develop appropriateness criteria and risk factors based on available evidence, further supplemented by the panel's opinion. Similar to the Delphi, it also involves searching for the present evidence with literature review and focus on clinical guidelines, followed by assessment of the patient scenarios by the panel. However, RAM differs from Delphi in that consensus is not the goal. In RAM, panelists represent diverse stakeholders, and between rounds of scoring clinical scenarios, panelists work with a moderator to openly discuss and derive refined answers in subsequent rounds.

Clinical Databases

The rising efforts to develop clinical databases comprising the clinical care data from multiple medical centers has given a big push toward the standardization of the delivery and quality of care. Focusing on the specialty of spine surgery, there are a number of databases, which can be used for risk stratification of the patient.

American College of Surgeons National Surgical Quality Improvement Program (ACS NSQIP)

The ACS NSQIP database is a multicenter registry which collects over 200 variables with regard to patient characteristics, comorbidities, operative variables, and 30-day postoperative events on patients undergoing major surgical procedures. This prospective database is maintained by onsite surgical clinical reviewers (SCR) at over 180 participating academic and private centers. To ensure high quality of data, the NSQIP uses an auditing system for quality control. Thus, risk models can be built based on the variables available for the patient profile and surgery.

Medicare [26]

The Medicare database is a nationwide registry, which has all the inpatient and outpatient utilization and cost data in the United States for each year. This administrative database has claims data from the Medicare Standard Analytic Files (SAFs) provided by the Centers for Medicare and Medicaid Services. The SAFs contain all medical claims for a randomly selected 5% cohort of Medicare beneficiaries enrolled in the Medicare fee-for-service program. SAFs include all medical claims for laboratory tests, inpatient hospital stays, outpatient care, physician care, skilled nursing facility care, home healthcare, durable medical equipment use, and hospice care. In addition, these claims also contain submitted charges, Medicare-allowed charges, and Medicare payments. Demographic characteristics (age, gender, race, etc.) are also linked to these claims.

Identification of population of interest can be done with International Classification of Diseases, Tenth Revision, Clinical Modification (ICD-10-CM) diagnosis code for a particular spine diagnosis of interest. Then, medical claims for this group can be linked via encrypted beneficiary identification numbers and followed longitudinally over time. Stratification can be done based on (a) claims for surgical treatment, (b) type of surgery and time from diagnosis until surgery (ICD-10-CM procedural codes), (c) Charlson comorbidity index (CCI; includes demographics and comorbidities and can be calculated using medical claims before the spine diagnosis), and (d) Medicare payments for all services, which can help determine the most cost-effective and durability of surgical care.

National Neurosurgery Quality and Outcomes Database (QOD) [26]
This is a nationwide, prospective longitudinal registry of spine care utilizing patient-reported outcome tools to systematically measure and aggregate surgical safety and 1-year postoperative outcome data. N2QOD avoids the use of administrative data proxies.

This registry has all the data required to build risk stratification models to ensure good quality and value of postoperative clinical outcomes and includes:

- Preoperative data: demographics, comorbidity data duration of symptoms, preoperative PROMs, diagnosis
- Operative data: ASA grade, LOS, length of surgery, intraoperative transfusion, etc.
- Postoperative data: postoperative PROMs, discharge location, readmission, return to work in 3 months and 12 months, etc.

From Risk Modeling to Risk Stratification

Combination of risk elements identified in previously described methodologies is used to create defined categories of risk. In the past, many different risk models for prediction of the quality and value of clinical outcome have been developed, and attempts have been made to stratify patients based on risk of a negative outcome.

Spine-Related Risk Stratification Efforts Related to Complications

McDonnell et al. [12]: This was a study of 447 patients who underwent anterior procedures of the spine with incidence of complications as an outcome. Age > 60 years, medical comorbidity, and diagnosis of neuromuscular scoliosis (NMS) were the significant predictive factors of perioperative complications in this population.

Schuster et al. [27]: This was a systematic review of 32 articles focusing on the influence of perioperative risk factors and therapeutic interventions on infection rates

Table 8.2 Multivariate regression model for prediction of major complications after spine surgery

Major complication	Odds ratio (95% CI)	*p*-value
Diagnosis of trauma	5.290 (3.236–8.648)	0.001
Diagnosis of infection	3.740 (1.946–7.185)	<0.001
Previous cardiac history	2.440 (1.423–4.182)	0.001
COPD	2.179 (1.157–4.100)	0.016
Hypertension	1.685 (1.059–2.680)	0.028
Surgical Invasiveness Score	1.064 (1.038–1.089)	<0.001
Age	1.033 (1.018–1.048)	<0.001

Data from: Lee et al. [16]
COPD chronic obstructive pulmonary disease

Table 8.3 Risk factors predictive of complications based on multivariate regression model

Risk factor	Odds ratio (95% CI)
Pre-op	
Preoperative transfusion	13.41 (8.19–21.95)
Inpatient	5.22 (4.17–6.53)
Disseminated cancer	4.97 (3.83–6.44)
Sepsis	4.49 (3.66–5.51)
Quadriplegia	4.15 (3.06–5.63)
Dependent functional status	3.72 (3.28–4.22)
Previous surgery <30 d	3.69 (3.02–4.50)
Contaminated wound	2.71 (2.28–3.22)
Not admitted from home	2.58 (2.36–2.83)
Diabetes mellitus on insulin	2.38 (2.11–2.69)
Age > 60	2.23 (2.04–2.44)
Intra-op	
Operative time > 4 h	4.60 (4.19–5.05)
Emergency case	3.35 (2.74–4.10)
Attending and resident in OR	2.70 (2.44–2.99)
ASA 3–5	2.59 (2.36–2.83)
Spinal fusion	2.50 (2.28–2.73)

Data from: Kimmel et al. [11]
P-value < 0.001 for all

after spine surgery. Age > 60 years, medical comorbidity, and blood transfusion were found to be the significant risk factors for infection after spine surgery.

Lee et al. [16]: This study of 1476 patients developed and validated a predictive model for medical complications after spine surgery on a prospective registry. Multivariate regression model for predicting major complications gave results as follows in Table 8.2.

Kimmell et al. [11]: This study was retrospective review of 22,430 spine surgeries from the NSQIP database. After identifying risk factors through the predictive model, a score predictive of complications was developed. Multivariate regression identified 20 factors predictive of complications with major ones mentioned in Table 8.3. By assigning 1 point for the presence of each risk factor, a risk model was developed with a score ranging from 0 to 13. The risk model successfully predicted complication rates, with complication rate of 1.2% for a score of 0 and 63.6% and 100% for scores of 12 and 13, respectively ($p < 0.001$).

Leven et al. [9]: This was a retrospective study of 1001 patients from NSQIP to determine if the modified frailty index (mFI) could be used to predict postoperative complications in ASD patients. mFI of 0.09 and 0.18 was an independent significant predictor of any complication and mortality, requiring a blood transfusion, pulmonary embolism/deep vein thrombosis, and reoperation.

Somani et al. [13]: This was a retrospective analysis of 5805 ASD patients included in the NSQIP database. Multivariate logistic regression revealed ASA class to be a significant risk factor for mortality (odds ratio [OR] = 21.0), reoperation within 30 days (OR = 1.6), length of stay ≥5 days (OR = 1.7), overall morbidity (OR = 1.4), wound complications (OR = 1.8), pulmonary complications (OR = 2.3), cardiac complications (OR = 3.7), intra-/postoperative red blood cell transfusion (OR = 1.3), postoperative sepsis (OR = 2.7), and UTI (OR = 1.6). ASA class was considered important for any risk stratification initiatives.

Piper et al. [28]: This was a retrospective review of 99,152 spine surgery patients in NSQIP database from 2012–2014. Wound complications were associated with the following preoperative characteristics: BMI ≥30, smoker, female, chronic steroid use, hematocrit <38%, infected wound, inpatient status, emergency case, and operation time > 3 h. A risk score was calculated based on the number of these characteristics that were applicable; >7 unweighted score versus 0 equates to 25-fold more likelihood of wound complication. This study developed a novel risk score for the development of wound dehiscence and SSIs.

Spine-Related Risk Stratification Efforts Related to Outcomes

Glassman et al. [10]: This was a retrospective review of prospectively collected data of 327 patients with lumbar degenerative disease who underwent lumbar spinal fusion. Stratification by diagnosis was done to compare clinical outcome measures between different groups. Preoperative diagnoses were disc pathology, spondylolisthesis, instability, stenosis, or scoliosis. For revision patients, the diagnoses were nonunion, adjacent level degeneration, or postdiscectomy revision. The percentage of patients reaching MCID for ODI at 2 years post-op ranged from 71% in spondylolisthesis to 34.8% in the nonunion subgroup. For SF-36 PCS, percentage of patients reaching MCID ranged from 63.6% in disc pathology to 25% in the nonunion subgroup. Diagnostic specificity was proven predictive of the quality of the clinical outcome.

Burkus et al. [29]: These were 2 prospective multicenter US FDA-approved studies of 277 patients with single-level lumbar degenerative disc disease, treated with either an open or laparoscopic procedure. Patients received rhBMP-2 on an absorbable collagen sponge with lumbar fusion cage implants. Significant improvement in ODI, SF-36 PCS, and VAS back and leg scores achieved at 6 weeks post-op is sustained at 6-year follow-up ($p < 0.001$). The percentage of patients who were working at 6 months (63%) was higher than preoperative percentage (52%), and this is sustained at 6 years (68%). This represents strong evidence of a desired outcome in spine care, where quality and value rose due to durability of clinical outcome at 6 years.

Weinstein et al. [7]: This is a Spine Patient Outcomes Research Trial (SPORT) trial of patients with degenerative spondylolisthesis with spinal stenosis who were offered enrollment in either randomized (304 patients) or observational cohorts (303 patients). Standard decompressive laminectomy (with or without fusion) was compared with non-operative care. Clinically relevant advantages of surgery versus non-op at 2 years were maintained at 4 years, with treatment effects of 15.3 (95% CI, 11 to 19.7) for bodily pain, 18.9 (95% CI, 14.8 to 23) for physical function, and 214.3 (95% CI, 217.5 to 211.1) for ODI. The study depicts durable clinical benefit even at 4 years making this intervention of great quality and value.

Glassman et al. [30]: This was a cost-effectiveness analysis for single-level instrumented fusion during a 5-year post-op period. A cumulative 0.69 QALY improvement during the 5-year interval was observed. Mean direct medical costs based on actual reimbursements for 5 years after surgery, including the index and revision procedures, were $22,708, with resultant cost per QALY gained at 5-year post-op of $33,018. The analogous mean direct cost based on Medicare reimbursement for 5 years was $20,669, with a resultant cost per QALY gained of $30,053. The mean total work productivity cost (indirect costs) for 5 years was $14,377. The total cost (direct and indirect) per QALY gained ranged from $53,949 to $53,914 at 5 years postoperatively. At 5-year follow-up, single-level instrumented posterolateral spine fusion was both effective and durable, resulting in a favorable cost/QALY gain compared to other widely accepted healthcare interventions.

Frailty: Canadian Study of Health and Aging (CSHA)

The CSHA included 10,263 people aged 65 or over, from 36 communities across Canada. Representative samples were assessed at intervals of every 5 years: in 1991, 1996, and in 2001. The objectives initially focused on the epidemiology of dementia. However, it also described patterns of disability, frailty and healthy aging, and utilization of health services for different diagnostic groups.

The Canadian Study of Health and Aging Frailty Index (CSHA-FI) derived from CSHA includes patient characteristics found in history and physical examination. Advancing the concept of risk stratification in spine care, the modified frailty index (mFI) was recently constructed based on the CSHA-FI using standard demographic variables of 18,294 patients in NSQIP database (2006–10) [31]. Sixteen preoperative clinical NSQIP variables were matched to eleven CSHA-FI variables (changes in daily activities, gastrointestinal problems, respiratory problems, clouding or delirium, hypertension, coronary artery and peripheral vascular disease, congestive heart failure, etc.). The outcomes assessed were 30-day occurrences of adverse events: any infection, wound-related complication, Clavien IV complications (life-threatening, requiring ICU admission), and mortality.

8.1% of patients with mFI of 0 developed at least one complication, versus 24.3% of patients with mFI of 0.27. mFI of 0 was associated with a mortality rate of 0.1%, versus 2.3% for an mFI of 0.27. mFI of 0 had a 1.7% rate of SSIs and 0.8% rate of Clavien IV complications, versus mFI of 0.27 with 4.1% and 7.1% rate of SSIs and Clavien IV complications, respectively. Multivariate analysis showed that the preoperative mFI and ASA III had a significantly increased risk of leading to Clavien IV complications and death. Thus, mFI is a useful instrument to improve risk stratification of spine surgery patients before the surgery.

The ACS NSQIP Surgical Risk Calculator

This risk calculator was developed [32] using standardized clinical data from 393 ACS NSQIP hospitals and 1,414,006 patients with 1557 unique CPT codes. Surgeons were asked to enter 21 preoperative factors (e.g., demographics, comorbidities, procedure) on a web-based tool. The universal model was compared to procedure-specific models. Regression models were developed to predict eight 30-day postoperative outcomes based on 21 preoperative risk factors. To include surgeon's input, a subjective Surgeon Adjustment Score (SAS), allowing risk estimates to vary within the estimate's confidence interval, was introduced and tested with 80 surgeons using 10 case scenarios. NSQIP risk calculator showed excellent performance for mortality (c-statistic = 0.944; Brier = 0.011[where scores approaching zero are better]), morbidity (c-statistic = 0.816, Brier = 0.069), and six additional complications (c-statistics>0.8). Predictions were similarly robust for the universal calculator vs. procedure-specific calculators (e.g., colorectal). The universal model was more accurate in 47.9% colon models presented. Among models with differences between colon-specific and universal model predicted rates of at least 0.01, the universal model was more accurate in 76.5%. Surgeons demonstrated considerable agreement on the case scenario scoring (80–100% agreement), suggesting reliable score assignment between surgeons.

With 21 predictive factors and 8 quality-of-life outcomes, this calculator assists surgeons in stratifying patients according to outcome. It provides empirically derived, patient-specific risks to guide clinicians in decision support and counseling regarding surgical care.

Putting the Full Concept Together

Meaningful endpoints are the basis for risk stratification. The endpoints need to be properly defined before proceeding to the construction of a risk model. The endpoint may be incidence of a major complication, 30-day reoperation, 30-day readmission, etc. Once the desired metric is established, data and experts are used to build a model of risk factors. In terms of the level of evidence, results from data analyses are considered superior to the decisions made by expert panels, but this may not always be true as demonstrated by RAM studies. Preoperative risk factors form the foundation of stratification into groups. This categorization divides patients ranging from high risk to low risk for the decided endpoint. Then, the risk calculator is applied to patients to compute the magnitude of risk and can be used for [32]:

- Risk mitigation if modifiable parameters are identified. Modifiable parameters would include smoking, anemia, uncontrolled DM, hyperlipidemia, osteoporosis, and psychiatric illness such as depression, anxiety, etc.
- Shared decision-making with patients. The physician can counsel the patient regarding the realistic improvement after the surgery.
- Algorithms for optimal care decisions. The magnitude of risk should call for an evaluation of the decision to perform surgery. An algorithm should be constructed to comprise the risk score, quality of life of the patient, invasiveness of surgery, chance of improvement in pain, etc. If indecisive, a discussion among colleagues from the same or different disciplines is recommended.
- Exclusion/inclusion of patients into a care pathway or bundled care program. After assessment, a need might arise to exclude a patient from a specific care pathway or switch to/from bundled care programs.
- Benchmarking of performance between clinicians/hospitals/programs. As data becomes more robust, surgeons may wish to provide patients with patient-specific estimates of postoperative complications. Recording these risk scores and actual outcomes achieved after surgery can allow comparisons between clinicians and hospitals. The era when the patients can compare their physician with respect to their colleagues and the national aggregate is not far.

Conclusion

Risk is inherent in medicine but has remained poorly defined or is trusted to the experience and knowledge of care providers. The emergence of large data sets and innovative methodologies permits the establishment of useful risk stratification. Demands on cost containment, proper allocation of resources, and quality care are driving factors of risk stratification and routine application in clinical spine care. Risk stratification holds promise to allow patient-centered care to improve value in health systems. With move to accountable healthcare, risk stratification can prove to be an excellent guiding tool for physicians to ensure optimal quality of care.

References

1. Engla NEW. Getting more performance from performance measurement. Perspective [Internet]. 2010;363(1):1–3. Available from: http://scholar.google.com/scholar?hl=en&btnG=Search&q=intitle:New+engla+nd+journal#0
2. Engla NEW. What is value in health care? Perspective [Internet]. 2010;363(1):1–3. Available from: http://scholar.google.com/scholar?hl=en&btnG=Search&q=intitle:New+engla+nd+journal#0
3. Rihn JA, Currier BL, Phillips FM, et al. Defining the value of spine care. J Am Acad Orthop Surg [Internet]. 2013 [cited 2014 November 17];21(7):419–26. Available from: http://www.ncbi.nlm.nih.gov/pubmed/23818029.

4. Godil SS, Parker SL, Zuckerman SL, et al. Determining the quality and effectiveness of surgical spine care: patient satisfaction is not a valid proxy. Spine J [Internet]. United States: Elsevier Inc; 2013 [cited 2017 March 7];13(9):1006–12. Available from: https://doi.org/10.1016/j.spinee.2013.04.008
5. Lilian Y, Chan Y-CL. Improving hospital cost accounting with activity-based costing. Health Care Manage Rev [Internet]. 1993;18(1):71–9. Available from: http://journals.lww.com/hcmrjournal/Abstract/1993/01810/Improving_hospital_cost_accounting_with.8.aspx
6. Keel G, Savage C, Rafiq M, et al. Time-driven activity-based costing in health care: A systematic review of the literature. Health Policy (New York) [Internet]. Elsevier Ireland Ltd; 2017;121(7):755–63. Available from: https://doi.org/10.1016/j.healthpol.2017.04.013
7. Weinstein JN, Lurie JD, Tosteson TD, et al. Surgical compared with nonoperative treatment for lumbar degenerative spondylolisthesis. four-year results in the Spine Patient Outcomes Research Trial (SPORT) randomized and observational cohorts. J Bone Jt Surg [Internet]. 2009 [cited 2014 June 3];91(6):1295. Available from: https://doi.org/10.2106/JBJS.H.00913
8. Herkowitz H, Andersson G, Albert T. NIH Public Access. 2012;36(24):2061–8.
9. Leven DM, Lee ÃNJ, Kothari ÃP, et al. Frailty index is a significant predictor of complications and mortality after surgery for adult spinal deformity. Spine. 2016;41(23):E1394–401.
10. Glassman SD, Carreon LY, Djurasovic M, et al. Lumbar fusion outcomes stratified by specific diagnostic indication. Spine J [Internet]. Elsevier Inc; 2009;9(1):13–21. Available from: https://doi.org/10.1016/j.spinee.2008.08.011
11. Kimmell KT, Algattas H, Joynt P, et al. Risk modeling predicts complication rates for spinal surgery. Spine (Phila Pa 1976). 2015;40(23):1836–41.
12. McDonnell MF, Glassman SD, Dimar JR, et al. Perioperative complications of anterior procedures on the spine. J Bone Joint Surg Am [Internet]. 1996;78(6):839–47. Available from: http://www.ncbi.nlm.nih.gov/pubmed/8666601%5Cn; http://content.wkhealth.com/linkback/openurl?sid=WKPTLP:landingpage&an=01241398-199701000-00052
13. Somani S, Di Capua J, Kim JS, et al. ASA classification as a risk stratification tool in adult spinal deformity surgery: a study of 5805 patients. Global Spine J. 2017;7(8):719–26.
14. McClellan M, McKethan AN, Lewis JL, et al. A national strategy to put accountable care into practice. Health Aff [Internet]. 2010;29(5):982–90. Available from: http://www.ncbi.nlm.nih.gov/pubmed/20439895
15. Tetreault LA, Kopjar B, Vaccaro A, et al. A clinical prediction model to determine outcomes in patients with cervical spondylotic myelopathy undergoing surgical treatment: data from the prospective, multi-center AOSpine North America study. JBJS. 2013;95:1659–66.
16. Lee MJ, Cizik AM, Hamilton D, et al. Predicting medical complications after spine surgery: a validated model using a prospective surgical registry. Spine J [Internet]. Elsevier Inc; 2014 [cited 2014 Apr 3];14(2):291–9. Available from: http://www.ncbi.nlm.nih.gov/pubmed/24239799
17. Chen H-N, Tsai Y-F. A predictive model for disability in patients with lumbar disc herniation. J Orthop Sci [Internet]. 2013;18(2):220–9. Available from: http://linkinghub.elsevier.com/retrieve/pii/S0949265815305236
18. Mathai KM, Kang JD, Donaldson WF, et al. Prediction of blood loss during surgery on the lumbar spine with the patient supported prone on the Jackson table. Spine J [Internet]. Elsevier Inc; 2012;12(12):1103–10. Available from: https://doi.org/10.1016/j.spinee.2012.10.027
19. Spratt KF, Keller TS, Szpalski M, et al. A predictive model for outcome after conservative decompression surgery for lumbar spinal stenosis. Eur Spine J. 2004;13(1):14–21.
20. Daubs MD, Hung M, Adams JR, et al. Clinical predictors of psychological distress in patients presenting for evaluation of a spinal disorder. Spine J [Internet]. Elsevier Inc; 2014 ;14(9):1978–83. Available from: http://www.ncbi.nlm.nih.gov/pubmed/24333833
21. Azimi P, Benzel EC, Shahzadi S, et al. Use of artificial neural networks to predict surgical satisfaction in patients with lumbar spinal canal stenosis. J Neurosurg Spine [Internet]. 2014;20(3):300–5. Available from: https://doi.org/10.3171/2013.12.SPINE13674
22. Scheer JK, Osorio JA, Smith JS, et al. Development of validated computer-based preoperative predictive model for proximal junction failure (PJF) or clinically significant PJK With 86%

accuracy based on 510 ASD patients with 2-year follow-up. Spine (Phila Pa 1976) [Internet]. 2016 [cited 2017 April 17];41(22):E1328–35. Available from: http://www.ncbi.nlm.nih.gov/pubmed/27831987
23. Okoli C, Pawlowski SD. The Delphi method as a research tool: an example, design considerations and applications. Inf Manag. 2004;42(1):15–29.
24. Mohandas A, Summa C, Worthington WB, et al. Best practices for outpatient anterior cervical surgery. Spine (Phila Pa 1976). 2017;42(11):E648–59.
25. Keshtkaran A, Bagheri MH, Ostovar R, et al. Developing criteria for lumbar spine magnetic resonance imaging (MRI) using RAND appropriateness method (RAM). Iran J Radiol. 2012;9(3):130–8.
26. Alluri RK, Leland H, Heckmann N. Surgical research using national databases. Ann Transl Med [Internet] 2016;4(20):393. Available from: http://atm.amegroups.com/article/view/12155/12517
27. Schuster JM, Rechtine G, Norvell DC, et al. The influence of perioperative risk factors and therapeutic interventions on infection rates after spine surgery: a systematic review. Spine (Phila Pa 1976) [Internet]. 2010;35(9 Suppl):S125–37. Available from: http://www.ncbi.nlm.nih.gov/pubmed/20407344
28. Piper KF, Tomlinson SB, Santangelo G, Van Galen J, DeAndrea-Lazarus I, Towner J, Kimmell KT, Silberstein H, Vates GE. Risk factors for wound complications following spine surgery. Surg Neurol Int. 2017;8:1–7.
29. Burkus JK, Gornet MF, Schuler TC, et al. Six-year outcomes of anterior lumbar interbody arthrodesis with use of interbody fusion cages and recombinant human bone morphogenetic protein-2. J Bone Jt Surgery-American Vol [Internet] 2009;91(5):1181–9. Available from: http://content.wkhealth.com/linkback/openurl?sid=WKPTLP:landingpage&an=00004623-200905000-00018
30. Glassman SD, Polly DW, Dimar JR, et al. The cost effectiveness of single-level instrumented posterolateral lumbar fusion at 5 years after surgery. Spine (Phila Pa 1976) [Internet]. 2012 [cited 2014 March 24];37(9):769–74. Available from: http://www.ncbi.nlm.nih.gov/pubmed/20489676
31. Ali R, Schwalb JM, Nerenz DR, et al. Morbidity and mortality from spine surgery. J Neurosurg Spine. 2016;25(October):537–41.
32. Kmiecik TE, Ko CY, Cohen ME. Development and evaluation of the universal ACS NSQIP surgical risk calculator: a decision aide and informed consent tool for patients and surgeons. J Am Coll Surg. 2014;217(2013):833–42.

Risk Adjustment Methodologies

9

Zach Pennington, Corinna C. Zygourakis,
and Christopher P. Ames

Introduction

Each year there are more than one million admissions for patients undergoing spine surgery [1]. This translates to roughly 149 non-instrumented decompressions and 143 spine fusions per 100,000 adults in the United States. The national costs of surgical spine care are enormous, estimated to be between $15.6 and $18 billion annually [2–4]. To effectively counsel patients undergoing spine surgery and to accurately compare outcomes across providers and facilities, it is essential to have risk adjustment tools that appropriately account for both patient and procedure-specific risk factors. For example, longer spine constructs and three-column osteotomies are both associated with higher complication rates [5], as is deformity surgery in general [6]. Comparisons between providers who specialize in one-level, minimally invasive procedures for healthy young adults and those performing multilevel deformity corrections in elderly populations may be flawed, as these procedures have very different risk profiles. Outcome comparisons between patients undergoing these disparate procedures may be misleading, and statistics gleaned from pooled populations provide data that may be unhelpful for specific patients.

There are several general risk stratification models for surgical patients, such as the American Society of Anesthesiology (ASA) or the Charlson Comorbidity Index (CCI), but these do not incorporate spine surgery-specific risk factors. As a result, there is increased emphasis on developing risk stratification systems tailored specifically to patients undergoing spine surgery. In this chapter, we describe risk

Z. Pennington · C. C. Zygourakis
Department of Neurosurgery, Johns Hopkins Hospital, Baltimore, MD, USA

C. P. Ames (✉)
Department of Neurosurgery, University of California San Francisco,
San Francisco, CA, USA
e-mail: Christopher.Ames@ucsf.edu

J. Ratliff et al. (eds.), *Quality Spine Care*,
https://doi.org/10.1007/978-3-319-97990-8_9

factors for poor outcomes after spine surgery, methodologies for risk adjustment, and the application of predictive analytics to enable providers to accurately counsel spine patients regarding their surgical risk based on the patient's individual risk factors and the specific surgery they are undergoing.

Why Is Risk Adjustment Important for Spine Surgery?

The majority of national surgical databases, such as the Nationwide Inpatient Sample (NIS) or the Centers for Medicare and Medicaid Services (CMS) databases, lump spine surgery patients into broad categories based on either DRG codes (e.g., DRG 473 "cervical spinal fusion without comorbidity or complication or major complication or comorbidity", DRG 460 "spinal fusion except cervical without major complication or comorbidity") or ICD-9/10 procedure and diagnosis codes. Unfortunately, these broad grouping systems may include patients undergoing very different surgeries. For example, DRG 473 may include a 40-year-old undergoing a one-level ACDF (anterior cervical discectomy and fusion), as well as a 70-year-old having a 6-level posterior cervical fusion. Similarly, DRG 460 may include a 30-year-old having a minimally invasive one-level TLIF (transforaminal lumbar interbody fusion) versus a 65-year-old undergoing an open eight-level posterior thoracolumbar fusion. These surgeries obviously have very different costs [7] (due to the actual procedure performed and implants used) as well as drastically different complication profiles, based on both procedural and patient-specific differences.

It is therefore of utmost importance to develop risk adjustment methodologies that account for patient comorbidities and procedural differences so that we can accurately compare/predict outcomes and healthcare costs across these heterogeneous populations and procedures [8].

Approaches to Risk Adjustment

The first step in formulating a risk-adjustment model for spine surgery is to identify preoperative factors predictive of poor outcome and increased episode-of-care cost. This includes risk factors associated with intraoperative and perioperative complications, which directly increase the cost of care [9, 10], as well as factors associated with reoperations and 30-day readmissions, which are tracked by the CMS.

Risk Factors for Spine Surgery Complications (Table 9.1)

Bone Mineral Density and Osteoporosis

Multiple studies demonstrate that low bone mineral density is associated with increased mechanical and medical complications after spine surgery [11–13, 32–34]. Guzman et al. [12] examined the 30-day outcomes of 32,557 patients from the

Table 9.1 Risk factors for spine surgery complications

Factor	Risk	References
Low bone mineral density	Hardware failure Pseudarthrosis Revision Surgery	Bredow (2016) [11] Guzman (2016) [12] Okuyama (2001) [13]
Smoking	1+ major complication Pseudarthrosis Surgical site infection	How (2018) [14] Kong (2017) [15] Purvis et al. (2017) [16]
Diabetes	Inpatient death Surgical site infection 30-day readmission	De la Garza-Ramos (2016) [17] Guzman (2014) [18] Qin (2016) [19]
Older age	1+ complication Inpatient mortality 30-day readmission	Deyo (2010) [20] Kaye (2015) [21] Patil (2008) [22]
Obesity	1+ complication Surgical site infection 90-day readmission	Bono (2017) [23] De la Garza-Ramos (2016) [14] Kalanithi (2012) [24] Puvanesarajah (2017) [25]
Baseline neurologic disease	1+ complication 30-day readmission	De la Garza-Ramos (2017) [26] Jain (2015) [27] McClelland (2017) [28]
Poor baseline functional status	1+ complication	De la Garza-Ramos (2017) [29] Deyo (2013) [30] Karhade (2016) [31]

Nationwide Inpatient Sample (NIS) that underwent surgery for degenerative cervical spine conditions. Osteoporotic patients were significantly more likely to require revision surgery and had longer average hospital stays, associated with 30% higher healthcare costs.

In terms of mechanical complications, several studies show that low bone density predisposes patients to implant subsidence, hardware failure, and pseudarthrosis. Subsidence may cause nerve root compression, generating pain and occasionally a functional radiculopathy requiring reoperation [35]. Additionally, in long-construct deformity operations, implant subsidence may lead to loss of correction and worsening coronal or sagittal imbalance. This is associated with significant pain and disability among patients and is a prime motivator for reoperation [36], itself an expensive complication that often exceeds $40,000 [37]. Similarly, hardware failure and pseudarthrosis often contribute to significant pain and require reoperation [38]. In the context of a bundled care system, these reoperations may go uncompensated, representing a financial risk for providers and healthcare systems.

Smoking History

Many spine surgeons consider current tobacco use a relative contraindication to surgery, especially in patients being considered for large deformity corrections. Smoking has several osteoporotic effects, including trabecular thinning of the cancellous bone, increased vertebral endplate porosity, and direct killing of osteoblasts [39]. This increases the risk for hardware pullout, implant subsidence, and fracture of the instrumented vertebra. In addition, smoking increases the risk of nonunion through inhibition of angioproliferation during the repair stage of osseous fusion.

Multiple retrospective series and systematic reviews have demonstrated the association of smoking with perioperative and postoperative complications in spine surgery [14–16, 40, 41]. In a study of 25,869 ACDF patients in the American College of Surgeons National Surgical Quality Improvement Program® (ACS-NSQIP), Purvis et al. [16] found that smoking significantly increased the risk of suffering one or more major medical complications, including death, myocardial infarction, and septic shock. Other studies, including those of Sebaaly [42] and Kong [15], have demonstrated an increased risk of surgical site infection (SSI) among smokers. Elsamidacy et al. [41] found that smokers undergoing spinal deformity surgery had a significantly higher rate of postoperative cellulitis and venous thromboembolic events, and another group reported that smokers undergoing anterior lumbar interbody fusion (ALIF) were 37 times more likely to experience pseudarthrosis and nearly eight times as likely to experience any surgical complication [40].

Diabetes and Insulin Insensitivity

Multiple single-institution and multicenter studies have demonstrated an increased risk for surgical site infections and overall infections in diabetic patients undergoing spine surgery [18, 19, 30, 43–51]. In their analysis of 15,480 lumbar fusion patients in ACS-NSQIP, Golinvaux and colleagues [46] found that both insulin- and non-insulin-dependent diabetics had an increased risk of wound infection relative to nondiabetic controls (RR = 3.1 and 2.3, respectively). Insulin-dependent diabetics had nearly three times higher 30-day all-cause mortality, in addition to higher rates of sepsis, septic shock, urinary tract infection, and 30-day readmission.

In another study with the NIS database, Guzman et al. [45] reported that uncontrolled diabetics undergoing surgery for degenerative lumbar spine disease had significantly higher inpatient mortality, cerebrovascular, respiratory, genitourinary, hemorrhagic, and cardiac complications, as well as deep vein thrombosis. These particular risks were significantly higher in uncontrolled as compared to controlled diabetics. Furthermore, average hospitalization costs were $5,000 or 25% higher for diabetics versus nondiabetics.

Patient Age

As with diabetes, many studies demonstrate an association between increased patient age and higher rates of postoperative complications, inpatient mortality, prolonged hospitalization, increased care costs, pseudarthrosis, surgical site infection, nonsurgical site infection, and 30-day readmission [14, 20–22, 52–57]. These include studies on patients operated at all spinal levels, including thoracolumbar fusion [14, 53], ACDF [21, 52, 57] and lumbar laminectomy [20, 30], and for multiple indications, such as lumbar stenosis [20, 30], lumbar spondylolisthesis [56], thoracolumbar deformity [14, 22, 53], and cervical spondylotic myelopathy [21, 52, 57].

Importantly, however, some studies have failed to document a relationship between age and surgical complications [17, 58]. Although these discrepancies may arise from statistical differences (e.g., using age as a continuous versus ordinal variable, grouping patients in different age groups), some authors suggest the discrepancy is more fundamental. They argue that age is only associated with complications in those studies where it acts as an effective proxy for patient frailty: a state defined by cachexia, sarcopenia, and decreased physical reserve [59] that is seen in 42–50% of elderly surgical candidates and thought to be related to changing cytokine levels. Increased age is often associated with greater frailty [59, 60], which may be more predictive of postoperative complications than age itself [61].

Obesity and BMI

Multiple studies document the association between obesity and higher rates of surgical site infection, cost of care, unplanned 30-day readmission, and longer hospitalization [23–25, 42, 47, 53, 62–70]. In an analysis of 56,338 lumbar fusion patients in the PearlDiver Patient Records Database, both obese and morbidly obese patients had significantly higher rates of any major medical complication, wound infection, and wound dehiscence. Additionally, morbidly obese patients (BMI > 40) had significantly longer hospitalizations, higher 90-day readmission rates, and an average direct healthcare cost that was $8,000 higher than for patients with BMI less than 40 [25].

All the above studies utilized BMI (body mass index) as a marker for obesity. However, this metric fails to account for the changes in circulating hormone (e.g., insulin, leptin) and cytokine levels seen in obese patients, especially those with higher visceral fat volumes. Consequently, it may be superior to include underlying cytokine or adipokine profiles when risk stratifying, as they represent the true mediators of a patient's medical risk profile [71, 72]. Additionally, just as all fat is not metabolically the same, the torque exerted by all fat masses on the spine are not equal. Abdominal obesity (android obesity) exerts significantly greater torque on a patient's lumbar spine relative to peripelvic or lower extremity fat (gynecoid obesity), which may increase the risk of screw pullout and hardware failure. As a result, future risk stratification tools may incorporate metabolic profile and physical distribution of fat stores, rather than just BMI as a marker for obesity.

Other Risk Factors

Neurological disorders and functional status have also been associated with postoperative complications and cost of care in spine patients. Patients with degenerative neurological disorders such as Parkinson's disease are at increased risk for falls, as well as postoperative wound issues due to cognitive decline-associated neglect. As a result, they often require additional assistance and experience higher postoperative complication rates, 30-day readmission rates, and episode-of-care costs [26–28].

In addition, patients with preoperative functional deficits are also at higher risk for postoperative complications after many types of spinal surgery [31, 49, 59, 73, 74]. These patients are more likely to require longer hospital stays and/or postoperative inpatient rehabilitation.

General Surgical Risk Stratification Tools (Table 9.2)

Charlson Comorbidity Index (CCI)

The Charlson Comorbidity Index was originally formulated in 1987 to quantify cumulative morbidity among patients enrolled in longitudinal trials [75]. It has been adapted to numerous populations and has become the most extensively validated measure of multiple chronic comorbidities [76]. It includes the following variables: congestive heart failure, myocardial infarction, peripheral vascular disease, cerebrovascular disease, dementia, chronic pulmonary disease, connective tissue disease,

Table 9.2 General surgical risk adjustment tools

		Application to spine surgery	
Index	Metrics	Pros	Cons
ACS-NSQIP	Surgical procedure (CPT code) Age Sex Functional status Emergent nature of case ASA Class Chronic steroid use Ascites <30d prior to surgery Systemic sepsis <48 h prior to surgery Ventilator dependent Disseminated cancer Diabetes HTN requiring medication CHF <30d prior to surgery Dyspnea Current smoker < 1 yr prior to surgery COPD Dialysis Acute renal failure BMI	Developed specifically for surgical populations based upon procedure Easy-to-use formula Provides absolute probability for each complication Developed using large sample population	Does not include several risk factors for spine surgery patients, such as osteoporosis Procedure codes (CPT) do not fully encompass diversity in spine procedures Some endpoints (e.g., functional status) are subjective

Table 9.2 (continued)

Index	Metrics	Application to spine surgery	
		Pros	Cons
ASA	Presence of systemic disease Severity of systemic disease Smoking Alcohol use Extent of functional limitations BMI Trauma	Designed specifically to assess risk of surgical complication Flexible grading system – allows inclusion of many different factors Part of routine care	Subjective factor grading Poor distinction between ASA classes Does not include several risk factors for spine surgery patients
CCI	*1 point* CHF MI PVD CVD Dementia Chronic pulmonary disease CTD PUD Diabetes (uncomplicated) *2 points* Hemiplegia Moderate/severe renal disease Diabetes w/ end-organ damage Any tumor w/o metastasis Leukemia Lymphoma *3 points* Moderate/severe liver disease *6 points* Metastatic cancer AIDS	Easy-to-use formula Linear scoring scale Multiple comorbidities considered Previously validated in multiple populations	Not all factors applicable to spine surgery List of included factors is cumbersome Some included factors poorly defined (e.g., PVD) Inclusion of age as ordinal variable Does not include several risk factors for spine surgery patients, such as smoking and osteoporosis
EFI	Cognition General health status Functional status/need for assistance with ADL Social support Medication use Nutrition Mood Continence	Easy to use formula Linear scoring scale Includes both clinical and social inputs Can be quickly completed during clinic visit/ consultation	Uses predominately subjective endpoints Not previously studied in spine surgery population

Key: *ACS-NSQIP* American College of Surgeons National Surgical Quality Improvement Program calculator, *ADL* activities of daily living, *ASA* American Society of Anesthesiology score, *BMI* body mass index, *CCI* Charlson Comorbidity Index, *CHF* congestive heart failure, *COPD* chronic obstructive pulmonary disease, *CTD* connective tissue disease, *CVD* cerebrovascular disease, *EFI* Edmonton Frailty Index, *HTN* hypertension, *PUD* peptic ulcer disease, *PVD* peripheral vascular disease

ulcer disease, and uncomplicated diabetes (all 1 point); hemiplegia, moderate or severe renal disease, diabetes with end-organ damage, any tumor, leukemia, and lymphoma (all 2 points); moderate or severe liver disease (3 points); and metastatic cancer or AIDS (4 points each). Many studies show that CCI is associated with higher postoperative complications in patients undergoing spine surgery [32, 37, 53, 77–79]. A recent study by Jain and colleagues [37] using 90-day Medicare claims data found that CCI was significantly associated with complication rate, hospital length of stay, and overall cost of care, with an increase of $697 per patient per point on the CCI. These three metrics are assessed by many value-based care models, suggesting that the CCI may be a valuable addition to both risk stratification and compensation models.

The CCI has many advantages as a risk stratification tool. Most notably, it considers many medical conditions, is easily calculated, has been previously validated, and is already in widespread use. However, it fails to include several factors previously associated with poor outcome in spine patients, such as osteoporosis and smoking [80], discussed in detail earlier in this chapter. As a result, the CCI may be a valuable addition to a spine risk stratification tool but cannot stand alone in this role.

American Society of Anesthesiology (ASA) Score

The ASA score was initially developed in 1941 as a means of assessing the operative risk of surgical patients based upon the surgical procedure and experience of the care team members [81]. The current incarnation, adopted in 1962, is composed of six classes, with class I designating a normal, healthy patient and class VI designating legally brain-dead patients undergoing organ donation procedures. Each increase in grade represents an increase in the estimated surgical risk and is based upon the estimated physical reserve of a patient. Multiple studies report an association between ASA status and complications in emergent or elective spine surgery [30, 31, 42, 54, 67, 77, 82–84]. For example, in their analysis of 12,154 spine patients, Deyo et al. reported that ASA score was significantly associated with 90-day mortality, risk of experiencing any major medical complication, and risk of a life-threatening complication [30].

The cumulative results of these studies suggest that ASA score should be included as part of risk stratification models for patients undergoing spine procedures. Like the CCI however, ASA score is not without its limitations. The ASA score does not incorporate several risk factors known to be associated with worse outcomes in spine surgery, such as smoking and osteoporosis. In addition, most studies demonstrate a correlation of ASA grade with complication rate when looking at ASA I–II versus ASA III–IV patients without differentiation within the groups. This suggests that the perceived quasi-linearity of the ASA score is not prognostically useful in spine patients and perhaps a modified ASA (e.g., ASA I/II versus ASAIII/IV) could be implemented.

ACS-NSQIP Calculator

The National Surgical Quality Improvement Program (NSQIP) is a prospectively gathered, multi-institutional, all-payor database coordinated by the American College of Surgeons. First instituted at 118 hospitals in 2005, it has grown to include more than 700 institutions providing care for millions of patients annually. As part of the program, the ACS developed a risk stratification calculator that assesses the patient's risk for multiple complications within 30 days of surgery, including surgical site infection, urinary tract infection (UTI), readmission, death, reoperation, pneumonia, cardiac complication, venous thromboembolism, and nonroutine discharge [85]. The ACS-NSQIP calculator uses the inputs shown in Table 9.2 (procedural, clinical, and health behavior components) to estimate the absolute probability that the patient will experience one of the aforementioned complications.

Several studies have examined the predictive ability of the NSQIP surgical risk calculator in patients undergoing elective spine surgery. Wang and colleagues looked specifically at a cohort of 242 patients older than 60 undergoing conventional laminectomy and decompression for lumbar stenosis. Patient information was entered in the NSQIP calculator, and the cumulative risk for each outcome was weighted to give a predicted risk profile for the cohort. This was then compared to the actual complication rates for each of these endpoints. The authors found that while the NSQIP calculator had good predictive value for death (Area under curve (AUC) = 0.972) and 30-day readmission (AUC = 0.783), it was only moderately predictive of the patient experiencing a complication or serious complication (AUC = 0.683 or 0.666, respectively) [86].

Veeravagu et al. determined the NSQIP calculator to have reasonable prognostic ability in their cohort of 446 patients undergoing elective spine procedures (receiver operative curve C-statistic = 0.669) [87]. The NSQIP calculator predicted complications with far greater accuracy than the Charlson Comorbidity Index (CCI), which is currently widely used in the spine literature.

Frailty Indices

As discussed previously, a major predictor of surgical morbidity is patient frailty, where frailty is defined as loss of physical and mental reserve [88]. Multiple frailty indices have been formulated [89–91]. One of the earliest, called the Clinical Frailty Scale [88], is a 70-item frailty index based on multiple conditions associated with cognitive deficit and chronic health identified in the Canadian Study of Health and Aging. This index has since been refined to an 11-item battery called the modified frailty index (mFI) that significantly predicts postoperative mortality and complication risk in adult spinal deformity patients [92]. More recently, Rolfson and colleagues developed the Edmonton Frail Scale, which was designed as a provider-friendly instrument capable of quickly assessing overall patient fragility on ten domains, including two performance-based tests [60]. Additionally, this measure can be accurately assessed by the nonclinical staff to provide the surgeon with a pre-visit assessment of the patient's frailty [60]. No published literature exists describing the predictive power of this index in patients undergoing spine surgery, but previous work in general and orthopedic surgery suggests that it predicts overall care costs [93], risk for early postoperative complication, and postoperative performance in activities of daily life [94].

Spine-Specific Risk Adjustment Tools (Table 9.3)

Although general predictive scales, such as the CCI, ASA, NSQIP calculator, and frailty indices can be helpful in stratifying spine patients, they are far from complete risk assessment tools. To more appropriately compare and predict outcomes and costs for spine patients, risk assessment tools need to incorporate specific aspects of spine surgery that are not captured in general risk adjustment tools. For example, most of the general tools do not include procedure in their risk stratification; and if they do (e.g., NSQIP), the procedure description is vague and glosses over major differences in spine surgery techniques that impact procedure length, estimated blood loss (EBL), complications, etc. These spine-specific surgical variables include:

- *The use and type of instrumentation*: Multiple studies have demonstrated increased complication rates [99] and 30-day readmission rates in patients undergoing fusion operations compared to decompression alone [20, 30, 100, 101].
- *Number of operated levels*: A greater number of operated levels and longer constructs require larger incisions and more extensive muscle dissections. These have been associated with longer operative times, larger EBL, higher complication rates, as well as higher rates of pseudarthrosis, wound infection, and reoperation [14, 28, 42, 83, 102, 103].
- *Revision vs index procedure*: Revision procedures have been associated with increased rates of wound site infection and incidental durotomy, as well as higher overall complication rates [20, 47, 53, 58, 104, 105].
- *Surgery level and approach*: Evidence suggests that complication profile is dependent upon the surgical level, with anterior cervical surgeries having the lowest complication rate and posterior thoracolumbar fusions having the highest rate of surgical site infection. Combined front-back surgeries also have higher perioperative complication rates [21, 47, 67, 83, 104, 106].
- *Osteotomy Use*: Osteotomies are necessary to achieve alignment correction in some spine patients, but they are not without risk. Previous studies have shown them to be associated with increased operative time and blood loss, as well as higher rates of incidental durotomy, wound infection, and overall complication rate [51, 105, 107]. These risks are largest for vertebral column resections and three-column osteotomies [53].

Table 9.3 Spine-specific risk adjustment tools

Scale	Adult Spinal Deformity Frailty Index [95, 96]	Cervical deformity frailty Index [97]	Spine surgical invasiveness index [98]
Metrics	Physician-reported >3 medical problems BMI < 18.5 or >30 Cancer Cardiac disease Currently on disability Current smoker Depression Diabetes Hypertension Liver disease Lung disease Osteoporosis Peripheral vascular disease Previous DVT/PE/ischemic stroke Patient-reported Bladder incontinence Bowel incontinence SF-36 Leg weakness Loss of balance LSDI ODI SRS-22r	Physician-reported >3 medical problems BMI < 18.5 or >30 Cancer Cardiac disease Cerebrovascular disease Currently on disability Dementia Depression Diabetes Liver disease Lung disease Neuromuscular disease Osteoporosis Pancreatic disease Rheumatoid arthritis Smoker Vascular disease Venous disease Unsteady gait Patient-reported Bladder incontinence Bowel incontinence EuroQol-5D EuroQol-VAS Leg weakness LSDI mJOA LSDI NDI SWAL-QOL	Number of vertebral levels receiving each of the following: Anterior decompression Anterior fusion Anterior instrumentation Posterior decompression Posterior fusion Posterior instrumentation
Pro	Many different comorbidities Physician- and patient-reported variables	Many different comorbidities Physician- and patient-reported variables Correlated with both complications and PRO	Applicable to multiple populations Easily calculated following surgical planning
Con	Specific to one population Formulated using a small number of patients Large number of variables → cumbersome for clinical use	Specific to one population Large number of variables → cumbersome for clinical use	Requires very detailed procedural data not available in most public/national databases Does not include patient-specific details

Key: *EQ-5D* EuroQol, five dimensions, *EQ-VAS* EuroQol visual analog scale, *LSDI* lumbar stiffness disability index, *mJOA* modified Japanese Orthopaedic Association scale, *NDI* Neck Disability Index, *ODI* Oswestry Disability Index, *PRO* patient-reported outcome, *SF-36* short-form 36 version 2, *SRS-22r* Scoliosis Research Society-22r questionnaire, *SWAL-QOL* quality of life in swallowing disorders questionnaire

- *Minimally invasive (MIS) versus open technique*: Systematic reviews and meta-analyses comparing MIS and open spine procedures have been equivocal, with some showing no difference between the two approaches [108, 109] and some showing lower morbidity in the MIS cohort [110, 111]. Similarly, evidence surrounding the cost-effectiveness of minimally invasive procedures is equivocal, with some studies finding lower costs with MIS procedures and others finding no significant difference [112–114].

Spine Surgical Invasiveness Index

The Spine Surgical Invasiveness Index (SII) is a predictive tool designed to describe the complexity of surgical intervention in order to allow fair comparisons of complication rates among patients undergoing a wide range of spine procedures with different providers and in different hospital settings. The SII is scored on a scale of 0–48 based upon the surgical approach, number of decompressed vertebral levels, number of fused levels, and number of instrumented levels [115]. In a recent study of 1,532 spine patients, surgical invasiveness was the strongest predictor of surgical site infection [116]. For lumbar spine patients, surgical invasiveness was significantly associated with cardiac, pulmonary, neurological, and hematological complications [117].

Spine-Specific Frailty Index

The International Spine Study Group (ISSG) has developed spine-specific frailty indices, including the Cervical Deformity Frailty Index [97] and Adult Spinal Deformity Frailty Index [95, 96]. The former index was created by Miller and colleagues using a population of 61 adults with significant cervical kyphoscoliosis. It includes both health comorbidities (e.g., diabetes, osteoporosis) and health-related quality of life (HRQoL) outcomes, such as EuroQoL-5D and modified Japanese Orthopaedic Association (mJOA), to classify patients as not frail, frail, or severely frail. Using the Cervical Deformity Frailty Index, Miller et al. showed a higher risk of any major complication among frail and severely frail patients relative to not frail patients, with severely frail patients being 43 times more likely to suffer a major complication than not frail patients [96].

The Adult Spinal Deformity Frailty Index (ASD-FI) was developed by the same group of investigators using a cohort of 417 patients who underwent surgery for adult spinal deformity [96]. Like the Cervical Deformity Frailty Index, it incorporates both medical comorbidities and HRQoL outcome measures. For adult spinal deformity patients, this spine-specific frailty index significantly predicts major postoperative complications, including reoperation, proximal junctional kyphosis, wound infection, and pseudarthrosis. A follow-up study by Reid and colleagues [95] demonstrated that patients classified as frail or severely frail by this index were also less likely to demonstrate clinically significant benefit on postoperative HRQoL measures such as the SF-36.

Taken together, the spine surgical invasiveness index and spine-specific frailty indices may be more accurate measures of risk stratification than general tools such as the CCI, ASA, ACS-NSQIP calculator, or Edmonton Frail Scale. Additionally, these tools can predict complications unique to spine surgery, such as proximal junctional kyphosis and pseudarthrosis, as well as general complications like wound infection and readmission. These spine-specific risk adjustment tools represent the future for spine surgery but require further validation in additional datasets before being adopted as standard of care.

Predictive Analytics

Many of the tools discussed to this point, including the ASD-FI, the ACS-NSQIP calculator, and the SII, were constructed using historical patient data to help predict the likelihood of perioperative and postoperative complications in surgically treated patients. As surgeons, it is essential for us to be able to prospectively identify patients who are at high risk of experiencing peri- and postoperative complications so that we can adjust our surgical plan and set appropriate expectations for our patients.

Predictive analytics is a relatively new field that uses computer algorithms to accomplish this goal by identifying patterns in patient data. Unlike older risk models, it has no need for a hypothesis and so can provide detailed and patient-specific information that can readily be applied when discussing risks during presurgical consultation with a patient. The first modern predictive model was advanced by Spratt and colleagues, who used a decision tree analysis to predict outcome following lumbar decompression [118]. Their model proved highly effective within their dataset, demonstrating a positive predictive value of 85.7% and sensitivity to successful outcome of 90.1%. However, it was limited by its small sample size. More recently, Daubs et al. used a similar analysis to accurately predict psychological distress among spine patients, with an overall accuracy of 92% [119]. Psychological distress has been associated with poor patient-reported outcomes, so this predictive tool enables preoperative identification of patients with psychological distress who are at higher risk for worse surgical outcomes. Lastly, Azumi and colleagues used an artificial neural network to predict 2-year surgical satisfaction in patients who underwent surgery for lumbar stenosis [120]. By accurately predicting satisfaction in 96.9% of patients, their model was superior to traditional logistic regression models.

The International Spine Study Group (ISSG) has recently developed two predictive analytic models for adult spinal deformity patients. They created one model using 234 adult spinal deformity patients from their multicenter prospectively enrolled cohort with the goal of predicting a minimum clinically important difference (MCID) in Oswestry Disability Index (ODI) at 2 years post-op. Forty-six variables, including patient demographics, radiographic parameters, surgical variables, and health-related quality of life metrics, were used to train the model. The final model had 11 variables that were most predictive of patient outcome: depression, ODI, number of posterior levels fused, presence of arthritis, presence of 1 or more comorbidities, presence of osteoporosis, three-column osteotomy, upper instrumented vertebra, leg pain, decompression (yes/no), and back pain. The final model had a C-statistic of 0.96 and overall accuracy of 85.5%, indicating that this may be a useful tool for preoperatively predicting a postoperative clinically important improvement in adult spinal deformity patients [98].

Using similar predictive analytic techniques, including decision trees, bootstrapping, and internal validation with 70/30 data split, Scheer et al. created a predictive model for adult spinal deformity patients having at least one major intraoperative or postoperative complication. Based on 557 ISSG patients and incorporating 45 variables in their model training, their final model had an accuracy of 87.6% and a C-statistic of 0.89, indicating a very good model fit for predicting major complications. The 20 variables determined to be the top predictors of complications were age, leg pain, ODI, number of decompression levels, number of interbody fusion levels, physical component summary of SF-36, Scoliosis Research Society coronal curve type, CCI, SRS activity, T-1 pelvis angle, ASA grade, osteoporosis, pelvic tilt, sagittal vertical axis, primary versus revision surgery, SRS pain, SRS total, use of bone morphogenic protein, use of iliac crest graft, and pelvic incidence-lumbar lordosis mismatch [32].

In the future, these predictive models can be translated into easy online calculators to allow spinal deformity surgeons to use surgery-specific risk adjustment tools to provide real-time, preoperative risk prediction for their patients.

Conclusion

In summary, the increased availability of big data, both from national databases like the Nationwide Inpatient Sample (NIS) and National Surgical Quality Improvement Program (NSQIP), as well as spine-specific registries like the ISSG, have allowed us to investigate the specific patient and surgical factors associated with poor outcomes and high costs in spinal surgery. It is critical for us to be able to appropriately risk-stratify our patients as we strive to better compare patient outcomes across surgeons and hospitals and as compensation models shift to bundled payment and value-based care models.

Many of these initial studies have been retrospective reviews utilizing basic regression techniques and generalized risk-adjustment tools, such as ASA, CCI, or frailty index, to show associations between certain patient factors and outcomes. In recent years, we have developed spine-specific risk adjustment tools, including the spine surgical invasiveness index and spine-specific frailty indices. Future work will also include application of novel predictive analytic techniques to more accurately predict complications and high cost in spine surgery.

References

1. Fingar KR, Stocks C, Weiss AJ, Steiner CA. Most frequent operating room procedures performed in U.S. hospitals, 2003–2012: Statistical Brief #186. 2014;186.
2. Martin BI, Turner JA, Mirza SK, Lee MJ, Comstock BA, Deyo RA. Trends in health care expenditures, utilization, and health status among US adults with spine problems, 1997–2006. Spine (Phila Pa 1976). 2009;34(19):2077–84.
3. Davis MA, Onega T, Weeks WB, Lurie JD. Where the United States spends its spine dollars: expenditures on different ambulatory services for the management of back and neck conditions. Spine (Phila Pa 1976). 2012;37(19):1693–701.
4. Weiss AJ, Elixhauser A, Andrews RM. Characteristics of operating room procedures in U.S. hospitals, 2011. Statistical Brief #170. Healthcare Cost and Utilization Project (HCUP) Statistical Briefs. 2014;170.
5. Kim HJ, Piyaskulkaew C, Riew KD. Comparison of Smith-Petersen osteotomy versus pedicle subtraction osteotomy versus anterior-posterior osteotomy types for the correction of cervical spine deformities. Spine. 2015;40(3):143–6.
6. Kim HJ, Bridwell KH, Lenke LG, Park MS, Song KS, Piyaskulkaew C, et al. Patients with proximal junctional kyphosis requiring revision surgery have higher postoperative lumbar lordosis and larger sagittal balance corrections. Spine. 2014;39(9):576.
7. Uddin OM, Haque R, Sugrue PA, Ahmed YM, El Ahmadieh TY, Press JM, et al. Cost minimization in treatment of adult degenerative scoliosis. J Neurosurg Spine. 2015;23(6):798–806.
8. Juhnke C, Bethge S, Mühlbacher AC. A review on methods of risk adjustment and their use in integrated healthcare systems. Int J Integr Care. 2016;16(4):4.
9. Yeramaneni S, Robinson C, Hostin R. Impact of spine surgery complications on costs associated with management of adult spinal deformity. Curr Rev Musculoskelet Med. 2016;9(3):327–32.
10. Culler SD, Jevsevar DS, Shea KG, McGuire KJ, Schlosser M, Wright KK, et al. Incremental hospital cost and length-of-stay associated with treating adverse events among medicare beneficiaries undergoing lumbar spinal fusion during fiscal year 2013. Spine. 2016;41(20):1613–20.
11. Bredow J, Boese CK, Werner CML, Siewe J, Löhrer L, Zarghooni K, et al. Predictive validity of preoperative CT scans and the risk of pedicle screw loosening in spinal surgery. Arch Orthop Trauma Surg. 2016;136(8):1063–7.
12. Guzman JZ, Feldman ZM, McAnany S, Hecht AC, Qureshi SA, Cho SK. Osteoporosis in cervical spine surgery. Spine. 2016;41(8):662–8.
13. Okuyama K, Abe E, Suzuki T, Tamura Y, Chiba M, Sato K. Influence of bone mineral density on pedicle screw fixation: a study of pedicle screw fixation augmenting posterior lumbar interbody fusion in elderly patients. Spine J. 2001;1(6):402–7.
14. How NE, Street JT, Dvorak MF, Fisher CG, Kwon BK, Paquette S, et al. Pseudarthrosis in adult and pediatric spinal deformity surgery: a systematic review of the literature and meta-analysis of incidence, characteristics, and risk factors. Neurosurg Rev. 2018. https://doi.org/10.1007/s10143-018-0951-3. [Epub ahead of print].
15. Kong L, Liu Z, Meng F, Shen Y. Smoking and risk of surgical site infection after spinal surgery: a systematic review and meta-analysis. Surg Infect (Larchmt). 2017;18(2):206–14.
16. Purvis TE, Rodriguez HJ, Ahmed AK, Boone C, De la Garza-Ramos R, Elder BD, et al. Impact of smoking on postoperative complications after anterior cervical discectomy and fusion. J Clin Neurosci. 2017;38:106–10.
17. De la Garza-Ramos R, Abt NB, Kerezoudis P, McCutcheon BA, Bydon A, Gokaslan Z, et al. Deep-wound and organ-space infection after surgery for degenerative spine disease: an analysis from 2006 to 2012. Neurol Res. 2016;38(2):117–23.
18. Guzman JZ, Skovrlj B, Shin J, Hecht AC, Qureshi SA, Iatridis JC, et al. The impact of diabetes mellitus on patients undergoing degenerative cervical spine surgery. Spine. 2014;39(20):1656–65.

19. Qin C, Kim JYS, Hsu WK. Impact of insulin dependence on lumbar surgery outcomes: an NSQIP analysis of 51,277 patients. Spine. 2016;41(11):687.
20. Deyo RA, Mirza SK, Martin BI, Kreuter W, Goodman DC, Jarvik JG. Trends, major medical complications, and charges associated with surgery for lumbar spinal stenosis in older adults. JAMA. 2010;303(13):1259–65.
21. Kaye ID, Marascalchi BJ, Macagno AE, Lafage VA, Bendo JA, Passias PG. Predictors of morbidity and mortality among patients with cervical spondylotic myelopathy treated surgically. Eur Spine J. 2015;24(12):2910–7.
22. Patil CG, Santarelli J, Lad SP, Ho C, Tian W, Boakye M. Inpatient complications, mortality, and discharge disposition after surgical correction of idiopathic scoliosis: a national perspective. Spine J. 2008;8(6):904–10.
23. Bono CM, Harris MB, Warholic N, Katz JN, Carreras E, White A, et al. Pain intensity and patients' acceptance of surgical complication risks with lumbar fusion. Spine (Phila Pa 1976). 2013;38(2):140–7.
24. Kalanithi PA, Arrigo R, Boakye M. Morbid obesity increases cost and complication rates in spinal arthrodesis. Spine. 2012;37(11):982–8.
25. Puvanesarajah V, Werner BC, Cancienne JM, Jain A, Pehlivan H, Shimer AL, et al. Morbid obesity and lumbar fusion in patients older than 65 years: complications, readmissions, costs, and length of stay. Spine. 2017;42(2):122–7.
26. de la Garza-Ramos R, Goodwin CR, Jain A, Martinez-Ramirez D, Karikari IO, Sciubba DM. Inpatient morbidity after spinal deformity surgery in patients with movement disorders. J Spine Surg. 2017;3:601–8.
27. Jain A, Puvanesarajah V, Menga EN, Sponseller PD. Unplanned hospital readmissions and reoperations after pediatric spinal fusion surgery. Spine. 2015;40(11):856–62.
28. McClelland S, Baker JF, Smith JS, Line BG, Errico TJ, Ames CP, et al. Impact of Parkinson's disease on perioperative complications and hospital cost in multilevel spine fusion: a population-based analysis. J Clin Neurosci. 2017;35:88–91.
29. De la Garza Ramos R, Goodwin CR, Elder BD, Boah AO, Miller EK, Jain A, et al. Preoperative functional status as a predictor of short-term outcome in adult spinal deformity surgery. J Clin Neurosci. 2017;39:118–23.
30. Deyo RA, Hickam D, Duckart JP, Piedra M. Complications after surgery for lumbar stenosis in a veteran population. Spine. 2013;38(19):1695–702.
31. Karhade AV, Vasudeva VS, Dasenbrock HH, Lu Y, Gormley WB, Groff MW, et al. Thirty-day readmission and reoperation after surgery for spinal tumors: a National Surgical Quality Improvement Program analysis. Neurosurg Focus. 2016;41(2):E5.
32. Scheer JK, Smith JS, Schwab F, Lafage V, Shaffrey CI, Bess S, et al. Development of a preoperative predictive model for major complications following adult spinal deformity surgery. J Neurosurg Spine. 2017;26(6):736–43.
33. Satake K, Kanemura T, Yamaguchi H, Segi N, Ouchida J. Predisposing factors for intraoperative endplate injury of extreme lateral interbody fusion. Asian Spine J. 2016;10(5):907–14.
34. Formby PM, Kang DG, Helgeson MD, Wagner SC. Clinical and radiographic outcomes of transforaminal lumbar interbody fusion in patients with osteoporosis. Global Spine J. 2016;6(7):660–4.
35. Nemani VM, Aichmair A, Taher F, Lebl DR, Hughes AP, Sama AA, et al. Rate of revision surgery after stand-alone lateral lumbar interbody fusion for lumbar spinal stenosis. Spine. 2014;39(5):326.
36. Glassman SD, Berven S, Bridwell K, Horton W, Dimar JR. Correlation of radiographic parameters and clinical symptoms in adult scoliosis. Spine. 2005;30(6):682–8.
37. Jain N, Phillips FM, Khan SN. Distribution and determinants of 90-day payments for multilevel posterior lumbar fusion: a medicare analysis. Clin Spine Surg. 2018;31:E197–203.
38. Adogwa O, Carr RK, Kudyba K, Karikari I, Bagley CA, Gokaslan ZL, et al. Revision lumbar surgery in elderly patients with symptomatic pseudarthrosis, adjacent-segment disease, or same-level recurrent stenosis. Part 1. Two-year outcomes and clinical efficacy: clinical article. J Neurosurg Spine. 2013;18(2):139–46.

39. Berman D, Oren JH, Bendo J, Spivak J. The effect of smoking on spinal fusion. Int J Spine Surg. 2017;11:29.
40. Phan K, Fadhil M, Chang N, Giang G, Gragnaniello C, Mobbs RJ. Effect of smoking status on successful arthrodesis, clinical outcome, and complications after Anterior Lumbar Interbody Fusion (ALIF). World Neurosurg. 2017;110:998–1003.
41. Elsamadicy AA, Adogwa O, Sergesketter A, Vuong VD, Lydon E, Behrens S, et al. Reduced impact of smoking status on 30-day complication and readmission rates after elective spinal fusion (≥3 levels) for adult spine deformity: a single institutional study of 839 patients. World Neurosurg. 2017;107:233–8.
42. Sebaaly A, Shedid D, Boubez G, Zairi F, Kanhonou M, Yuh S, et al. Surgical site infection in spinal metastasis: incidence and risk factors. Spine J. 2018. pii:S1529-9430(18)300004-4.
43. Shamji MF, Mroz T, Hsu W, Chutkan N. Management of degenerative lumbar spinal stenosis in the elderly. Neurosurgery. 2015;77(Suppl 4):68.
44. Phan K, Rogers P, Rao PJ, Mobbs RJ. Influence of obesity on complications, clinical outcome, and subsidence after Anterior Lumbar Interbody Fusion (ALIF): prospective observational study. World Neurosurg. 2017;107:334–41.
45. Guzman JZ, Iatridis JC, Skovrlj B, Cutler HS, Hecht AC, Qureshi SA, et al. Outcomes and complications of diabetes mellitus on patients undergoing degenerative lumbar spine surgery. Spine. 2014;39(19):1596–604.
46. Golinvaux NS, Varthi AG, Bohl DD, Basques BA, Grauer JN. Complication rates following elective lumbar fusion in patients with diabetes: insulin dependence makes the difference. Spine. 2014;39(21):1809–16.
47. Fei Q, Li J, Lin J, Li D, Wang B, Meng H, et al. Risk factors for surgical site infection after spinal surgery: a meta-analysis. World Neurosurg. 2016;95:507–15.
48. Epstein NE. Predominantly negative impact of diabetes on spinal surgery: a review and recommendation for better preoperative screening. Surg Neurol Int. 2017;8:107.
49. Cook C, Tackett S, Shah A, Pietrobon R, Browne J, Viens N, et al. Diabetes and perioperative outcomes following cervical fusion in patients with myelopathy. Spine. 2008; 33(8):254.
50. Browne JA, Cook C, Pietrobon R, Bethel MA, Richardson WJ. Diabetes and early postoperative outcomes following lumbar fusion. Spine. 2007;32(20):2214–9.
51. Abdul-Jabbar A, Takemoto S, Weber MH, Hu SS, Mummaneni PV, Deviren V, et al. Surgical site infection in spinal surgery: description of surgical and patient-based risk factors for postoperative infection using administrative claims data. Spine. 2012;37(15):1340–5.
52. Boakye M, Patil CG, Santarelli J, Ho C, Tian W, Lad SP. Cervical spondylotic myelopathy: complications and outcomes after spinal fusion. Neurosurgery. 2008;62(2):462.
53. Smith JS, Klineberg E, Lafage V, Shaffrey CI, Schwab F, Lafage R, et al. Prospective multicenter assessment of perioperative and minimum 2-year postoperative complication rates associated with adult spinal deformity surgery. J Neurosurg Spine. 2016;25(1):1–14.
54. Pugely AJ, Martin CT, Gao Y, Mendoza-Lattes S. Causes and risk factors for 30-day unplanned readmissions after lumbar spine surgery. Spine. 2014;39(9):761–8.
55. Patil CG, Lad SP, Santarelli J, Boakye M. National inpatient complications and outcomes after surgery for spinal metastasis from 1993–2002. Cancer. 2007;110(3):625–30.
56. Kalanithi PS, Patil CG, Boakye M. National complication rates and disposition after posterior lumbar fusion for acquired spondylolisthesis. Spine. 2009;34(18):1963–9.
57. Buerba RA, Giles E, Webb ML, Fu MC, Gvozdyev B, Grauer JN. Increased risk of complications after anterior cervical discectomy and fusion in the elderly: an analysis of 6253 patients in the American College of Surgeons National Surgical Quality Improvement Program database. Spine. 2014;39(25):2062–9.
58. Leven D, Passias PG, Errico TJ, Lafage V, Bianco K, Lee A, et al. Risk factors for reoperation in patients treated surgically for intervertebral disc herniation: a subanalysis of eight-year SPORT data. J Bone Joint Surg Am. 2015;97(16):1316–25.
59. Partridge JSL, Harari D, Dhesi JK. Frailty in the older surgical patient: a review. Age Ageing. 2012;41(2):142–7.

60. Rolfson DB, Majumdar SR, Tsuyuki RT, Tahir A, Rockwood K. Validity and reliability of the Edmonton Frail Scale. Age Ageing. 2006;35(5):526–9.
61. Joseph B, Pandit V, Zangbar B, Kulvatunyou N, Hashmi A, Green DJ, et al. Superiority of frailty over age in predicting outcomes among geriatric trauma patients: a prospective analysis. JAMA Surg. 2014;149(8):766–72.
62. Sebastian A, Huddleston P, Kakar S, Habermann E, Wagie A, Nassr A. Risk factors for surgical site infection after posterior cervical spine surgery: an analysis of 5,441 patients from the ACS NSQIP 2005-2012. Spine J. 2016;16(4):504–9.
63. Ou C, Lee T, Lee T, Huang Y. Impact of body mass index on adjacent segment disease after lumbar fusion for degenerative spine disease. Neurosurgery. 2015;76(4):402; quiz 402.
64. Manoharan SR, Baker DK, Pasara SM, Ponce B, Deinlein D, Theiss SM. Thirty-day readmissions following adult spinal deformity surgery: an analysis of the National Surgical Quality Improvement Program (NSQIP) database. Spine J. 2016;16(7):862–6.
65. Lingutla KK, Pollock R, Benomran E, Purushothaman B, Kasis A, Bhatia CK, et al. Outcome of lumbar spinal fusion surgery in obese patients: a systematic review and meta-analysis. Bone Joint J. 2015;97-B(10):1395–404.
66. Lim S, Edelstein AI, Patel AA, Kim BD, Kim JYS. Risk factors for postoperative infections after single-level lumbar fusion surgery. Spine. 2018;43(3):215–22.
67. Lee NJ, Shin JI, Kothari P, Kim JS, Leven DM, Steinberger J, et al. Incidence, impact, and risk factors for 30-day wound complications following elective adult spinal deformity surgery. Global Spine J. 2017;7(5):417–24.
68. De la Garza Ramos R, Nakhla J, Nasser R, Schulz JF, Purvis TE, Sciubba DM, et al. Effect of body mass index on surgical outcomes after posterior spinal fusion for adolescent idiopathic scoliosis. Neurosurg Focus. 2017;43(4):E5.
69. Buerba RA, Fu MC, Gruskay JA, Long WD, Grauer JN. Obese Class III patients at significantly greater risk of multiple complications after lumbar surgery: an analysis of 10,387 patients in the ACS NSQIP database. Spine J. 2014;14(9):2008–18.
70. Abdallah DY, Jadaan MM, McCabe JP. Body mass index and risk of surgical site infection following spine surgery: a meta-analysis. Eur Spine J. 2013;22(12):2800–9.
71. Cornier M, Després J, Davis N, Grossniklaus DA, Klein S, Lamarche B, et al. Assessing adiposity: a scientific statement from the American Heart Association. Circulation. 2011;124(18):1996.
72. Romero-Corral A, Somers VK, Sierra-Johnson J, Thomas RJ, Collazo-Clavell ML, Korinek J, et al. Accuracy of body mass index in diagnosing obesity in the adult general population. Int J Obes. 2008;32(6):959–66.
73. Sing DC, Yue JK, Metz LN, Winkler EA, Zhang WR, Burch S, et al. Obesity is an independent risk factor of early complications after revision spine surgery. Spine. 2016;41(10):632.
74. Bohl DD, Ahn J, Tabaraee E, Ahn J, Jain A, Grauer JN, et al. Urinary tract infection following posterior lumbar fusion procedures: an American College of Surgeons National Surgical Quality Improvement Program Study. Spine. 2015;40(22):1785–91.
75. Charlson ME, Pompei P, Ales KL, MacKenzie CR. A new method of classifying prognostic comorbidity in longitudinal studies: development and validation. J Chron Dis. 1987;40(5):373–83.
76. Charlson M, Wells MT, Ullman R, King F, Shmukler C. The Charlson comorbidity index can be used prospectively to identify patients who will incur high future costs. PLoS One. 2014;9(12):e112479.
77. Whitmore RG, Stephen JH, Vernick C, Campbell PG, Yadla S, Ghobrial GM, et al. ASA grade and Charlson Comorbidity Index of spinal surgery patients: correlation with complications and societal costs. Spine J. 2014;14(1):31–8.
78. Shen Y, Silverstein JC, Roth S. In-hospital complications and mortality after elective spinal fusion surgery in the United States: a study of the nationwide inpatient sample from 2001 to 2005. J Neurosurg Anesthesiol. 2009;21(1):21–30.
79. Howe CR, Agel J, Lee MJ, Bransford RJ, Wagner TA, Bellabarba C, et al. The morbidity and mortality of fusions from the thoracic spine to the pelvis in the adult population. Spine. 2011;36(17):1397–401.

80. Lovy AJ, Guzman JZ, Skovrlj B, Cho SK, Hecht AC, Qureshi SA. Prevalence, comorbidities, and risk of perioperative complications in human immunodeficiency virus-positive patients undergoing cervical spine surgery. Spine. 2015;40(21):1128.
81. Fitz-Henry J. The ASA classification and peri-operative risk. Ann R Coll Surg Engl. 2011;93(3):185–7.
82. Somani S, Capua JD, Kim JS, Phan K, Lee NJ, Kothari P, et al. ASA classification as a risk stratification tool in adult spinal deformity surgery: a study of 5805 patients. Global Spine J. 2017;7(8):719–26.
83. Pugely AJ, Martin CT, Gao Y, Ilgenfritz R, Weinstein SL. The incidence and risk factors for short-term morbidity and mortality in pediatric deformity spinal surgery: an analysis of the NSQIP pediatric database. Spine. 2014;39(15):1225–34.
84. Phan K, Kim JS, Lee NJ, Kothari P, Cho SK. Relationship between ASA scores and 30-day readmissions in patients undergoing anterior cervical discectomy and fusion. Spine. 2017;42(2):85–91.
85. Bilimoria KY, Liu Y, Paruch JL, Zhou L, Kmiecik TE, Ko CY, et al. Development and evaluation of the universal ACS NSQIP surgical risk calculator: a decision aid and informed consent tool for patients and surgeons. J Am Coll Surg. 2013;217(5):3.
86. Wang X, Hu Y, Zhao B, Su Y. Predictive validity of the ACS-NSQIP surgical risk calculator in geriatric patients undergoing lumbar surgery. Medicine (Baltimore). 2017;96(43):e8416.
87. Veeravagu A, Li A, Swinney C, Tian L, Moraff A, Azad T, et al. Predicting complication risk in spine surgery: a prospective analysis of a novel risk assessment tool. J Neurosurg Spine. 2017;27(1):81–91.
88. Rockwood K, Song X, MacKnight C, Bergman H, Hogan DB, McDowell I, et al. A global clinical measure of fitness and frailty in elderly people. CMAJ. 2005;173(5):489–95.
89. Fried LP, Tangen CM, Walston J, Newman AB, Hirsch C, Gottdiener J, et al. Frailty in older adults: evidence for a phenotype. J Gerontol A Biol Sci Med Sci. 2001;56(3):M157.
90. De la Garza Ramos R, Goodwin CR, Jain A, Abu-Bonsrah N, Fisher CG, Bettegowda C, et al. Development of a metastatic spinal tumor frailty index (MSTFI) using a nationwide database and its association with inpatient morbidity, mortality, and length of stay after spine surgery. World Neurosurg. 2016;95:555.e4.
91. Ahmed AK, Goodwin CR, de la Garza-Ramos R, Kim RC, Abu-Bonsrah N, Xu R, et al. Predicting short-term outcome after surgery for primary spinal tumors based on patient frailty. World Neurosurg. 2017;108:393–8.
92. Leven DM, Lee NJ, Kothari P, Steinberger J, Guzman J, Skovrlj B, et al. Frailty index is a significant predictor of complications and mortality after surgery for adult spinal deformity. Spine. 2016;41(23):E1401.
93. Eamer GJ, Clement F, Pederson JL, Churchill TA, Khadaroo RG. Analysis of postdischarge costs following emergent general surgery in elderly patients. Can J Surg. 2018;61(1):19–27.
94. Kua J, Ramason R, Rajamoney G, Chong MS. Which frailty measure is a good predictor of early post-operative complications in elderly hip fracture patients? Arch Orthop Trauma Surg. 2016;136(5):639–47.
95. Reid DBC, Daniels AH, Ailon T, Miller E, Sciubba DM, Smith JS, et al. Frailty and health-related quality of life improvement following adult spinal deformity surgery. World Neurosurg. 2018;112:e548–54.
96. Miller EK, Neuman BJ, Jain A, Daniels AH, Ailon T, Sciubba DM, et al. An assessment of frailty as a tool for risk stratification in adult spinal deformity surgery. Neurosurg Focus. 2017;43(6):E3.
97. Miller EK, Ailon T, Neuman BJ, Klineberg EO, Mundis GM, Sciubba DM, et al. Assessment of a novel adult cervical deformity frailty index as a component of preoperative risk stratification. World Neurosurg. 2018;109:e806.
98. Oh T, Scheer JK, Smith JS, Hostin R, Robinson C, Gum JL, et al. Potential of predictive computer models for preoperative patient selection to enhance overall quality-adjusted life years gained at 2-year follow-up: a simulation in 234 patients with adult spinal deformity. Neurosurg Focus. 2017;43(6):E2.

99. Iyer S, Klineberg EO, Zebala LP, Kelly MP, Hart RA, Gupta MC, et al. Dural tears in adult deformity surgery: incidence, risk factors, and outcomes. Global Spine J. 2018;8(1):25–31.
100. Sato S, Yagi M, Machida M, Yasuda A, Konomi T, Miyake A, et al. Reoperation rate and risk factors of elective spinal surgery for degenerative spondylolisthesis: minimum 5-year follow-up. Spine J. 2015;15(7):1536–44.
101. Onyekwelu I, Glassman SD, Asher AL, Shaffrey CI, Mummaneni PV, Carreon LY. Impact of obesity on complications and outcomes: a comparison of fusion and nonfusion lumbar spine surgery. J Neurosurg Spine. 2017;26(2):158–62.
102. Pereira BJ, de Holanda CVM, Ribeiro CA, de Moura SM, de Carvalho Galvão PE, Quidute BSQ, et al. Impact of body mass index in spinal surgery for degenerative lumbar spine disease. Clin Neurol Neurosurg. 2014;127:112–5.
103. Patel N, Bagan B, Vadera S, Maltenfort MG, Deutsch H, Vaccaro AR, et al. Obesity and spine surgery: relation to perioperative complications. J Neurosurg Spine. 2007;6(4):291–7.
104. Leckie S, Yoon ST, Isaacs R, Radcliff K, Fessler R, Haid R, et al. Perioperative complications of cervical spine surgery: analysis of a prospectively gathered database through the Association for Collaborative Spinal Research. Global Spine J. 2016;6(7):640–9.
105. Ishikura H, Ogihara S, Oka H, Maruyama T, Inanami H, Miyoshi K, et al. Risk factors for incidental durotomy during posterior open spine surgery for degenerative diseases in adults: a multicenter observational study. PLoS One. 2017;12(11):e0188038.
106. Passias PG, Poorman GW, Jalai CM, Line B, Diebo B, Park P, et al. Outcomes of open staged corrective surgery in the setting of adult spinal deformity. Spine J. 2017;17(8):1091–9.
107. ter Gunne P, Albert F, van Laarhoven CJHM, Cohen DB. Surgical site infection after osteotomy of the adult spine: does type of osteotomy matter? Spine J. 2010;10(5):410–6.
108. Sidhu GS, Henkelman E, Vaccaro AR, Albert TJ, Hilibrand A, Anderson DG, et al. Minimally invasive versus open posterior lumbar interbody fusion: a systematic review. Clin Orthop Relat Res. 2014;472(6):1792–9.
109. Jin-Tao Q, Yu T, Mei W, Xu-Dong T, Tian-Jian Z, Guo-Hua S, et al. Comparison of MIS vs. open PLIF/TLIF with regard to clinical improvement, fusion rate, and incidence of major complication: a meta-analysis. Eur Spine J. 2015;24(5):1058–65.
110. Xie Q, Zhang J, Lu F, Wu H, Chen Z, Jian F. Minimally invasive versus open Transforaminal lumbar Interbody fusion in obese patients: a meta-analysis. BMC Musculoskelet Disord. 2018;19(1):15.
111. Khan NR, Clark AJ, Lee SL, Venable GT, Rossi NB, Foley KT. Surgical outcomes for minimally invasive vs open transforaminal lumbar interbody fusion: an updated systematic review and meta-analysis. Neurosurgery. 2015;77(6):874; discussion 874.
112. Lubelski D, Mihalovich KE, Skelly AC, Fehlings MG, Harrop JS, Mummaneni PV, et al. Is minimal access spine surgery more cost-effective than conventional spine surgery? Spine. 2014;39(22 Suppl 1):65.
113. Phan K, Rao PJ, Kam AC, Mobbs RJ. Minimally invasive versus open transforaminal lumbar interbody fusion for treatment of degenerative lumbar disease: systematic review and meta-analysis. Eur Spine J. 2015;24(5):1017–30.
114. McGirt MJ, Parker SL, Lerner J, Engelhart L, Knight T, Wang MY. Comparative analysis of perioperative surgical site infection after minimally invasive versus open posterior/transforaminal lumbar interbody fusion: analysis of hospital billing and discharge data from 5170 patients. J Neurosurg Spine. 2011;14(6):771–8.
115. Mirza SK, Deyo RA, Heagerty PJ, Turner JA, Lee LA, Goodkin R. Towards standardized measurement of adverse events in spine surgery: conceptual model and pilot evaluation. BMC Musculoskelet Disord. 2006;7(1):53.
116. Cizik AM, Lee MJ, Martin BI, Bransford RJ, Bellabarba C, Chapman JR, et al. Using the spine surgical invasiveness index to identify risk of surgical site infection: a multivariate analysis. J Bone Joint Surg Am. 2012;94(4):335–42.
117. Lee MJ, Cizik AM, Hamilton D, Chapman JR. Predicting medical complications after spine surgery: a validated model using a prospective surgical registry. Spine J. 2014;14(2):291–9.

118. Spratt KF, Keller TS, Szpalski M, Vandeputte K, Gunzburg R. A predictive model for outcome after conservative decompression surgery for lumbar spinal stenosis. Eur Spine J. 2004;13(1):14–21.
119. Daubs MD, Hung M, Adams JR, Patel AA, Lawrence BD, Neese AM, et al. Clinical predictors of psychological distress in patients presenting for evaluation of a spinal disorder. Spine J. 2014;14(9):1978–83.
120. Azimi P, Benzel EC, Shahzadi S, Azhari S, Mohammadi HR. Use of artificial neural networks to predict surgical satisfaction in patients with lumbar spinal canal stenosis: clinical article. J Neurosurg Spine. 2014;20(3):300–5.

Suggested Reading

Bekelis K, Desai A, Bakhoum SF, Missios S. A predictive model of complications after spine surgery: the National Surgical Quality Improvement Program (NSQIP) 2005–2010. Spine J. 2014;14(7):1247–55.
Neuman BJ, Ailon T, Scheer JK, Klineberg E, Sciubba DM, Jain A, et al. Development and validation of a novel adult spinal deformity surgical invasiveness score: analysis of 464 patients. Neurosurgery. 2017;82:847–53.

Part III

Healthcare Systems

Healthcare Systems in the United States 10

Luis M. Tumialán

Abbreviations

ACA	Patient Protection and Affordable Care Act
AHA	American Hospital Association
AMA	American Medical Association
CCMC	Committee on the Cost of Medical Care
CHIP	Children's Health Insurance Program
CMS	Centers for Medicare and Medicaid Services
CPT	Current Procedural Terminology
GDP	gross domestic product
HMO	health maintenance organization
ICD-10	*International Statistical Classification of Diseases and Related Health Problems, 10th Revision*
OECD	Organization for Economic Cooperation and Development
PPO	preferred provider organization
POS	point of service
RVU	relative value unit
WHO	World Health Organization

L. M. Tumialán
Department of Neurosurgery, Barrow Neurological Institute,
St. Joseph's Hospital and Medical Center, Phoenix, AZ, USA
e-mail: neuropub@barrowneuro.org

J. Ratliff et al. (eds.), *Quality Spine Care*,
https://doi.org/10.1007/978-3-319-97990-8_10

Introduction

The United States stands alone among industrialized nations as the only healthcare system without a nationwide single-payer or state healthcare system. But the United States is far from a homogenous private sector—financed market. Private, employer-based insurance programs insure only 60–65% of the population. Another 20–25% of the population is insured by a combination of social welfare insurance (Medicaid) and societal healthcare (Medicare). Prior to the passage of the Patient Protection and Affordable Care Act (ACA) in 2010, 13% were uninsured. That legislation created a federal marketplace with state involvement where any individual could seek coverage with a government subsidy, if necessary. The objective of the marketplace in conjunction with the individual mandate provision of the ACA was to insure the remaining 47 million Americans who did not have health insurance prior to 2010 [1]. Despite the passage of the ACA, equal access to healthcare in the United States remains problematic. Compared to the universal coverage offered in other industrialized nations, the US system has inherent inequities regarding access. It is only through a view of the historical context of the evolution of the current US healthcare system that one can explain the existence of the current system. The focus of this chapter is to present the US healthcare system from its origins at the turn of the nineteenth century, through the initiation of Medicare in the mid-1960s, up to the passage of the ACA in 2010. As the emphasis in the United States shifts from a fee-for-service system to a value proposition defined by quality over cost, the quality assessment reviewed later in this text becomes especially germane in the realm of spine care in any healthcare system.

International policymakers in a variety of countries draw from comparisons with other healthcare systems to make recommendations to modify their own approaches [2]. In each circumstance, the population density, the geography, and especially the political climate have had an equal share in forging the framework of each country's respective system. National healthcare systems are determined as much by their history and geography as they are by politics.

Analysis of the US healthcare system must first consider that, if one were to design a national healthcare system from the ground up, it would look nothing like the US system today. There are significant inefficiencies built into the system that seem to have obvious solutions and redundancies that have no apparent purpose. Buried within the Byzantine framework of the US healthcare system is the indelible political history of a country influenced by its expansive geography, considerable population, and general distrust of the federal government and the distinctive American spirit of self-determination and self-reliance. The reaction to the ACA's individual mandate provision is an example of the impact of these elements.

A careful examination of these agents may explain how the United States stands alone among industrialized nations as the only country without a nationwide single-payer or state healthcare system. The balance between the federal mandates and state governance over healthcare issues has been the topic of vigorous debate for the past century, which continues to this day. The ACA's mandate to expand Medicaid defines this tenuous relationship between the states and the federal government.

That mandate ultimately yielded a US Supreme Court ruling allowing states to opt out of Medicaid expansion and define their own path toward insuring the uninsured citizens within their states [3].

A second observation about the US healthcare system is its cost. By almost every metric and by every ranking method, the United States has the most expensive healthcare system in the world. Currently, the United States spends 17% of its gross domestic product on healthcare, and, despite the passage of the ACA, that percentage will likely reach 19.9% by 2025 [4]. Critics have juxtaposed the cost of healthcare in the United States with the overall quality of healthcare measured by the World Health Organization (WHO) and the Organization for Economic Cooperation and Development (OECD) and have concluded that Americans pay more for their healthcare than citizens of any other industrialized country and in return receive the lowest quality of care. A recent Commonwealth Fund report ranked the United States last among 11 industrialized nations [5].

One glance at that report and it would seem that no one should ever consider having an elective spine operation within the borders of the United States. But built into the metrics of that ranking system are the heavily weighted parameters of access to care, along with efficiency and equity of care. The universal coverage in Canada and the countries of Europe will always trump the private commercial and employer-based insurance models in those categories. Whereas the United States hovers in the 80–85% range for healthcare coverage of its citizens with private, employer-based, and government-insured (Medicare and Medicaid) coverage, those countries with universal coverage consistently approach 100%.

There is little question that the populations of these countries have an impact on the capacity to administer healthcare by a governmental system. The population of the United States alone exceeds the combined populations of Australia, Canada, England, France, and Germany. A universal single-payer system administering to a relatively homogenous population of 36 million in Canada may have logistical challenges, but attempting to scale such a system to a heterogeneous population almost ten times that size raises significant logistical issues. The smaller populations in European countries allow for a degree of centralization that lends itself to more efficient care. Citizens of these countries have accepted the expanded role of government in their lives, which furthers the efficiency and limits expenditures. The larger population in the United States, the desire of states to retain control of healthcare within their borders, and the general reluctance to expand the role of government will make it difficult for the United States to fare any better in such rankings in the years to come. However, even with these self-imposed limitations in the US healthcare system, few would deny the capacity of the current US system to foster an environment conducive to innovation, safety, and progress. It should be noted that the United States ranks first in spending on research and development, far beyond what any other industrialized nation invests [2].

The WHO and Commonwealth Fund rankings notwithstanding, the United States remains one of the leading countries in the world in which to undergo the most advanced, most innovative, and safest spinal surgical procedures. The current ranking systems do not seem to have the capacity to capture that aspect of the US healthcare experience.

The value proposition in the US healthcare system of tomorrow will begin to make inroads into the practice of medicine. While a single-payer system remains unlikely in the near term, a more centralized system, similar to the European and Canadian models, does not. A continued evolution will come to the current model of fee-for-service, but what form that system will take is not clear at present. What is certain is that US physicians now practice medicine in an era with the ACA as their backdrop. Legislators, insurers, and physicians alike should explore modifications to the current system to insure more people at less cost within a marketplace environment that has made high quality a top priority at a low cost. The quality assessment metrics presented in this text (Part IV) will play an increasingly important role in that new environment. An analysis of outcome measures of a procedure relative to its cost will guide the spinal procedures in an environment with an unsustainable current trajectory of expenditure. Spine surgery will be impacted by an analysis of the quality measured relative to the cost of the procedure. Weaving the quality metrics into the reimbursement element of the US healthcare system offers the promise of bending the unsustainable cost curve. The goal of this chapter is to provide a historical context to the current US healthcare system, to describe its current form and structure, and to discuss its future trajectory.

Classifying Healthcare Systems

It may be helpful to examine the classification of healthcare systems in general terms by component parts and their roles. As defined by Quadagno [6], a healthcare system may be described as an organization that delivers care and medical services while administering and financing the delivery of those services. Working within that definition, multiple permutations are possible. Employed physicians work for the state, hospital, or care organizations. Private physicians work independently or in large groups. For-profit hospitals, not-for-profit hospitals, state-owned hospitals, and clinics represent the delivery arm of the medical services. The administration and funding of those services may come from government, state, or local communities or from private insurance companies.

In applying this model to the current healthcare systems of industrialized nations, Quadagno created three general categories: private, state, and societal healthcare systems. In practice, each system blurs the lines that distinguish it from other systems. It is difficult to demarcate one particular system into one pure category. For instance, most economists and healthcare policy wonks would consider the United States a classic example of a private healthcare system. But the US system contains elements of all three models. Let us take the healthcare administered to active duty men and women and veterans of the various armed service branches as an example of a state system. The US Military Health System (MHS) is a federally funded, federally employed, and federally administered healthcare system. Composed of the Army, Air Force, Navy, and Coast Guard (Marines fall under the care of the Navy), the MHS has a $50 billion annual budget to provide healthcare services to 1.2 million active duty military personnel and their dependents (approximately 8 million additional beneficiaries). Those 9–10 million beneficiaries are cared for in 65 hospitals and 412 clinics, which are federally owned and operated by 137,000 federal employees. The healthcare professionals are all employed, either on active duty themselves or as government service workers. If we were to add the 9 million veterans who seek their care in the Veterans Health Administration system, the combined population serviced by these two federal entities now approaches 20 million, which is two-thirds of the population of Canada (36 million), almost equal to the population of Australia (24.5 million), and far exceeding the population of many European countries that provide universal coverage. Unlike Medicare, where only one person in ten relies solely on Medicare for coverage, active duty military personnel have no other health insurance coverage. In its purest form, the MHS is a state healthcare system that offers universal coverage for active duty military personnel and their dependents not unlike the state-sponsored universal coverage systems of Canada, Denmark, the United Kingdom, Sweden, Italy, and Ireland.

The 44 million Americans (15% of the population) who obtain their healthcare through Medicare mirror the societal healthcare systems of Austria, Belgium, France, Germany, and Luxembourg. The universality of Medicare is based on age. Medicare is available for any American 65 years of age and older, and it also covers persons with a diagnosis of amyotrophic lateral sclerosis or renal failure requiring dialysis. Like their European counterparts, Medicare patients are expected to pay only a modest out-of-pocket copayment, with the remainder funded by a Medicare tax, analogous to the healthcare tax in European countries.

The universally insured British and Canadian citizens find themselves enrolling in private insurance to cover the cost of supplementary benefits (e.g., dental care, drug coverage) not covered by their universal insurance. About two-thirds of Canadians purchase private supplemental insurance policies or use an employer-sponsored plan, similar to those available to Americans, to cover such uncovered services. The purchase of additional insurance in a single-payer system is an example of convergence, whereby elements of one healthcare system infiltrate those of another. These examples of convergence among the various systems reflect a trend that allows particular system in one country to evolve by embracing a functional element of another system in another country. Convergence will be a constant theme that surfaces through this analysis.

From the examples provided above, the convergence of healthcare systems makes the analysis of a single individual system a tenuous exercise. However, if we were to view the US healthcare system through the lens of the private payer, an unambiguous analysis between a competitive marketplace and universal coverage model may be examined. The first logical question is how the United States arrived at the current fee-for-service system in place today that is funded in large part by employer-sponsored insurance supplied by private payers. A greater understanding of the current healthcare system begins with a review of its historical evolution.

A Brief History of Health Insurance in the United States

While Germany was already exploring universal coverage under Prince Otto von Bismarck in 1884 and the British were making their first futile attempt at National Health Insurance under Prime Minister Lloyd George in 1911, the nineteenth- and twentieth-century Americans remained firmly in the fee-for-service model of medicine [7]. With limited technology and diagnostic capability, the role of the hospital in the general welfare of the population was minimal. Most patients who had the means to do so were cared for at home by a physician. Nineteenth-century hospitals were more for the indigent, whose expenses were covered primarily by charities. And so, with the majority of general healthcare not requiring a hospital admission, medical expenses would be limited to the physician's fee, medical supplies, and medication.

The earliest forms of health insurance in the United States were workplace accident insurance products intended for persons working in the railroad, lumber, and steamboat industries [8]. The workers in these industries were uniquely susceptible to injury, prompting employers to offer coverage for medical expenses and lost wages in the event of a mishap. Medical interventions at the time were quite limited. The majority of the compensation was more for lost wages because of the resulting inability to work than for medical expenses.

The technological advances in the twentieth century expanded the role of the hospital. The introduction of radiography, aseptic techniques for surgery, and antibiotics began to shift medical care from the home to the hospital. As the role of the hospital increased, so did the charges that were billed to the patient. By the mid-1920s, it became clear that the cost of healthcare was becoming increasingly difficult for patients to afford, largely due to the cost of hospital admissions. One hospital administrator took notice of this trend and offered a solution that would usher in the modern era of insurance coverage.

Justin Ford Kimball was in his first year as the vice president of Baylor Hospital in Dallas, Texas, when he took notice of a growing number of unpaid hospital bills. Kimball identified this trend especially among teachers in Dallas [9]. As a former educator himself, he was sensitive to the earnings of teachers and the increasing cost of healthcare. In 1929, Kimball mimicked the prepayment plans offered to railroad and lumber workers and began offering teachers in Dallas a hospital insurance plan for $0.50 a month or $6.00 a year that would cover a 21-day inpatient stay. In doing so, Kimball created the first employer-sponsored health insurance plan. The American Hospital Association (AHA) quickly took notice of Kimball's work and propagated it to other hospitals. The prepayment plans were immensely popular and hospital-based insurance flourished. By 1939, the AHA consolidated many of these plans and began to fund care not only in the hospital but also with providers. The AHA insignia at the time was a blue cross. Companies developing healthcare insurance plans soon appropriated the descriptive name of the AHA insignia and ultimately developed into Blue Cross insurance plans, which still exist today [9].

The increasing cost of healthcare and the expanding role of hospital stays did not escape the policymakers in Washington, DC. In 1927, the Committee on the Costs of Medical Care (CCMC) was established to conduct the country's first comprehensive study of medical economics [10]. The committee studied the various forms of coverage in European countries and considered the capacity to apply one of those models to the US healthcare system. After considering a variety of models, the committee favored a private insurance model and went against the various European models that the committee members had reviewed as part of their report. The rationale behind their decision was that the United States had a higher standard of living and therefore had a better chance of making a voluntary private insurance system successful. The committee believed that the European models ran counter to the American spirit, which prided itself on freedom and private enterprise. This opinion arose before the 1929 stock market crash and the start of the Great Depression.

When Franklin D. Roosevelt was elected president in 1932, the United States found itself in the worst economic disaster in its history. With 13 million Americans out of work and general distrust of big business and Wall Street, the belief in individualism and self-reliance was shaken. Americans began to accept the concept of an interdependence with the federal government. Roosevelt spoke in perfect pitch to a downtrodden population when he said, "One of the duties of the State is that of caring for those of its citizens who find themselves the victims of such adverse circumstances as makes them unable to obtain even the necessities for mere existence without the aid of others. The responsibility is recognized by every civilized nation… To these unfortunate citizens aid must be extended by Government—not as a matter of charity but as a matter of social duty" [10].

A federally funded healthcare system was part of the Roosevelt platform. If there ever was a time for passage of such legislation, it was when a country was suffering the worst economic downturn in its history. But passage of healthcare legislation did not come easy, even for Roosevelt. A stalwart resistance to government involvement in healthcare is a constant theme that future occupants of the Oval Office would also encounter. Roosevelt was genuinely surprised by the acrimony involved in this debate, in which the American Medical Association (AMA) was especially vociferous. Subsequent presidents would encounter similar sentiments from the AMA.

The father-in-law of the president's son was none other than Harvey Cushing. Through a series of meetings, Cushing would weigh in heavily on the debate for a national health insurance program [11]. In the end, Roosevelt expended his political capital on the Social Security Program and deferred delving into the healthcare arena.

With the federal government unable to solidify support for a national healthcare program, along with a tacit endorsement from the CCMC to have private insurers become the financing arm of healthcare, private payers found fertile ground for the development of their commercial products. A fee-for-service model funded by private insurers became firmly entrenched into the US healthcare system over the next several decades and continues to this day. Employer-sponsored healthcare coverage was the next chapter in the evolution of the US healthcare system.

The Rise of Employer-Sponsored Healthcare Coverage

The need for active duty military personnel fighting simultaneously in the Pacific and Atlantic theaters during World War II created a shortage of workers for factories stateside. An increased demand for products and a tightened labor pool forced employers to seek ways to attract and keep workers. Federally imposed wage and price controls prohibited manufacturers and other employers from raising wages enough to attract workers. But a loophole existed in the benefits that employers could offer prospective employees. Federal mandates did not restrict employer-sponsored health insurance. Logically, employers offered expanded and increasingly competitive insurance packages to attract and keep workers [12]. Many of these prospective workers were women now providing for their families, while the fates of their husbands at war remained uncertain. Over time, employer-sponsored healthcare coverage became another element firmly entrenched in the US healthcare system, with 60% of Americans today obtaining their health insurance through an employer-sponsored program [8].

The Passage of Medicare

In 1945, President Harry S. Truman became the first sitting president to formally introduce the concept of national health insurance coverage. The concept of government entering the healthcare arena was now gradually becoming part of the national conversation. Truman's plans for a voluntary national health service encountered the same inimical response that Roosevelt's had a decade earlier. It would have the same tones as the arguments that would reach the ears of future Presidents Clinton and Obama decades later. Truman scuttled the plan after the AMA labeled his efforts "socialism" [10]. Even though the concept was popular with Americans, it became apparent that the legislation would involve a long and costly political battle with little likelihood of passage.

Over the ensuing decades, there was a progressive increase of government involvement in healthcare that would ultimately yield the Centers for Medicare and Medicaid Services (CMS). In 1961, President John F. Kennedy furthered the conversation by advocating for national health insurance coverage for the elderly. The employer-based model of health insurance functioned only when the individual was working. If it was not part of a pension plan for their retirement years, the elderly had no viable alternative for health insurance. On July 30, 1965, President Lyndon B. Johnson signed Medicare into law amid the backdrop of Independence, Missouri, with former President Truman at his side [13]. With passage of that law, Truman's vision of a national health service for the elderly was realized, and the US government became inextricably tied to healthcare policy and the reimbursement of physicians. The passage of Medicare changed the healthcare insurance market in the United States from solely a private market-based system to a system that includes societal health insurance for the elderly.

Types of Health Insurance in the US Healthcare System

The political influences in the evolution of the US healthcare system may explain how the United States stands alone as the only industrialized nation without a single payer that universally covers its citizens. But the current system is far from static. The various types of health insurance coverage are a component of the continued evolution of the US healthcare marketplace.

On the most basic level, health insurance exists in two forms: traditional indemnity insurance and managed care insurance. In an indemnity insurance plan, a patient seeks care from a provider, pays for that encounter, and then submits a claim to the insurance carrier. If the service was covered by the patient's agreed-upon benefits, the insurance company reimburses (or indemnifies) the patient for the service provided. At one point, indemnity insurance was a common form of coverage, but there was little in the way of cost containment. Instead, it was the responsibility of the individual policyholder to navigate the complicated medicine landscape. The cost associated with such insurance prompted the development of various managed care options, which decreased cost to the patient and the insurer alike. Over the past several decades, indemnity insurance has continued to decline and now represents less than 2% of the insurance products offered nationwide. Managed care options represent the majority of the insurance products offered by employers.

There are three main forms of managed care options: health maintenance organization (HMO), preferred provider organization (PPO), and point-of-service (POS) plans [14]. Each form of managed care has its own unique structure, with the intent of controlling the ever-increasing costs of healthcare.

HMO, PPO, and POS Plans

An HMO is a managed care health plan that forms a network to deliver healthcare services. The network is formed by contracts negotiated between the HMO and the hospitals and physicians within the community. The individual patient cannot select a provider that is outside the network, and in that manner, the HMO contains costs. Contracted rates are such that hospitals and providers believe that the volume offered by the captive patient population enrolled in the HMO will provide an adequate flow of patients to offset a lower reimbursement rate. At the same time, the HMO negotiates rates that they believe will allow adequate coverage of beneficiaries without losing money. If an individual patient goes outside the HMO network, the cost is not covered. In some systems, the HMO owns the facilities (i.e., hospitals and clinics) and employs the physicians (e.g., Kaiser Permanente system). More, HMOs contract with the hospitals, physicians, and physician groups within a community.

HMOs can be restrictive regarding the patient's choice of physicians and access to specialists. Choices for providers and facilities are limited by the network that was negotiated. Most HMOs require a referral by a primary care physician prior to being seen by a specialist, a remnant of the gatekeeper model introduced in the 1980s [15]. Although the gatekeeper concept was never a popular component of the HMO, vestiges of it still exist. HMOs maintain their popularity by having lower premiums and no deductibles. The limiting nature of the HMO prompted insurers to offer another less restrictive model at an additional cost: the PPO.

A PPO is a managed care arrangement that shares several characteristics of an HMO but is more flexible overall. These plans allow a greater choice of providers, offer an out-of-network benefit, and do not require a referral from a primary care physician to see a specialist. However, the greater choice and flexibility come at an increased cost. PPO premiums are generally higher, and the plans often have a deductible that must be met before coverage begins.

The third type of managed care health plan is the POS. This plan is a hybrid of an HMO and a PPO. Like an HMO, the POS has no deductible and requires only a modest copayment due at the time of service. But like a PPO, the POS offers greater freedom of choice for the patient in choosing providers. Collectively, these three managed care models make up approximately 90% of the commercial health insurance market [8, 14].

Commercial Insurance Market Versus Universal Coverage

As mentioned previously, the US healthcare system is not one homogenous entity. There are elements of state-sponsored health insurance (the military), societal health insurance (Medicare), and social welfare insurance (Medicaid and CHIP [Children Health Insurance Program]). With the military providing health insurance coverage for 10 million beneficiaries, Medicare covering 44 million elderly citizens, Medicaid covering 35 million adults, and CHIP covering 35 million children, 124 million people in the United States have some governmental form of health insurance. That number far exceeds the individual populations of Canada (36 million), England (55 million), France (66 million), and Germany (82 million). There are inherent challenges to the administration of healthcare to such a large population by the federal and state government. It would be difficult to conceive the impact of adding 180 million Americans who are currently insured through employer-sponsored health insurance to some federally funded universal coverage arrangement like that common in European countries and in Canada.

A logical question arises as to the ability of a privately insured model versus a universal coverage model to administer healthcare to an entire population. The juxtaposition of the American, Canadian, and European systems allows for a rational analysis of that question. Based on an examination of data on these systems, possible conclusions could be that privately funded healthcare leads to gross inequity in access to care, to more expensive care, and to an inferior quality of care. But reliable measures of access are unavailable. The insured status of the individual therefore becomes an indirect surrogate for access to care. By any measure, insured status is a poor indicator of access to care. No uninsured person who walks into an emergency department in the United States will be deprived of care; therefore it is not possible to accurately determine how the limited health insurance coverage in the United States affects the health status of the population and true access to healthcare. Nor is there an accurate measure of the impact that long wait times to see specialists have on persons who are insured in universal coverage models [16].

Cost of Healthcare in the United States

Proponents of the Canadian healthcare system tout both the lower cost of healthcare and the universal coverage available to the Canadian populace, whereas proponents of the US healthcare system express their trepidation with having their healthcare system turn into a "socialist" system with inherent bureaucratic inefficiency [2]. Defenders of the current US healthcare system qualify their argument by citing long wait times for Canadians to see a specialist and even longer wait times for surgical procedures.

Acknowledging the long waits and challenges to see specialists, some Canadians seek a more for-profit delivery of specific healthcare services [2]. Defenders of the current Canadian system argue that allowing such an enterprise would result in inefficiencies and inequities that currently characterize the market-based healthcare system in the United States. The high cost of administering numerous health plans that exist in the United States further corroborates the argument against for-profit episodes of care.

The Impact of the ACA on the Uninsured Population

The framers of the ACA conceived the legislation so that affordable insurance would be available to all Americans. Acknowledging that most Americans received health insurance through their employer (60%) or from Medicare (15%), policymakers needed to identify a mechanism through which to insure the remaining 25% (44 million inhabitants of this country, 33 million of whom were citizens). Two main vehicles were used to accomplish this goal: Medicaid expansion and government-subsidized support for the individual purchase of private insurance in federal or state marketplaces. In theory, if the risk pool were increased, the cost to administer the whole enterprise would be more fiscally viable. Thus, an individual mandate was added to the legislation. After full enactment of the ACA, the number of uninsured Americans decreased from 44 million to 28 million in 2017 [17].

The Cost of Health Insurance in the United States

Even before the passage of the ACA, the vast majority of Americans were insured. Approximately 84% of the population (270 million Americans) was covered by government insurance or private commercial insurance. Of the private commercial insurance, approximately 60% was employer-based insurance, with the individual obtaining health insurance through the employer with shared contributions to cover the annual premium. According to a Kaiser Foundation study, the average annual premium in 2017 for a family would be $18,764, of which $13,049 (70%) would be paid by the employer and $5,714 (30%) would be paid by the employee [18].

Nearly 26% of the US population is covered by public health insurance (i.e., Medicare and Medicaid). Medicare consists of two parts: Part A for inpatient hospital care and Part B for physician services and outpatient hospital services. A Medicare tax, similar to the Social Security tax, funds Part A, whereas monthly premiums (25%) and general taxes (75%) fund Part B.

Reimbursement Process

Perhaps the most defining element of the single-payer systems in Canada and Europe is that all providers and facilities are paid through a single publicly financed system. Public finance does not necessarily mean government employment, nor does it exclude supplemental insurance for patients, but it does centralize the payment process. Aside from Medicare, the US healthcare system has no such uniform platform. A multi-payer system, along with a complex tax code, fosters a combination of for-profit, not-for-profit, and governmental (military and Veterans Administration) facilities. Healthcare providers reflect the institution where they work (i.e., private physicians practice in private hospitals, HMO-employed physicians work in HMO-owned and HMO-operated hospitals, and military physicians essentially practice as employed physicians in military hospitals since they are on active duty).

There is a perception that countries with single-payer national health insurance systems have a lower administrative burden than their US counterpart. However, there are some striking similarities between all healthcare systems regarding diagnosis and procedural coding. The countries of Canada, Denmark, Sweden, and Norway all have single-payer national health insurance. The administration of that health insurance is orchestrated by the government. All costs related to healthcare are paid for with tax dollars, but physicians are not employed by or salaried through the government. For the most part, physicians work in private practice, submitting claims with diagnostic and procedural codes just as their American counterparts do. The main advantage of the single-payer national health insurance system is that all claims go through provincial health authorities. A centralized process lends itself to increased efficiency.

In England, all physicians are salaried and all hospitals are publicly owned. The National Health Service funds all healthcare through taxes. Wait times associated with the National Health Service have fostered the development of a private healthcare marketplace, where diagnostic and procedural codes are the mechanism for reimbursement.

US physicians submit their diagnoses using ICD-10 (*International Statistical Classification of Diseases and Related Health Problems, 10th Revision)* and their procedures using Current Procedural Terminology (CPT), an AMA coding system that evolved alongside Medicare. The use of CPT codes allows for a uniform platform that reimburses physicians for specific procedures at a rate defined by the value of the code submitted. Each code carries with it a relative value unit (RVU) as determined by a representative body of physicians within the AMA. The RVU of a code is then multiplied by a conversion factor. Physicians negotiate that conversion factor with private insurance companies, whereas the US Congress determines the conversion factor for Medicare [19].

US National Health Expenditures

A snapshot of current US National Health Expenditure (NHE) data provides perhaps the most accurate reflection of the current US healthcare system. The NHE distribution demonstrates the heterogeneity of private-payer, tax-subsidized societal healthcare, and social welfare healthcare in the United States. In 2016, the NHE totaled $3.3 trillion, or $10,348 per person [4]. That amount accounted for 17.9% of the US gross domestic product (GDP). In 2016, Medicare spending totaled $672.1 billion (20% of NHE), Medicaid spending was $565.5 billion (17% of NHE), and private health insurance reached $1.123 trillion (34% of NHE). In contrast, out-of-pocket spending by Americans totaled $352.5 billion (11% of NHE). Hospital expenditures topped $1.082 trillion. Physician and clinical services were $664.9 billion, and prescription drug spending accounted for $328.6 billion.

In total, the federal government funded 28.3% of total national healthcare spending and individual households funded 28.1% [4]. The private business share of healthcare spending accounted for 19.9% of the overall total, while state and local governments accounted for 16.9%. The distribution of funding sources perfectly reflects the heterogeneous nature of the US healthcare system.

If the current trajectory continues, healthcare spending is projected to grow 1.2% faster than the GDP per year during 2016–2025, and the healthcare share of the GDP will rise from 17.9% in 2016 to 19.9% by 2025. Continued efforts to bend this trajectory with quality reporting outcome data will be essential. Defining what spinal procedures offer the greatest value to the population through quality assessments will ensure the viability of those procedures. Equally important will be a thoughtful examination of those procedures with high cost but without quality metrics that demonstrate benefit to the patient. Such procedures are detrimental not only to the patient but also to the population. The viability of unsubstantiated procedures in the future healthcare landscape will be tenuous.

Conclusions

The US healthcare system offers the most advanced, highest-quality medical and surgical care in the world. But the increasing cost of that care and providing equal access to it for all Americans remain continuing issues despite the passage of the ACA. The distinct advantages of healthcare delivery through a government-provided single-payer system are the centralization of the administration of the system and the standardization of the care delivered. From that standpoint, there has been convergence in the US healthcare system toward a more centralized organization. Instead of a direct government-initiated effort, the recent trend in centralization in the US healthcare system has been more of an indirect consequence of legislative efforts, namely, the ACA. Market forces reacting to the legislative resolves of the ACA have resulted in the consolidation of hospital groups, physician groups, and commercial payers. The hope of consolidation is a decrease in administrative costs and standardization of healthcare delivery.

The market competition model with for-profit insurers and hospitals administering healthcare in the United States has no shortage of critics. Data exist for these critics to note an inferior healthcare experience at a greater personal cost to the US population, such as reduced life expectancy, increased infant mortality, and increased disability. However, when these numbers are reconciled with the socioeconomic differences among the respective countries, the disparities among these healthcare systems become dampened. Americans have access to the world's best healthcare. While high cost and limited access may be fair criticisms, the gradual shift from a fee-for-service system to a system based on quality outcomes measures should begin to remedy these shortcomings.

Regardless of the system (single-payer, state-funded, or competitive private payer), healthcare systems face the same economic challenges: insuring more people at a lower cost in an aging population with a diminishing workforce. Regardless of the system, legislators, physicians, and healthcare administrators alike are aligned in the desire to achieve the highest quality of care at the lowest cost. In the management of spine care, the registry efforts mentioned in this text will supply clinicians in all systems with the necessary context to evaluate the role of surgical intervention. The data generated across all healthcare systems in all industrialized nations will offer a path for even greater convergence among healthcare systems to achieve higher-quality care at a lower cost.

Acknowledgments The authors thank the staff of Neuroscience Publications at Barrow Neurological Institute for assistance with manuscript preparation.

References

1. Health Insurance Coverage of the Total Population. http://kff.org/other/state-indicator/total-population/. Accessed 15 Jan 2018.
2. Globerman S, Hodges H, Vining A. Canadian and the United States' health care systems performance and governance: elements of convergence. Appl Health Econ Health Policy. 2002;1(2):75–88.
3. Blumenthal D, Abrams M, Nuzum R. The affordable care act at 5 years. N Engl J Med. 2015;373(16):1580. https://doi.org/10.1056/NEJMc1510015.
4. Services CfMaM. National health expenditure fact sheet. 2016. cms.gov. Accessed 15 Jan 2018.
5. Davis K, Stremikis K, Squires D, Schoen C. Mirror, mirror on the wall: how the performance of the U.S. health care system compares internationally. New York: The Commonwealth Fund; 2014.
6. Quadagno J. Institutions, interest groups, and ideology: an agenda for the sociology of health care reform. J Health Soc Behav. 2010;51(2):125–36. https://doi.org/10.1177/0022146510368931.
7. Smoot D. Socialized medicine. The Freeman: Ideas on Liberty. 1960;9–11.
8. Health Insurance Association of America. Fundamentals of health insurance, Part A. Washington: HIAA Insurance Education; 1997.
9. Kimball MD, Ford J. Handbook of Texas Online. https://tshaonline.org/handbook/online/articles/fki09. Accessed 14 Jan 2018.
10. Corning PA. The second round: 1927 to 1940. In: The evolution of medicare: from idea to law. Washington: Office of Research and Statistics, Social Security Administration; 1969.
11. Rovit RL, Couldwell WT. No ordinary time, no ordinary men: the relationship between Harvey Cushing and Franklin D. Roosevelt, 1928–1939. J Neurosurg. 2001;95(2):354–68. https://doi.org/10.3171/jns.2001.95.2.0354.
12. Buchmueller TC, Monheit AC. Employer-sponsored health insurance and the promise of health insurance reform. Cambridge, MA: National Bureau of Economic Research; 2009.
13. Goldfield N. National health reform advocates retrench and prepare for Medicare. Physician Exec. 1993;19(3):7–13.

14. Lynch ME. Health insurance terminology. Washington, DC: Health Insurance Association of America; 1992.
15. Catlin RF, Bradbury RC, Catlin RJ. Primary care gatekeepers in HMOs. J Fam Pract. 1983;17(4):673–8.
16. Beckfield J, Olafsdottir S, Sosnaud B. Healthcare systems in comparative perspective: classification, convergence, institutions, inequalities, and five missed turns. Annu Rev Sociol. 2013;39:127–46. https://doi.org/10.1146/annurev-soc-071312-145609.
17. Cohen RA, Zammitti EP. Health insurance coverage: early release of estimates from the National Health Interview Survey, January–March 2017.
18. Claxton G, Rae M, Long M, Damico A, Whitmore H, Foster G. Health benefits in 2017: stable coverage, workers faced considerable variation in costs. Health Aff (Millwood). 2017;36(10):1838–47. https://doi.org/10.1377/hlthaff.2017.0919.
19. Thorwarth WT Jr. CPT: an open system that describes all that you do. J Am Coll Radiol. 2008;5(4):555–60. https://doi.org/10.1016/j.jacr.2007.10.004.

The National Health Service (NHS) in England: Trying to Achieve Value-Based Healthcare

11

Ashley A. Cole, Lee M. Breakwell, and Michael James Hutton

Introduction

Seventy years ago, on July, 5 1948, the NHS was launched by the Minister for Health, Aneurin Bevan, with the principles that it would meet the needs of everyone, be free at the point of delivery and be based on clinical need and not the ability to pay. Advances in treatment options, an agieng population and increasing expectations have resulted in increasing demand for healthcare with spiralling costs.

The important factors associated with improving quality in spinal surgery in the UK are the same as those seen in other countries: improving patient outcomes, improving patient experience and improving safety. However, within the National Health Service (NHS), this also means that a quality service also needs to consider equity of access and timeliness.

This chapter reviews the ways in which changes can be made across the NHS to improve the quality and cost-effectiveness of spinal care. This is mostly due to system change rather than using scientific evidence to influence change, although there are mechanisms to implement findings from scientific research nationally in a quick and effective way.

There is an increasing emphasis on achieving a high-quality service with excellent patient safety, outcomes and experience at an affordable cost. A quality service needs longevity, and building a service based on quality alone without considering financial stability is not logical in a system with increasing healthcare demand and costs. A recent report from the Institute for Fiscal Studies and the Health Foundation (https://www.health.org.uk/publication/securing-future-funding-health-and-social-care-2030s) suggests NHS funding will need to increase between 3.3% each year just to maintain current levels of service. For spinal surgery, this means that

A. A. Cole (✉) · L. M. Breakwell
Sheffield Children's Hospital, Sheffield, UK
e-mail: ashley.cole4@nhs.net

M. J. Hutton
Princess Elisabeth Orthopaedic Centre, Royal Devon & Exeter Hospital, Exeter, UK

J. Ratliff et al. (eds.), *Quality Spine Care*,
https://doi.org/10.1007/978-3-319-97990-8_11

procedures with little or no evidence of cost-utility will become less likely to be commissioned by the NHS.

Commissioning of Spinal Services in England

In 2013, the NHS divided many areas of treatment into 'specialised' and 'nonspecialised'. For all areas, including spinal surgery, specialised surgery is commissioned and paid for by NHS England which is a central commissioning structure for England organised through ten regional commissioning hubs. Nonspecialised spinal surgery is commissioned by the Clinical Commissioning Groups (CCGs). There were originally 211 CCGs, but these have reduced to 195 following mergers (Fig. 11.1). They are clinically led groups each as an independent legal entity responsible for planning and commissioning local healthcare services. The CCG populations are between 84,000 and 884,000.

Specialised spinal surgery is commissioned and paid for by NHS England. The division between specialised and nonspecialised spinal surgery is as follows:

Specialised Spinal Surgery
All anterior lumbar surgery
All posterior lumbar instrumented fusions more than two levels
All thoracic spinal surgery
All instrumented cervical surgery (except anterior cervical discectomy and fusion)
All spinal deformity surgery

Payment for Spinal Surgery in the NHS

To understand how a service is commissioned, we must understand how it is funded. The NHS pays hospitals to deliver surgical procedures. If quality-adjusted life years (QALYs) are considered the measure of quality, the cost per QALY is defined as 'cost-utility'. If these costs can be minimised whilst not adversely affecting quality, then the cost-utility of spinal surgery may fair well when competing for scarce national resources.

In England all hospital inpatient episodes are coded, recording diagnosis using ICD-10 codes and any interventional procedures using OPCS v4.8 codes. These codes with other demographic- and admission-related data form the Hospital Episode Statistics which is the basis of many large analyses of NHS healthcare. The codes are entered in a software programme, the Local Payment Grouper, which applies a set of rules to give each inpatient episode a Healthcare Resource Group (HRG). These HRGs have been developed by groups of clinicians (Expert Working Groups) so that each inpatient episode contained within it should be approximately of equal cost. Every year, all NHS providers must submit their cost for providing the care for each HRG. These are called 'reference costs'. These costs are usually not

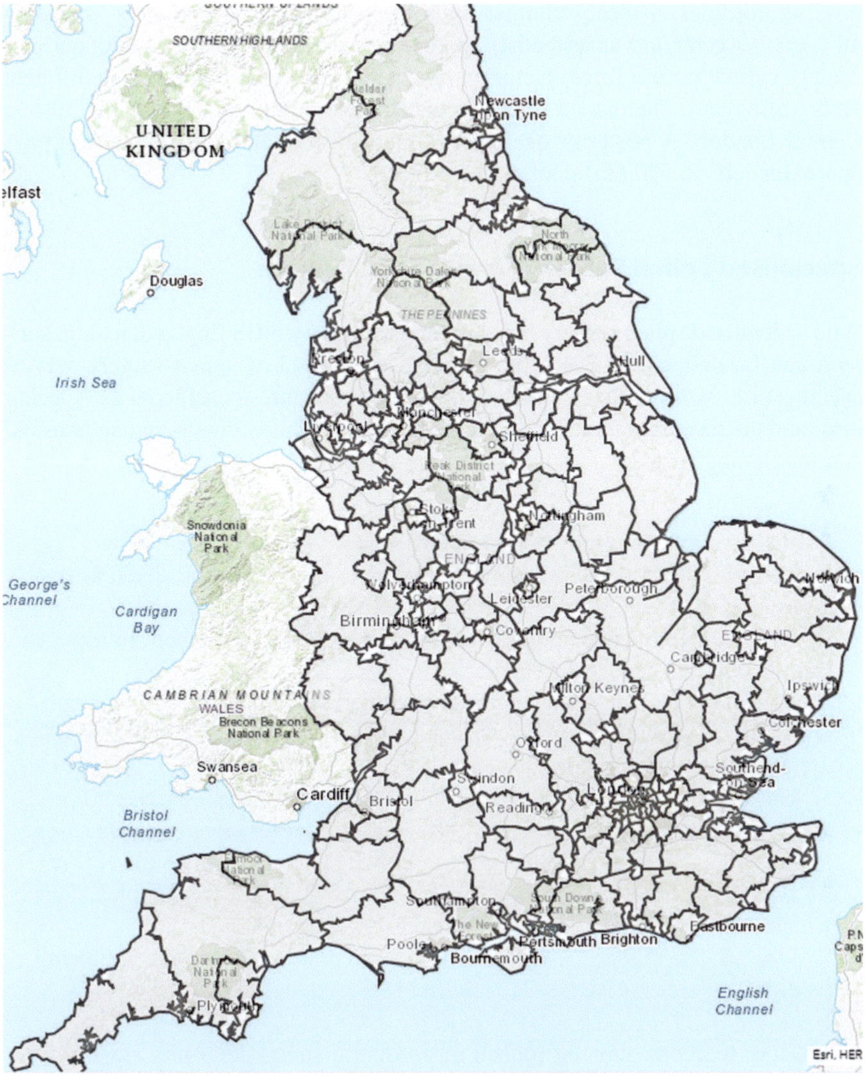

Fig. 11.1 Map of Clinical Governance Groups (CCGs) in England

calculated at patient level, and their accuracy has been questioned. This can be seen from the wide variation of costs for each HRG by different providers.

These reference costs are used to inform the price (tariff) for each HRG which is set every 1–2 years. This becomes a self-regulating system as providers attempt to reduce the cost of providing care so that they can achieve their budget. This reduced cost is fed back as the reference cost thereby reducing the tariff in the next cycle.

For spinal surgery, the Local Payment Grouper produces a payment and who should pay (NHS England or CCG) depending on the procedure performed. Admissions without a procedure are paid by the CCG. Currently, for a patient with no co-morbidities, an elective lumbar microdiscectomy pays the provider (including all costs, surgeon and anaesthetist) approximately £3,300 plus an additional percentage called 'market forces factor' to reflect the cost of providing care in different parts of England. The market forces factor ranges from 0% in Cornwall to 30% in Central London. A posterior one-level primary instrumented lumbar fusion pays approximately £6,500 plus market forces factor.

Specialised Spinal Surgery Service Specification

With specialised spinal surgery being commissioned by NHS England, national criteria can be defined. In 2013, the 'specialised (complex) spinal surgery service specification' was produced which defined the procedures considered as 'specialised' and the resources required to deliver the service (https://www.england.nhs.uk/commissioning/spec-services/npc-crg/group-d/d03/).

Paediatric Spinal Deformity Service Specification

It is proposed that paediatric spinal deformity surgery be considered as two types:

Type I: Instrumented spinal deformity correction in ambulant, otherwise healthy children aged 9–18 years

Type II: All other spinal deformity surgery including surgery on non-ambulant children, those with associated medical problems and younger children with congenital deformity

This distinction has the advantage of allowing existing spinal centres operating on paediatric spinal deformity who currently refer more complex cases to larger units to continue offering the service. This will reduce travel times for patients and provide a valuable outpatient service for more complex cases which will be referred to type II centres if surgery is required.

Type II Paediatric Spinal Deformity Centres require the following facilities:

- More than one surgeon trained in paediatric spinal deformity surgery to allow adequate case discussion and joint operating where necessary.
- A mentoring system should be in place for newly appointed consultants including joint operating and case monitoring until it is felt to be no longer required by both sides.
- At least one surgeon should be available at all times (regardless of leave or other commitments) when there are inpatients that have had spinal deformity surgery.
- Staffing of the unit should enable two spinal surgeons to work together if it is felt to be in the patient's interests.
- Regular spinal unit meeting attended by all spinal surgeons and anaesthetists to discuss operative cases, other relevant specialists (radiologists, paediatric

respiratory physicians, paediatric cardiologists, paediatric neurologists) should attend to discuss cases where their expertise is required.

- Surgery should be performed in the spinal centre on a regular basis to maintain skills and familiarity for the whole team.
- Paediatric intensive care and high-dependency facilities must be available including the ability for prolonged post-operative ventilation.
- Spinal cord monitoring supported by neurophysiology or medical physics. Currently somatosensory evoked potential monitoring is considered adequate for all cases. Motor evoked potential monitoring or combined monitoring may detect changes in spinal cord function more quickly and therefore may become the 'Standard of Care'.
- Collection of diagnosis, surgical procedure, complications and patient-reported outcome measures (PROMs). The British Spine Registry and Spine Tango allow this process. It is only by taking part in multicentre audit of outcome for surgery can a consistently high level of service provision be ensured, maximising patient satisfaction and facilitating service development.
- A clinical specialist nurse/physiotherapist is recommended to improve communication with patients and their families, provide information, co-ordinate preoperative assessment and help reduce avoidable surgical cancellations and facilitate outcome data collection.
- Specialist paediatric anaesthetist familiar with the problems associated with this surgery.
- Adequate and timely access to blood products including cell salvage.
- On-site 24 h access to sterile spinal implants including removal instruments for all recently implanted implants.
- On-site 24 h access to MR scanning or CT myelography with radiologists to perform and interpret these images.
- On-site 24 h access to paediatric medical care.
- Paediatric pain management service.
- Access to paediatric neurosurgeon, paediatric neurologist, paediatric cardiologist, paediatric respiratory physician and paediatric surgeon. These do not need to be on-site but should be available for urgent opinions and possible patient transfer if required. For patients with associated medical co-morbidities where it is felt that the paediatric physician/surgeon for that condition is required to be on-site, then the patient should be transferred to a spinal centre where that can be obtained.
- Ability to take high-quality long cassette radiographs in standing and sitting positions and appropriate flexibility radiographs. Access to picture archiving and communication system (PACS) for preoperative planning and in the outpatient clinic and theatre. Measurement tools for measuring angles and distances should be integrated into the PACS. All imaging must be stored long term for these patients as surgery in adult life may be required.

- Preoperative assessment facilities including respiratory function, paediatric echocardiography, bone mineral density measurement, physiotherapy and occupational therapy support.
- Policies for venous thromboembolism prophylaxis, pregnancy testing and transition of care to adult services.
- Appropriate paediatric environment for both inpatient and outpatient facilities including teachers and play-specialists whilst inpatients.
- Orthotic services as required by the local spinal service.
- To maintain high-quality decision-making, each patient should ideally be reviewed by the Consultant Paediatric Spinal Deformity Surgeon on a minimum of alternate clinic visits.
- Access to a local wheelchair service and good communication links with service providers in the geographical catchment area for those patients requiring seating adjustments or post-operative assessments.

Type I Paediatric Spinal Deformity Centres require all the facilities above except on-site paediatric intensive care and the ability for short-term post-operative ventilation.

Complex (Specialised) Spinal Surgery Service Specification (NHS England) 2013

Listed above are the facilities required for paediatric spinal deformity surgery. The service specification only defined the service requirements rather than the providers, and in the early years of this new system, it has proven difficult to regulate providers to ensure they meet all the requirements.

The new Specialised Spinal Surgery Service Specification defines the co-dependent services and facilities required to deliver the service. Quality measures are also identified from national data sources to produce a national dashboard of spinal surgery. Data sources will include hospital self-reporting through a national Quality Surveillance Information System, HES data and data from the British Spine Registry. Hospitals failing to meet the required standards for spinal surgery will be identified and systems triggered including peer review to ensure they make changes to meet the requirements. Hospitals will be defined that can be commissioned for the various areas of specialised spinal surgery. For example, a hospital may meet all the requirements to deliver an adult spinal deformity service but may not meet the requirements to deliver a paediatric spinal deformity service. They will therefore only be commissioned for the specialised services where the requirements are met.

NHS England Spinal Services Clinical Reference Group (CRG)

Advice on spinal surgery comes from the Spinal Services Clinical Reference Group (CRG). This group also advises on spinal cord injuries and is composed of clinicians, commissioners, patients and a representative from Public Health England. The Chair, where necessary, acts as the National Clinical Director. This committee can advise on nonspecialised spinal surgery, but the CCGs as independent legal entities make their own decisions regarding commissioning priorities for their local area. The Spinal Services CRG is responsible for any changes to the service specification, developing policies on new treatments or controversial areas and reviewing the national dashboard and quality indicators. Policies on new treatments are based on evidence reviews and consideration of cost-effectiveness. Current policies include:

- Non-invasively lengthened spinal rods for scoliosis (currently MAGEC)
- Cervical disc replacement
- Bone morphogenetic protein-2 in spinal fusion
- Vertebral Body Tethering (in progress)
- Lumbar disc replacement (in progress)

Policies clearly define inclusion and exclusion criteria which ensure that treatments are not expanded beyond the limits of their scientific evidence. A good example is the policy for 'non-invasively lengthened spinal rods for scoliosis' with inclusion criteria:

- The consultant paediatric spinal surgeon feels that an instrumented spinal fusion will result in an unacceptable reduction in final height and respiratory function.
- Between the ages of 2 and 11 for girls and 2 and 13 for boys. Some children are not as skeletally mature as their chronological age so a radiograph confirming bone age within the acceptable age limits is satisfactory.
- And exclusion criteria:
- Infection or pathologic conditions of the bone such as osteopenia which would impair the ability to securely fix the device.
- Metal allergies and sensitivities.
- Patient with pacemaker or similar implantable device.
- Patient requiring MRI imaging during the expected period device will be implanted.
- Patients younger than 2 years old.
- Patients weighting less than 25 lb. (11.4 kg).
- Patients and/or families unwilling or incapable of following post-operative care instructions.

Whilst in theory these criteria should allow controlled introduction of a new technology or procedure, in practice, these are difficult to police, and more automated systems are being considered. For all policies, where a clinician feels a patient would benefit from a particular treatment, even though they do not meet the criteria, an application for funding can be placed as an Individual Funding Request (IFR).

Advice for Commissioning Spinal Services

The Spinal Services CRG and NHS commissioners (NHS England and CCGs) also get advice on commissioning priorities from other sources. The next five sections are the other sources of advice referred to in this sentence.

National Institute for Health and Care Excellence (NICE)

NICE was established in 1999 with an aim to reduce variation in the quality of treatment and care and to resolve uncertainty about which treatments work best and which represent best value for the NHS.

For spinal surgery, NICE guidance can take several forms:

- Health Technology Appraisals: These review the clinical and cost-effectiveness of health technologies including procedures, devices and diagnostic agents. NHS England and the CCGs must comply with recommendations from these appraisals within 3 months. There has been one Health Technology Appraisal for spinal surgery evaluating percutaneous vertebroplasty and kyphoplasty for osteoporotic fractures (https://www.nice.org.uk/guidance/ta279).
- NICE guidelines: These make evidence-based recommendations on a wide range of topics often related to managing specific conditions. Two recent NICE guidelines affecting spinal surgery are:
  - Low back pain and sciatica in over 16 s: assessment and management (NG59) November 2016 (https://www.nice.org.uk/guidance/ng59)
  - Spondyloarthritis in over 16 s: diagnosis and management (NG65) June 2017 (https://www.nice.org.uk/guidance/ng65)
- Interventional procedures guidance: These assess the clinical effectiveness and safety of interventional procedures without considering cost-effectiveness. Many of these are relevant to spinal surgery (https://www.nice.org.uk/guidance/conditions-and-diseases/musculoskeletal-conditions/spinal-conditions)
- Medical technologies guidance: These are requested by manufacturers of new devices and technologies and compare them with existing treatments looking at clinical and cost-effectiveness. The only spinal example is MAGEC for children with scoliosis (https://www.nice.org.uk/guidance/mtg18). Medtech Innovation Briefings review the role and evidence of new technology and state the cost but without evaluation against existing treatments.

Right Care

The 195 Clinical Commissioning Groups (CCGs) commission nonspecialised spinal surgery, and most of their advice comes from Right Care. Right Care is an NHS England supported national programme to analyse available data at local level (CCG) and to benchmark nationally and against CCGs with similar population demographics. The data comes from a variety of national data sets including HES data (see above). The analysis is done across a range of services allowing CCGs to identify priority areas. Right Care will also support innovation such as shared decision-making tools and pathways. They will work with CCGs to identify the best opportunities for improving value, what to change to improve patient experience and outcome and how to change in a systematic way.

Care Quality Commission (CQC)

The CQC is an independent regulator of health and social care in England. They are largely responsible for 'safety'. As part of their remit, they inspect all hospitals against the standards:

- Care and treatment meet the needs and preferences of the individual patient.
- All patients are treated with dignity and respect.
- Consent is required before any treatment is given.
- Care is safe with patients not put at risk of harm which could be avoided.
- Care is delivered by staff with the required qualifications, competencies and skills.
- Patients must be safe from abuse or improper treatment with no inappropriate limits on freedom.
- Enough food and drink to keep good health.
- Premises and equipment must be clean, suitable and looked after.
- There must be a system in place to manage complaints and take action if required.
- Governance standards must be met to ensure quality and safety of care and help the service improve.
- Enough suitably qualified, competent and experienced staff with adequate support, training and supervision to ensure they can meet standards.
- Strong recruitment processes and checks to ensure employment of staff who can provide care and treatment appropriate for their role.
- Duty of candour: The provider must be transparent about care and treatment and inform patients if something goes wrong providing support and apologise.

Each hospital is assessed against five questions:

1. Is it safe?
2. Is it effective?
3. Is it caring?
4. Is it responsive to people's needs?
5. Is it well led?

Against each of these five questions, they are rated as Outstanding, Good, Requires Improvement or Inadequate. Each hospital must display their CQC rating.

The CQC performs detailed inspections of all health and social care facilities and their ratings receive significant media attentions. There is a statutory requirement to notify the CQC about certain events such as a duty of candour.

Francis Report

The Francis report, published in 2013, was the result of a public inquiry chaired by Robert Francis to look at the systematic failure of the Mid Staffordshire NHS

Foundation Trust. This was commissioned by the Secretary of State for Health and is an unusual but important mechanism for improving quality in healthcare. It was concerned with mortality and quality of patient care across a hospital rather than spinal services directly, and the report had far-reaching consequences for the NHS with improved CQC inspections and more attention paid to patient feedback resulting in significant service change across the NHS [1].

Specialist Societies

The British Association of Spine Surgeons has produced a series of information leaflets and consent guidance for common spinal conditions (http://www.spinesurgeons.ac.uk/patients-area/). These have been widely adopted.

Improving Spinal Care Project

National Back and Radicular Pain Pathway

In 2014, a group of 31 stakeholders were brought together by an NHS England project to develop a National Back and Radicular Pain Pathway (NBRPP) detailing the management of patients with low back and/or radicular pain. At each step entry and exit criteria, competencies, assessment and interventions are carefully defined. One of the key features of the pathway is that all patients are referred to a single point of access where their care is co-ordinated by a Spinal Triage Practitioner. This Pathway is referred to in the recent Lancet article on prevention and treatment of low back pain [2].

Initial poor uptake of the Pathway by the CCGs and long NHS waiting lists for spinal surgery resulted in NHS England supporting the Improving Spinal Care Project led by the Spinal Services CRG with the support of the Spinal Societies which started in January 2016. The aim of the project was twofold:

- Encourage implementation of the National Back and Radicular Pain Pathway
- Develop Regional Spinal Networks

Over 2 years later, implementation of the National Back and Radicular Pain Pathway with almost 200 CCGs has proven difficult, and we estimate that about 50 have a functioning pathway. A Pathway implementation day in 2017 resulted in the formation of a National Back Pain Clinical Network which is a Society with aims of implementing, evaluating and improving the National Back and Radicular Pain Pathway. There are regional representatives to aid local discussions with CCGs.

Results from the pathway in two Regions have shown approximately 1–2% of the adult population are referred into the service each year, 13% have an MRI scan, 6% are referred on to spinal surgery in secondary care and 1.5% to pain management [3].

When NICE updated guidelines on Low Back and Radicular Pain in November 2016 (https://www.nice.org.uk/guidance/ng59), the Guidance Development Group revised the National Back and Radicular Pain Pathway to include the 41 NICE recommendations and the new Pathway was endorsed by NICE in June 2017. Right Care is integrating it into their implementation plans for musculoskeletal services. Although it is felt by clinicians to be an effective and high-quality pathway for managing these patients, there is no national mechanism for implementation. Where there has been implementation of the Pathway, funding has rarely been found for a Combined Physical and Psychological programme for managing some patients with low back pain. This has proven difficult to fund even where the rest of the Pathway has been implemented.

Regional Spinal Networks

Regional Spinal Networks (RSNs) have been supported by clinicians for many years. The aim is to develop 14 RSNs to co-ordinate emergency and elective spinal care in each region and ensure equality of service provision. The hospital providing the 24/7 emergency service is the spinal hub. Other hospitals are either a spinal partner if they have spinal surgeons or a non-spinal partner if they have an emergency department and therefore take emergency spinal patients. The spinal hub and spinal partners are developing pathways and policies for emergency spinal care. The network approach combined with the commissioning rules regarding specialised and nonspecialised spinal surgery ensures more complex surgery is sent to the centres with the facilities and surgical team capable of producing the best outcomes. For elective spinal surgery, there is support for all surgeons through multidisciplinary meetings to ensure that the correct surgery is performed in the best location. Nonspecialised spinal surgery (lumbar decompressions and discectomies and anterior cervical discectomy and fusion) forms most of the surgery, and to manage capacity, the spinal partner hospital activity is essential.

The RSNs have defined operating principles and responsibilities:

- Implementation of regional pathways, guidelines and policies for elective and emergency spinal care including those from national organisations: Spinal Services CRG, NICE and spinal societies.
- Produce a 'directory' of pathways, guidelines and policies for the region to be made available nationally.
- Confirm that all spinal consultants are entering all cases on the British Spine Registry.
- Ensure resources are available to collect and analyse the network monitoring data.
- Review the monitoring data and produce a plan to implement any changes.
- Review clinical governance issues (deaths, serious untoward incidents, never events, duties of candour, root cause analysis and risk management issues). Implement any lessons learnt or changes and collate for national review.
- Keep a record of any audits, service evaluations or research presented at the Regional Network Meeting with any changes to clinical practice or service delivery. Ensure these changes have been implemented.

- Identify areas for service improvement and ensure spread of good practice throughout the Network.
- Review educational and research opportunities.
- Review activity data and targets, working with commissioners to ensure equality of access across the region.
- Keep a record of the spinal workforce and services in the region. These will include Triage Services, availability of MRI imaging and spinal consultants. Anticipate and plan for potential problems which may affect service delivery.
- Review the Network Objectives and Work Plan.
- Compile and review a Network Risk Register.
- Discussion of complex spinal cases to produce a plan for future management.

It is hoped that this network approach will smooth waiting lists across regions, improve and share clinical governance and reduce successful litigation.

Getting It Right First Time (GIRFT)

Methodology

GIRFT was a project devised by Professor Tim Briggs CBE, currently the National Director of Clinical Quality and Efficiency. GIRFT aims to reduce unwarranted variation in clinical practice to improve patient care and outcome. The process is clinically led and, after an initial trial of the methodology in 2014 and 2015, is now in progress for 15 surgical and 20 non-surgical specialties. The Spinal Surgery GIRFT is led by Mike Hutton (with support from Justin Nissen for visits to neuro-surgical centres). The methodology involves:

- Defining many relevant data items from existing data sources. These can include numbers of procedures, length of stay, implant costs, repeat procedures such as injections, readmission rates and return to surgery rates.
- Producing a report for hospitals providing the service. This will compare them with other similar services often using funnel plots.
- Local clinicians review the report.
- Visit from the GIRFT clinical lead. For spinal surgery the clinical lead has visited all hospitals in England. At the visit, the data is reviewed with the local clinical and management team to discuss any identified variation. It is accepted that the data sources have some limitations and is there to inform discussion.
- A report is produced by the GIRFT team following the visit with agreed action points.
- Repeat visits are performed to ensure the actions have been delivered. Sometimes, GIRFT has revealed problems across a whole region which have resulted in regional GIRFT meetings.

- GIRFT has an implementation process where a regional representative is responsible for ensuring all GIRFT recommendations are being implemented across all the specialities.

The Spinal GIRFT report is expected later in 2018.

Assessment of a Spinal Service for Quality

This national audit process is a very powerful tool to identify what a good service looks like and equally demonstrate services that have areas requiring improvement. Any improvement in patient care is usually associated with a reduction in the cost of care episodes. Improvements may lead to increased capacity within clinical service lines to provide care to more patients.

The data itself from a national audit gives an idea where an individual spinal unit fits in the overall national picture, but consideration should be made for population and case risk adjustment wherever possible.

When assessing a spinal service, consideration should be made to the following:

1. Management of emergency spinal conditions: How easily can patients with potential emergency spinal conditions access the service? How quickly are patients investigated with potential emergency spinal conditions? When a patient has an emergency spine condition how quickly can that service deal with the problem and when they do so are the outcomes optimal?
2. Emergency spinal services can be broadly categorised into the management of:
   (a) Cauda equina syndrome
   (b) Spinal trauma and traumatic spinal cord injury
   (c) Spinal infection/epidural abscess
   (d) Symptomatic metastatic spinal cord compression
   (e) Others

   Management of Elective Spinal Conditions: Elective spine pathways should be assessed from first presentation to a medical practitioner through to secondary care provision of specialist pain services and spinal surgical services. The initial assessment of these patients should ensure that serious conditions are identified and that patients with symptoms and signs of potential serious spinal pathology are managed by the correct emergency pathways. Patients with non-emergency spinal conditions should be managed by pathways that respect the often-favourable natural history of spinal conditions. These pathways such as the National Back and Radicular Pain Pathway should also accommodate non-emergency but urgent conditions such as progressive myelopathy or severe radicular pain. Patients who do not respond to primary medical treatment (e.g. analgesia, advice and observation) may be referred to an interface/triage and treat service for further assessment and onward referral to an appropriate secondary care service, investigation or further conservative measures such as manual therapy. Care must be taken interpreting spinal surgery conversion rate

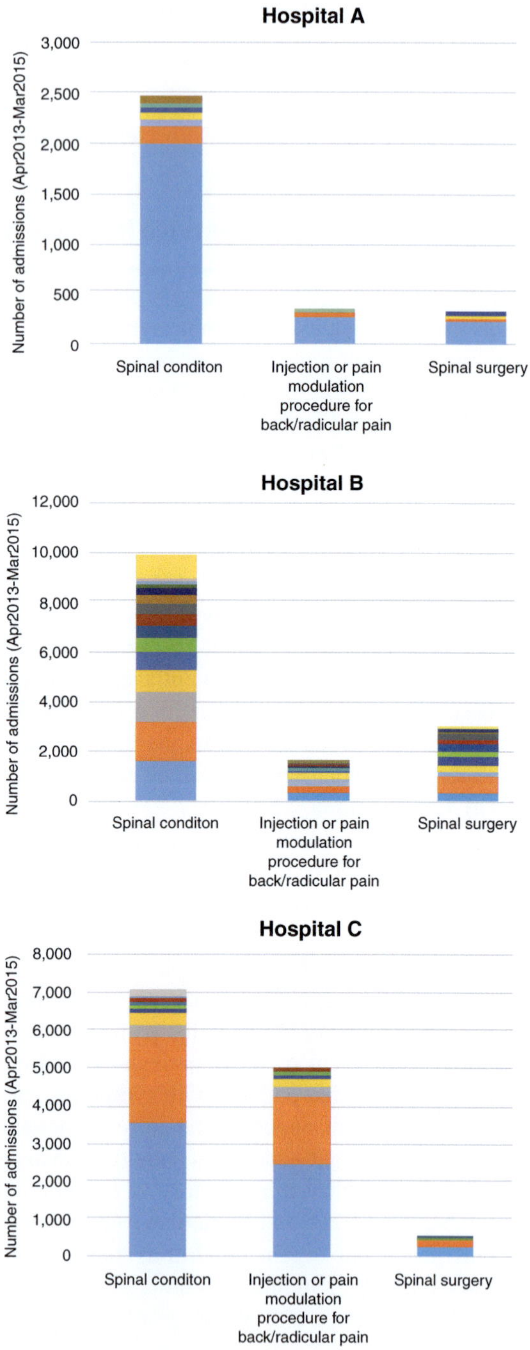

Fig. 11.2 Number of patients receiving injection/pain modulation or surgery in three hospitals within 40 miles of each other in England. Note the number of injections/pain modulation in Hospital C. Colours represent different CCGs. (Source: Hospital Episodic Data April 2013–March 2015. Admission at Trust, by CCG)

data at a secondary care level as it is very dependent on the 'filtering' effect of primary care and the interface service. If all services in a geographical region have the same interface service, then an assessment of what percentage of patients with an elective spinal condition is receiving an intervention can be compared (Fig. 11.2).

3. Costs: For NHS spinal services, costs should be evaluated in terms of:
   (a) How many patients can be seen safely per hour in an outpatient setting?
   (b) Are relevant investigations available for this consultation, most triage services will have established this.
   (c) What percentage of patients are being recycled within the system with no definitive management plan?
   (d) How many procedures are performed in an 8 h operating list?
   (e) What are the costs of consumables/implants in procedures?
   (f) What proportion of operating lists are not utilised?
   (g) Length of stay.

   We are still some way from being able to accurately quantify the savings that spinal surgery makes to society in terms of return to work, work productivity and other healthcare savings such as analgesia and pain management.
4. Infection rates: Any infection following a spinal procedure has significant impact on a patient's life and is also very costly. Spinal surgical services should have an idea of what their unit infection rate is and take measures to keep this as low as possible. Benchmarking infection rates at a national level has many methodological pitfalls and should be performed carefully. Infection rates must be adjusted for spinal pathology, procedure performed and patient risk factors such as diabetes. It is sensible in this context to look at specific surgical sites/operations on a comparative basis, e.g. elective single level discectomy or decompression.
5. Litigation rates: Spinal services are heavily litigated against in parts of the world where an adversarial legal system exists. The estimated cost for spinal services in England of litigation is £100 million per year (NHS Resolution). This is against a total NHS cost for spinal surgery (excluding consultations) of £325 million per year. Services should be reviewed both on the number of claims made against them and the total cost of those claims. This data if aggregated on a national basis allows themes to emerge that may allow better understanding of the causes of litigation and how to avoid them.

Data Sources in Spinal Surgery

Many of the processes already described from commissioning spinal services to the GIRFT project rely on national data. Usually many different data sources are available to a national audit. Part of planning a national audit should be mapping what data sources are available, how accurate the data contained within them is likely to be, how useful that data is in assessing provision of service and how valid conclusions drawn from the audit can be made.

The simplest rule in large databases is that the quality of the data extracted is only as good as the quality of data that is inputted. A useful exercise is to list all potential data sources and then correlate with the standards that the audit wishes to look at. Will they allow triangulation of a potential problem to the actual cause? For example, if a centre performs a very high volume of facet joint injections, this in isolation is not particularly meaningful. If the same unit provides all facet joint injections for a defined population and the rate of injection per 100,000 for that population is more than three standard deviations from the mean, then the unit has a high intervention rate.

The level and depth to which data is interpreted in part dictate its accuracy. In general, the date a patient is admitted to a hospital, the day that they had an intervention and the date they went home are recorded accurately (Hospital Episodic Statistics in the UK). Diving deeper into this data will unfortunately increase inaccuracy. Trying to establish exactly what procedure was undertaken (OPCS codes), why it was undertaken (diagnosis, ICD-10 codes) and the technique utilised and variables such as blood loss, time taken and post-procedure analgesia will be inaccurate unless there is a database with the information recorded compulsorily by all centres. This high-level data source does not exist in most circumstances, and therefore one of the primary goals in establishing a national audit should be a common approach to data collection. This has been recognised for many years in the UK, and once the British Spine Registry was developed, much political work has gone in to making its use mandatory.

What to Measure (Metrics) in Primary Care

For an overall picture of a patient's journey, the starting point for assessment may be their first contact with a medical practitioner. It is useful to calculate the observed and expected elective referrals and emergency referrals from a primary care practice into secondary care (Fig. 11.3). Practices can be observed in close geographical boundaries trying to minimise local demographic variation as cause for referral practice. Obvious variance from expected referral patterns can then be investigated more closely.

What to Measure (Metrics) in Secondary Care

Reviewing spinal services nationally in a comparative fashion should initially focus on common spinal conditions and common procedures. It should also identify how difficult it is to access these services. As a suggestion common metrics utilised are:

- Median time from referral to first clinic appointment, over and under 18
- Median time from referral to procedure (where procedure performed) over and under 18
- Median time from time placed on waiting list to procedure over and under 18
- Numbers of procedures performed
- Rate of intervention per 100,000 population for common procedures

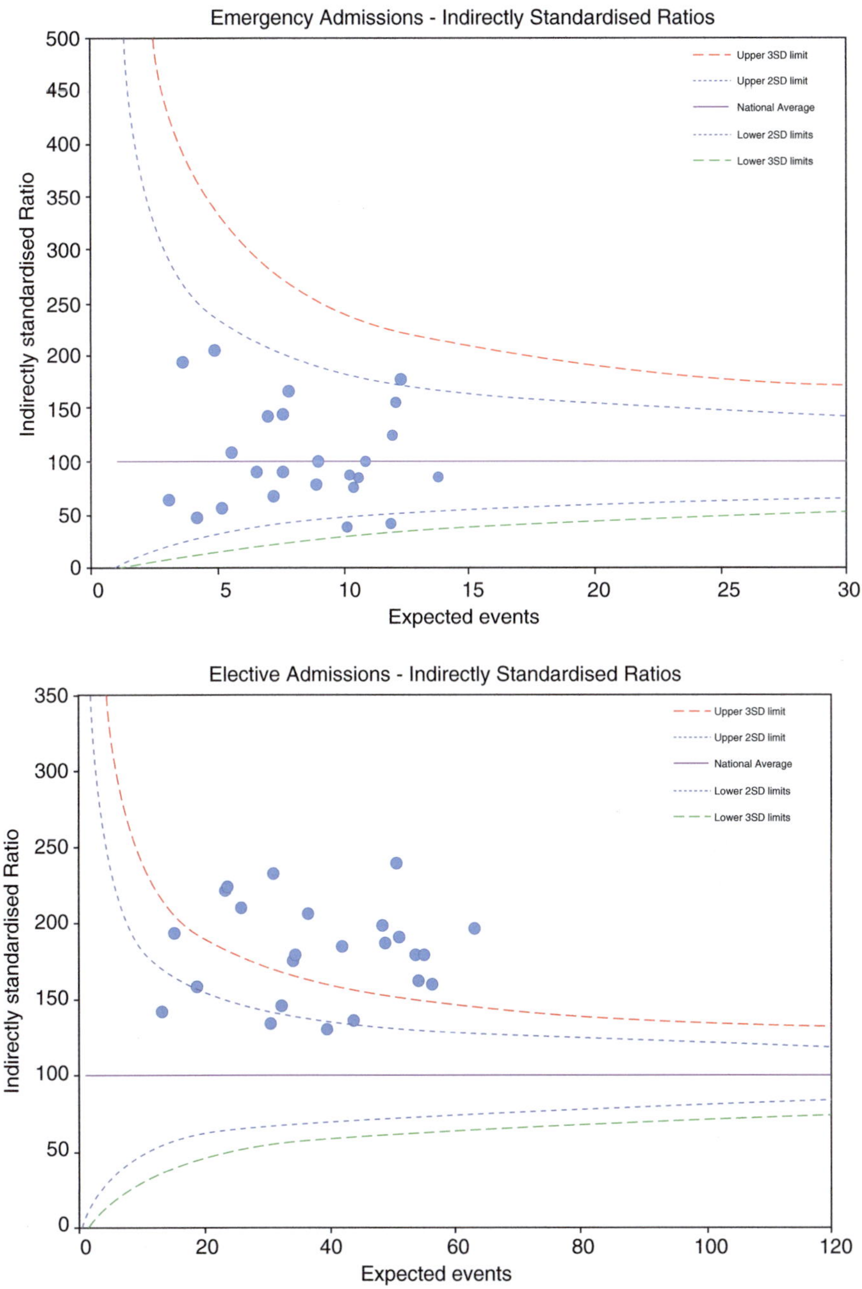

Fig. 11.3 Primary care emergency and elective admissions to spinal services in a single geographical commissioning group (CCG). Each dot represents a primary care unit. Note the unexpected elective referral pattern driven by a secondary care provider. (Source: Hospital Episodic Data April 2013–March 2015)

- Emergency readmission at 30 days
- Return to theatres same body site 90 days and 2 years for common spinal operations
- Median length of stay for elective common operations, e.g. single-level discectomy/decompression
- Implant and consumable expenditure
- Infection rate for elective single level discectomy/decompression
- Infection rate for elective posterior adolescent scoliosis correction
- Infection rate for elective posterior cervical spine instrumented decompression
- Number and cost of litigation claims over and under 18 years of age
- Patient-reported outcome data for common spinal operations

For some conditions requiring specialised spinal surgery, it is very difficult to know the catchment population and therefore difficult to calculate a rate of surgery per 100,000 population. In England, there are some clinical commissioning groups (CCGs) which are geographically based around a centre performing this surgery and therefore all patients from that CCG (with a known population) will be referred to the one centre. The rate of surgery for patients from that CCG done at the hospital can be calculated and compared against other hospitals performing that surgery. Whilst it would not be proof of high or low volume surgery, it would certainly start a conversation about indications. This has been done for paediatric spinal deformity surgery.

Data Validation

Having established what measurements will be made, it is a useful exercise to run the data where practice is already known. Variance may not necessarily be a bad thing, and it is important to check that the data run will identify things that are already established. For instance, a quick glance of the data will establish what type of approach to the spine is utilised at a unit for lumbar spinal fusion. A unit may be known for using an anterior lumbar approach which the data should identify. Supra-regional networks (e.g. for primary spine tumours) may have been established; the data should reflect this practice. Spinal units may be of different known sizes (e.g. major trauma receiving centres), and this should be clear in the data when comparing with non-trauma units.

Data Interpretation

Data is often not normally distributed in health provision. When it is not, it is imperative to look at both the national median and mean. Variation will always occur in a

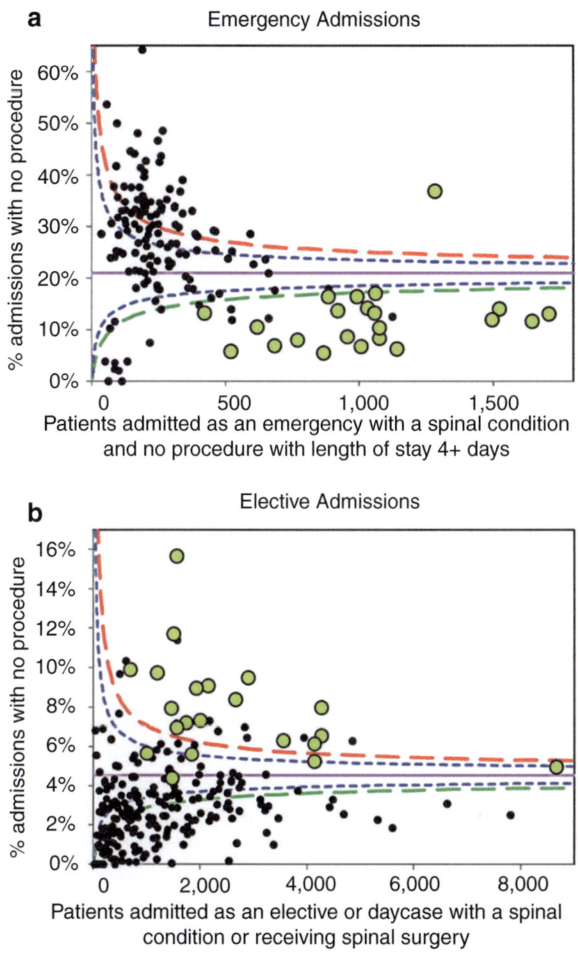

Fig. 11.4 Data Patterns. Each dot represents a unit offering spinal services in England. Green dots are centres providing major trauma care/24 h MRI cover. (**a**) Such centres have very high volume of emergency admissions, but patients do not stay in the hospital long as often they are just transferred for an MRI scan out of hours. In other centres, they have a lower volume of emergency admissions, but patients who do not require any intervention stay in the hospital for more than 4 days with far more frequency. X-axis, patients admitted as an emergency with a spinal condition and no procedure; y-axis, % admissions with a length of stay 4+ days. (**b**) An unfortunate consequence is major trauma centres/24 h MRI have very high rates of on-the-day cancellations for non-emergency spinal procedures because they have no bed capacity as they are often occupied by emergency admissions. X-axis – patients admitted as an elective or day case with a spinal condition planned to receive spinal surgery. Y-axis – % admissions with no procedure. (Source: Getting it Right First Time, NHS Improvement 2016)

population. Any variation from the national picture should be looked at not just statistically but if it has clinical importance. As an example, a unit may have an unacceptable mortality rate that has not reached statistical significance.

Once data has been run at a national comparative level, it is useful to look at groups of services establishing patterns and highlighting stories within the data such as the high on-day elective cancellation rate for spinal services in a major trauma centre (Fig. 11.4).

Financial Considerations

Savings can be attributed to any improvements in several ways.

Length of Stay

If the cost of a stay in bed is known per day (estimated to be £330 per day for orthopaedics in the NHS), a saving is generated if median length of stay for a procedure is improved. The number of bed days saved per annum multiplied by cost of a bed day will estimate the annual saving. Unplanned readmission can be considered in a similar way.

Operating Room Time

NHS operating room time for orthopaedics is estimated at £1400 per hour for a standard 8 h operating day. OR cost in the NHS does not just depend on length of the procedure but also on OR list utilisation. A 6 h operation with no additional procedure costs 8 h of OR time, whilst adding an additional case taking 2 h will reduce the cost attributable to each procedure. Unplanned return to the OR is clearly an additional cost and should be added to the cost of the original procedure.

Implant and High-Cost Consumables

Most services have a good repository of data that records the cost of implants and consumables. If this data is collected, comparison can be made between the cost of different implants and consumables used for the same purpose and the same implants and consumables used at different hospitals. This transparency has had a very powerful effect of driving down these costs.

Patient level costing is becoming mandatory in the NHS with many hospitals already reporting this data. Currently, the quality of this data remains in question.

Closing the Loop

All good surgical audits involve a process whereby having implemented change, the effects of that change are reviewed. The date of change in practice should be noted. Most databases will have a time lag in updating their data of at least 3 months. It is imperative that this is considered when deciding the timeframe of re-audit. Equally

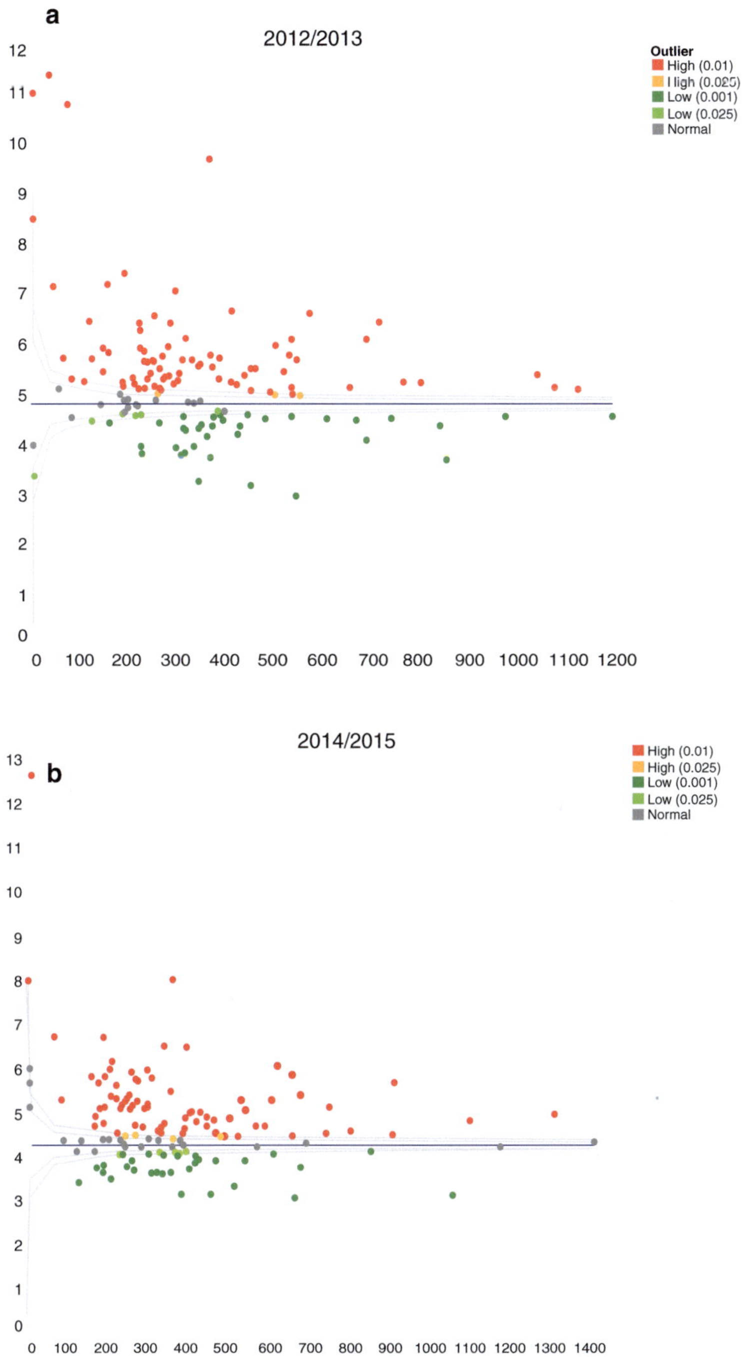

Fig. 11.5 Primary total hip replacement median length of stay in English orthopaedic units April 2012–April 2013 (**a**) and then after national audit and unit visits April 2014–April 2015 (**b**). Note the reduction in variance and the overall reduction in median length of stay. (Source: Getting it Right First Time, Elective Orthopaedics. Prof. Tim Briggs CBE)

the change in practice should be given enough time to have become established. Metrics should be re-analysed and any changes observed at both local and national levels. Figure 11.5 shows the effect of national audit in length of stay for primary hip replacement in England.

In conclusion, national audit of spinal services, if performed carefully and collaboratively with the services involved, can be an invaluable tool in improving the quality of healthcare provided to patients with spinal conditions.

British Spine Registry

Since the first surgeries performed, surgeons have recorded operative and outcome data on their patients. This has enabled development and improvement of surgical care to the high-tech and large volume healthcare systems present in developed countries today. The demands of the legal system and the advent of value-based healthcare [4] necessitate increasingly detailed contemporaneous data capture.

Care Quality Registers (CQRs) in the modern sense can be traced to 1970s Sweden, where in 1979 the Swedish Hip Register began the era of orthopaedic data capture on a population level with significant benefit to patients and to the national health system [5]. CQRs are enshrined in the Swedish system, and the Health Act defines them as 'An automated and structured collection of personal data that were initiated with the purpose to systematically and continuously develop and safeguard quality of care. A national or regional Quality Registry refers to one in which personal data have been collected from several caregivers and which allows for comparisons within healthcare at a national or regional level' [6].

The lumbar spine database subsequently followed in Sweden, with similar benefits [7]. It has since been recognised that a high volume, comprehensive, highly compliant registry is as good as a randomised controlled trial at assessing management outcomes in single disease, single procedure situations [8–10].

The UK

Political pressure in the publicly funded NHS in the UK has engendered a call for surgeon league tables. An increasing recognition of the existence of significant unwarranted variation in outcomes, and growing desires for patient centred healthcare, fuelled this effort.

The UK spinal societies recognised the need for procedure and outcome recording whilst maintaining concerns that without appropriate case-mix and complexity stratification, raw surgeon-level data can be misleading. Several league tables have already been published. However well-intentioned, these efforts have led to issues of individual career damage and may produce major problems with future workforce recruitment [11].

The British Orthopaedic Association supports the publication of data at hospital level. At individual surgeon level, data must be robust, include all surgeons and be sensitive to case-mix stratification to allow adequate comparisons. There must also be a robust variance analysis policy.

British Spine Registry (BSR)

In 2010, with the goal of achieving healthcare benefits and improved value, the British Association of Spine Surgeons (BASS) resolved to develop a modern, fit-for-purpose CQR. The advent of fast, secure and accessible web-based technology served to provide an ideal approach to the data capture and handling aspects of a register.

Perhaps the most relevant peer project to those in the UK at that time was the first multi-national spine registry, Spine Tango from the Spine Society of Europe [12]. At that time this project had only been adopted, albeit very successfully, by a handful of units. Spine Tango proved that with appropriate surgeon commitment and a fully funded administrative support team, data compliance including relevant outcome scores with prolonged follow-up could exceed 80%.

The nascent system, the British Spine Registry (BSR), (http://www.britishspineregistry.com/) was conceived as a surgeon-owned and controlled data repository of patient-centred and pathology-specific information. The initial aim was to monitor the outcomes of spinal procedures, collecting clinically relevant data including diagnostic and procedural information, complications and patient-reported outcome and experience measures (PROMs and PREMs). This differs from the initial aims of the arthroplasty registers, which were to monitor revision and mortality. By creating a web-based portal to the BSR, it was envisaged that individual surgeons and their teams would be empowered to collect accurate prospective data in a convenient and timely manner with access to the system wherever and whenever they wished. There was also the ability to use the Registry for multicentre research studies including RCTs.

A subcommittee of the Society was formed, led by Ashley Cole and Lee Breakwell, Consultant Spinal Surgeons, Sheffield Children's Hospital NHS Foundation Trust, UK, to define the data set and registry structure and to create a competitive IT industry proposals process. Bluespier International (Droitwich, UK) was the chosen partner; they worked with the BASS registry committee to design and launch the BSR on the Amplitude platform in May 2012.

Information governance and protection of patient health information are significant concerns, with regular headline grabbing episodes of security breaches across the globe [13]. Bluespier International demonstrated many years of secure data control within the NHS system, and their data storage facilities have NHS level security. The BSR is registered with the Information Commissioner's Office (ICO) and the Healthcare Quality Improvement Partnership (HQIP).

Consent remains the legal basis for data processing. Each patient is consented either by paper or through the patient portal with supplemental patient information. Legal advice has been sought regarding the wording of the consent and patient information. Failure at this stage may limit the ability to continue to hold and analyse data in the future. Different countries have different issues regarding holding personal data. In Europe, the General Data Protection Regulations (GDPR) now applies.

Designing a purpose-built register presented as many challenges as it did opportunities. It was recognised early on that spinal surgery offers a different proposition to that of joint arthroplasty. Examples of best practice were gleaned from existing registries, such as the Swedish Spine and Arthroplasty projects, as well as the well-established UK-based National Joint Registry (NJR). Advice was sought and received from many experienced sources.

Long-term outcomes capture requires accurate recording of patient demographics at the beginning of treatment. A multitude of methods for data capture were envisaged from paper forms like Spine Tango, kiosk input as seen in airports, through to email completion all enabling timely yet convenient questioning of spinal patients after surgery. Robust demographic collection was encouraged as part of the embedded consent process to ensure all subsequent capture options remained available.

British Spine Registry (BSR) Pathways

Lumbar degenerative
Cervical and thoracic degenerative
Tumour
Trauma
Infection
Deformity
Intra-dural

The complexity of registry data in spinal surgery is shown by the fact that different procedures may be performed for a single diagnosis, whilst conversely a specific operation may be undertaken for several distinct pathologies. To achieve a patient-focussed approach to data, a disease-centred pathway concept was imagined and embedded as the core strategy for database design.

Seven distinct pathways were created covering the scope of spinal surgery from the common, high volume areas, to the much rarer specialist niches. These pathways are separated by the different data sets and PROMs.

Once the disease-specific pathway was defined, relevant details of the presenting clinical symptoms and signs, information on co-morbidities and other conditions were agreed to define the patient-level pathology being treated. Design of the database aimed to capture reliable, reproducible details of the presenting complaint whilst allowing risk stratification of the subsequent results.

Arguably the most important part of any surgical register is the information defining the procedure performed. For each Pathway, the procedure form collects an 'operative log' detailing Surgeon, Hospital, Payer and a series of conditional questions defining the surgical procedure, approach, levels, implants and intraoperative complications. A comprehensive search tool was created to enable rapid lookup of the implants available in the UK market for the specific procedure in question, with a view to long-term implant surveillance.

As recognised previously, the success or failure of a CQR is largely based on the routine capture of large volumes of reliable data on a set of procedures. Initially, the BSR had no mandatory data set as there was concern this would affect uptake. Mandatory fields have now been introduced to ensure standard collection of these items which will be essential for future analysis. The principle of a mandatory data field is that the surgeon must know the answer at the end of surgery without having to measure or search for the information. Most of the mandated data points relate to patient demographics, basic presenting symptomatology, risk stratification information (e.g. co-morbidities) and surgical details. The surgical procedure is broken down into groupings to aid later comparison. In this regard, a procedure to release a nerve would be coded as decompression with or without discectomy. The details of the specific decompression performed can be easily recorded by tabulation, with an example of a central and lateral recess decompression at L4/5 demonstrated in Fig. 11.6. This enables reliable and reproducible recording of the levels and types of surgery without lengthy notation or the risk of typographical error. Single or multi-select boxes are preferred to drop down lists to reduce the number of mouse clicks and make it easier to use on a touchscreen device.

Any implant utilised can be similarly captured using the lookup facility, enabling surveillance of new and existing technologies. In the light of previous well-documented [14, 15] implant-related problems, registries are welcomed as a potential method of improving patient safety at a population level. National bodies in the UK have embraced the BSR as a system through which the delivery and vigilance of innovation can be achieved [16].

A major feature of the BSR is patient-reported outcome and experience measures (PROMs and PREMs). Each patient pathway allows collection of data, using validated scores:

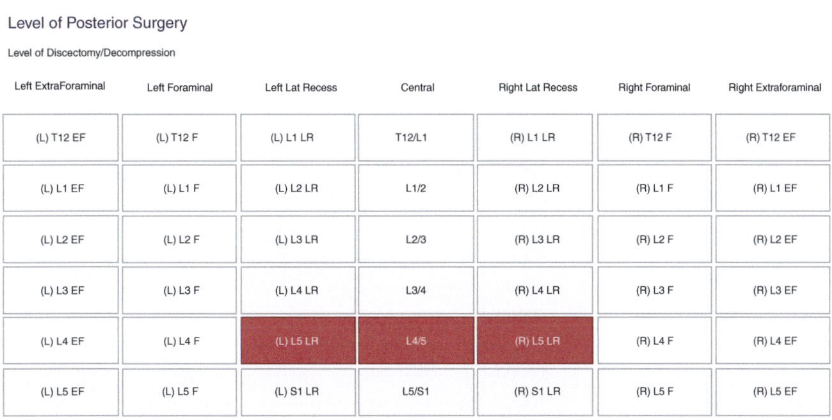

Fig. 11.6 BSR screenshot of level selection tabulation by push button

- Lumbar degenerative pathway: Visual analogue score for leg and back pain, Oswestry Disability Index [17] and EuroQoL 5D-5L [18]
- Cervical and thoracic degenerative pathway: Visual analogue score for arm and neck pain, Neck Disability Index [19] and EuroQoL 5D-5L
- Deformity: SRS-22 [20]

Additional questionnaires can be added to the pathway of a patient either due to diagnosis, e.g. the European Myelopathy Score for patients with cervical myelopathy, or for patients in specific multicentre research trials. All the questionnaires are sent by email to the patients at time-points designated by the Pathway. These are usually before surgery and at 6 weeks, 6 months, 1 year and 2 years after surgery. The email contains a link to the patient portal so they can complete their questionnaires. Reminders are sent and users can look at compliance reports.

Once surgeon registration is complete, they can nominate co-workers who can obtain access to act as 'delegates' and can enter patient data. This could be a secretary entering demographic data, a practice manager chasing missing PROMs or a resident completing an operative form or inserting information about post-operative complications. This follows the recognition as seen in Spine Tango practice that teamworking is required for quality data capture.

Since its launch, the BSR has grown organically (Fig. 11.7) predominantly due to early adopter enthusiasm and peer pressure. The stated aim of the spinal societies was to achieve full compliance with data enrolment, but without enforcement powers, this has proved difficult. Several initiatives have aided increased compliance, including the mandatory BSR data entry required by the NHS England Specialised Spinal Surgery Service Specification.

In April 2019, it is likely that a Best Practice Tariff will exist for completing the form for diagnostic and procedure details for all patients having elective and non-elective spinal surgery (excluding injection). This will be an additional payment to providers for achieving required data entry rates into the BSR. This will dramatically increase the compliance with the BSR as hospitals will ensure it is performed and adequate assistance for data entry is given. We are expecting more than 85% of the spinal surgical procedures to be entered onto the BSR.

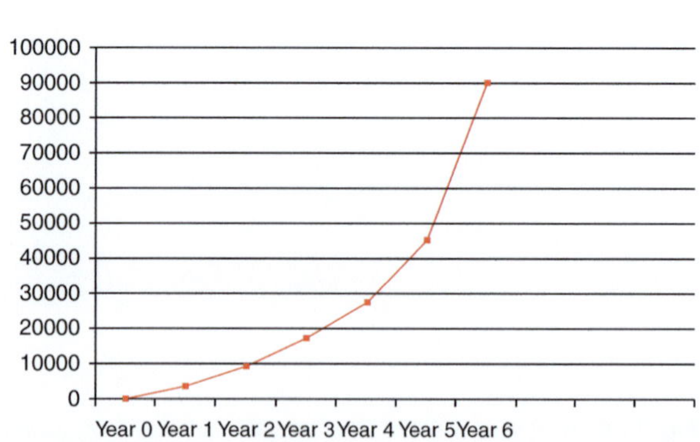

Fig. 11.7 Cumulative number of procedures on the BSR

Recently the inclusion rate for surgery for idiopathic scoliosis has increased to 75% across the nation in the 2017 audit. In early 2018, the BSR has over 1500 registered surgical team users with more than 120,000 enrolled patients.

Whilst the compliance rate still lies below the required level, the power of this volume of data means individuals can interrogate their data, with surgical outcomes, including complication rates by procedure type. The societies are beginning to be able, for the first time, to create real-time accurate population figures on spinal surgery in the UK.

The Future

It is suspected that surgical procedures without demonstrated cost-utility will gradually be stopped through the commissioning process, and this is being observed in nonspecialised spinal surgery where facet joint injections have been defined by the CCGs as 'procedures of limited clinical value (POLCV)' following the NICE guidelines in 2016. Facet joint injections are easily identified by a single OPCS code (V544), and their reduction is easy to monitor. It will be difficult in a few years to explain why spine surgery does not have cost-utility data on the procedures commonly performed such as lumbar microdiscectomy or ACDF. It is beholden upon our profession to collect and analyse large volumes of data to inform the decisions of both clinicians and purchasers to ensure the best and most cost-effective spinal care is available to our patients. The BSR will enable this on large volume real-life data.

Summary

A national commissioning system has the advantage of protecting against unwarranted variation in spinal practice. Care must be taken to continue to encourage innovation. Current data sources do not adequately describe the spinal work performed either in procedure codes (OPCS) or diagnostic codes (ICD-10). A mandatory spinal register like the British Spine Registry will allow long-term collection of clinically relevant data including complications and patient outcomes. It can also serve as an implant register and can collect data for multicentre research studies. Case-mix variables including a frailty index can also be collected before surgical procedures, and cost-utility analysis should also be an objective.

References

1. The Mid Staffordshire NHS Foundation Trust Public Inquiry – Chaired by Robert Francis QC. Final Report. Wednesday 6 February 2013 [online]. Accessed at: http://webarchive.nationalarchives.gov.uk/20150407084231/http://www.midstaffspublicinquiry.com/report
2. Foster NE, Anema JR, Cherkin D, Chou R, Cohen SP, Gross DP, Ferreira PH, Fritz JM, Koes BW, Peul W, Turner JA, Maher CG. Prevention and treatment of low back pain, evidence, challenges and promising directions. Lancet. 2018;391(10137):2368–83.

3. Withers S, Cole A, Athanassacopoulos M, Breakwell L, Chiverton N, Ivanov M, Michael R, Tomlinson J, Lachlan S, Wilson H. Triage and treat service for back and radicular pain: 3-year results. Spine J. 2017;17(3 suppl):S9.
4. Gray M. Value based healthcare. BMJ. 2017;356:j437.
5. Kärrholm J. The Swedish hip arthroplasty register. Acta Orthop. 2010;81(1):3–4.
6. Emilsson L, Lindahl B, Köster M. Review of 103 Swedish healthcare quality registries. J Intern Med. 2015;277:94–136.
7. Strömqvist B, Fritzell P, Hägg O, Jönsson B. The Swedish spine register: development, design and utility. Eur Spine J. 2009;18(Suppl 3):294–304.
8. Benson K, Hartz AJ. A comparison of observational studies and randomized, controlled trials. N Engl J Med. 2000;342(25):1878–86.
9. Concato J, Shah N, Horwitz RI. Randomized, controlled trials, observational studies, and the hierarchy of research designs. N Engl J Med. 2000;342(25):1887–92.
10. Cole AA. Fusion for lumbar spinal stenosis? BMJ. 2016;353:i3145.
11. Westaby S, Baig K, De Silva R, Unsworth-White J, Pepper J. Recruitment to UK cardiothoracic surgery in the era of public outcome reporting. Eur J Cardiothorac Surg. 2015;47(4):679–83.
12. Melloh M, Staub L, Aghajev E, Zweig T, Barz T, Theis J-C, Chavanne A, Grob D, Aebi M, Roeder C. The international spine registry SPINE TANGO: status quo and first results. Eur Spine J. 2008;17(9):1201–9.
13. National Audit Office (NAO). Investigation: WannaCry cyber attack and the NHS. 27 October 2017 [online]. Accessed at: https://www.nao.org.uk/report/investigation-wannacry-cyber-attack-and-the-nhs/
14. NHS. Fears of faulty 'toxic' hip replacement implant. Monday January 30 2012 [online]. Accessed at: https://www.nhs.uk/news/2012/01January/Pages/hip-implant-fears.aspx
15. Muirhead-Allwood SK. Lessons of a hip failure. If we want improved prostheses we must regulate their use. BMJ. 1998;316(7132):644.
16. National Institute for Health and Care Excellence (NICE). The MAGEC system for spinal lengthening in children with scoliosis. June 2014 [online]. Accessed at: https://www.nice.org.uk/guidance/mtg18/chapter/3-Clinical-evidence
17. Fairbank JC, Pynsent PB. The Oswestry disability index. Spine. 2000;25(22):2940–52.
18. EuroQol Group. EuroQol – a new facility for the measurement of health-related quality of life. Health Policy. 1990;16(3):199–208.
19. Vernon H, Mior S. The neck disability index: a study of reliability and validity. J Manip Physiol Ther. 1991;14:409–15.
20. Asher M, Min Lai S, Burton D, Manna B. The reliability and concurrent validity of the scoliosis research society-22 patient questionnaire for idiopathic scoliosis. Spine. 2003;28(1):63–9.

12 Quality Spine Care in Australasia

Bryan Ashman and John Chen Li Tat

Healthcare in Australia and Singapore

Population Demographics

In 2016 there were 23 million people in Australia with a population density of just 3 people per square kilometre due to the large landmass of the island (7.6 million square km) and the sparsely populated centre of the country. About 90% live in urban centres within 100 kilometres of the coastline, and of these three quarters live in the five mainland capital cities. Two thirds of the population are aged between 15 and 65 years and 15% are older than 65. Detached houses are home to 75%, while the rest live in apartments. The average household has 2.6 people and an income of AU$650 per capita per week [1].

Singapore is also an island nation with over 5 million people living in just 700 square kilometres, a population density of 7000 per square km. Three quarters are aged between 15 and 65, and only 9% are older than 65 years. The population is completely urbanised with more than 80% living in high-rise apartments and an average household size of 3.3 people. The average income is SG$1400 per capita per week [2].

Australian Healthcare System

Australia has a universal healthcare system called Medicare which provides free medical care and subsidised medicines to Australian residents. There is also a

B. Ashman (✉)
Division of Surgery, Canberra Hospital, Garran, ACT, Australia
e-mail: bryan.ashman@act.gov.au

J. Chen Li Tat
Department of Orthopaedic Surgery, Singapore General Hospital, Singapore, Singapore

J. Ratliff et al. (eds.), *Quality Spine Care*,
https://doi.org/10.1007/978-3-319-97990-8_12

private health industry providing access to care through private hospitals, clinics and insurance. Spending on healthcare in Australia in 2016 was almost 10% of the national gross domestic product, about AU$120 billion or AU$5000 per capita. The majority of the funding is provided by governments, national and state, with about one third from the private sector. Of the total, about 50% is spent on hospital-based care, 20% on visits to a doctor, 15% on pharmaceuticals and a further 15% on community public health and aged care [3].

Singapore Healthcare System

In Singapore, the health system is also universal but not free of charge. The government provides subsidies for public healthcare by compulsory nationalised health insurance (Medisave). These subsidies vary from small out-of-pocket expenses to very large gaps between fees and rebates. The private health system provides services to those who can afford private treatment and is utilised by the government to reduce waiting lists in the public system. Spending on healthcare in Singapore in 2015 was 5% of GDP, about SG$20 billion or SG$4000 per capita. The government component of this was only 2% of GDP due to the low subsidies compared to out-of-pocket expenses [4]. In 2014, the Singapore health system was rated as the world's most efficient by Bloomberg [5].

Spinal Disorders as a Population Health Problem in Australasia

The Australian Institute of Health and Welfare reported in 2017 on the incidence of musculoskeletal conditions in the Australian population [6]. These were predominantly chronic arthritis and spinal pain, each about 50%, and accounted for 10% of the burden of disease (defined as 'living with illness and injury or dying prematurely'). Only cancer (20%), cardiovascular disease (15%) and mental or substance abuse disorders (12%) ranked higher. The unit of measurement was disability-adjusted life years (DALYs) and was derived from the self-reported disability from a national census of health conducted by the Australian Bureau of Statistics in 2015. When considering only living with disability and not premature death, chronic arthritis and back pain were second only to mental health problems as a cause of difficulties with self-care, work or social enjoyment. Patients with spinal pain were more likely to rate their condition as severe (50%) than those with arthritis (40%). Risk factors associated with disability were obesity for arthritis (45%) and occupational exposure to lifting for spinal pain (20%). Chronic spinal pain affected about 20% of the Australian population during 2015 and accounted for AU$1.2 billion of healthcare expenditure and an estimated AU$3.5 billion in lost productivity due to 80% of sufferers being of working age [7].

The Singapore Burden of Disease and Injury Working Group published data in 2014 [8]. Musculoskeletal diseases were responsible for 5.6% of the total disease and injury burden in Singapore up to 2010, with only 5% of this burden due to premature mortality. Between 2004 and 2010, there was a 28.5% increase in musculoskeletal disease burden: 29.8% increase in disability burden and 7.1% increase in premature mortality burden. Crude and age-standardised overall burden per head of population increased by 18.8% and 5.4%, respectively. Rheumatoid arthritis was by far the largest contributor, accounting for 43% of the overall burden from musculoskeletal disease followed by osteoarthritis (27%). Rheumatoid arthritis was the 12th leading cause in overall burden and ranked 7th in overall DALYs for women. Osteoarthritis was the 16th leading cause in overall burden and was the 15th leading cause of overall burden in women.

Low back and neck pain maintained its rank as a leading health problem with the most disability second only to ischaemic heart disease. The rates of years lived with disability (YLDs) from 2005 to 2016 for low back and neck pain increased 25.5% during this period.

The annual years of healthy life lost per 100,000 people from low back pain in Singapore has increased by 21.6% since 1990, an average of 0.9% a year, and in 2016 had reached an average of 498 years lost for all age groups. The health burden of low back pain peaks at age 80+ and for men was 714 lost years in 2013, with women having an even higher rate of 1053 lost years.

Measuring the Quality of Health Care

In 1990 the US Institute of Medicine defined quality in healthcare as 'the degree to which health services for individuals and populations increase the likelihood of desired health outcomes' [9]. This definition encompasses all healthcare professionals in all settings of care and implies that not all individuals or groups have equitable access to healthcare and not all outcomes are good. Whether an outcome is desired or not depends on the value placed on it by the individual. Undesired outcomes can be avoided by minimising errors and choosing care that is appropriate, safe and evidence-based using current technology.

To decide if care is appropriate and safe, measurements of quality are required. At the healthcare provider level, quality measures can be considered under the categories of *structure* (capacity to deliver care), *process* (actual care delivery) or *outcomes* (the result of the care) [10]. For funders of healthcare, measures of effectiveness, efficiency and equity are important. At the level of the individual, though, measures of safety, timeliness, getting better and returning to health are more relevant [11].

Outcome measures are related to the delivery of care and the results of that care. Although it can be argued that the quality of care delivery is actually a process issue, the occurrence of adverse events directly related to care delivery is more appropriately measured as an outcome. Adverse event data can be obtained from medical records or from patient reports. Metrics like mortality rates, complication rates and readmissions are the usual data reported by healthcare providers. Direct measures of care quality rely on patient-reported experience measures (PREMs), like timeliness and coordination of care, and outcome measures (PROMs) such as pain, limitation of function and quality of life. The effectiveness of healthcare can therefore be measured both by negative indicators (adverse outcomes) reported by health providers and by positive indicators (reduced pain, reduced disability and improved quality of life) reported by patients themselves.

Quality Reporting of Healthcare in Australasia

The first report on adverse events in Australian hospitals was published in 1995 [12]. This study reviewed the medical records of over 14,000 admissions to 28 hospitals in 1992 and found that about 17% of these admissions were associated with an adverse event caused by the healthcare delivery which either resulted in a disability or prolonged the hospital stay for the patient. One in seven of these adverse events led to a permanent disability and a further 5% of the patients died. The authors estimated that more than half of the adverse events were probably preventable. The mean increase in length of stay was 7 bed-days.

Subsequent studies in hospitals in New Zealand, Japan, Singapore, the UK and Denmark showed an average rate of 10% of hospital admissions associated with adverse events and a WHO study in 2012 of developing countries showed a similar finding [13]. As a result of the outcome study in Australia, the Australian Commission on Safety and Quality in Health Care was established in 2000 and currently accredits every hospital in Australia against ten safety and quality standards on a triennial basis. It has published a range of tools to help analyse routine data collected by individual hospitals, including a classification of Hospital-Acquired Diagnoses (CHADx) which relate complications and adverse events to subgroups of patients or clinical units [14].

A separate organisation, the Australian Council on Healthcare Standards, reports annually on 360 healthcare indicators. In the years 2005–2012, more indicators improved than worsened, and in the latest report (2009–2016), this trend continued with 71 indicators improving and 42 deteriorating. Significant improvements were seen in reduced adverse events for day surgery patients, reduced complications of colonoscopy, less deep infections after CABG surgery and an increase in peer review of serious adverse events in maternity services to almost 100%. Notable worsening in indicators occurred in hypothermia in the post-anaesthetic recovery period, major viscus injury during gynaecological surgery and the use of physical restraint for mental health patients [15].

Surgical death audits are carried out in all states in Australia under the Royal Australasian College of Surgeons' Australian and New Zealand Audit of Surgical Mortality. Any surgical death occurring during hospitalisation is referred for analysis by the treating surgeon, and results are published annually. In a recent report based on the Victorian audits since 2007, Chen et al. identified that about 15% of surgical deaths were potentially preventable [16].

Alternative ways of measuring healthcare are to look at appropriateness of care and variability in care provision. Both of these approaches have been the subject of research and reporting in Australia. Appropriate care implies compliance by healthcare providers with evidence-based or consensus-based guidelines and variability in care suggests factors such as geographic location, socioeconomic status or provider preference influence the provision of healthcare.

In 2012, a study called CareTrack Australia reported on a sample of over 35,000 health encounters by 1100 patients with 22 common conditions in 2009–2010 and determined the percentage of encounters at which appropriate care had been recommended [17]. This study was based on a previous US study which found that overall only 55% of patients had received appropriate care in 1999 [18]. In the Australian study, the best compliance was seen for coronary artery disease (90% in 131 patients with 769 encounters) and one of the worst was antibiotic use (19% for 78 patients with 153 encounters).

The Australian Commission on Safety and Quality in Health Care released the first Australian Atlas of Healthcare Variation in 2015 which clearly showed geographical variation in six clinical areas that appeared unwarranted in that it exceeded the variation expected by health conditions in different populations or personal preferences [19]. The key findings were:

- An 11 times difference in antibiotic prescribing rates in areas with the highest to areas with the lowest and for amoxicillin alone a 20 times difference.
- A 30 times difference in colonoscopy rates
- An inappropriately high number of CT scans for low back pain and a ten times difference from highest to lowest rates
- A nine times difference in prostatic biopsy rates
- A five times variation in knee arthroscopy rates and over 30,000 procedures done for osteoarthritis in people over 55 years old during 2012–2013
- Five hundred thousand prescriptions for psychotropic medication for children with ADHD and a 75 times variation in rates
- Fifteen million prescriptions for antidepressants for adults with high rates in the over 65 years of age group
- Fourteen million prescriptions for narcotic analgesics with a ten times variation in rates

A second Atlas was published in 2017, and in the surgical category, lumbar spinal fusions and decompressions had the highest rates of variability [20]. This will be discussed below.

Measuring the Quality of Spine Care

Outcome measures for the treatment of low back pain are numerous and in general unstandardised. Clement et al. [21] defined a set of outcome metrics for low back pain using a Delphi technique involving an international group of experts (including a former spinal surgery patient). They identified that for comparison purposes, any outcome set should be available in multiple languages, allow for case-mix adjustments for specific disease groups and reflect what matters most to patients. They focussed on degenerative lumbar conditions and recommended a specific set of patient-reported outcome metrics (Table 12.1) and adverse clinical events (Table 12.2).

The expert group also recognised the importance of documenting pre-existing risk factors such as smoking status, BMI and medical comorbidities and, for surgical patients, the anaesthetic status and any previous surgery. Finally, while acknowledging the impact of psychosocial factors on treatment for LBP, they did not recommend formal psychometric testing, suggesting that these indicators are captured in some of the domains of the disability and quality of life tools.

Reports on spine care outcomes using PROMs and adverse events are almost exclusively restricted to research study publications. The implication is that low level evidence based on small case numbers or biased results cannot be generalised to whole populations of similar patients.

Spine Registries

Registries of spine care exist in many countries and are described in a separate chapter of this book. Although evidence is now available from one of the longest established registries (SweSpine) that patient outcomes can be influenced by utilising registry data, most registries have a high likelihood of being perceived as biased

Table 12.1 Patient-reported outcome measures

Outcome	Measurement tool	Definition
Pain	Numeric rating score	Average pain over last week (back and leg) rated 0 to 10
Disability	Oswestry disability index	Ten domains, six options from 'no problem' to 'severe impairment'
Quality of life	EQ5D-3L	Five domains, three options from 'no problem' to 'severe impairment'
Work status	Normal hours and duties, reduced hours or duties, not at work	Current status and time off due to LBP
Analgesic use	Narcotic or non-opioid	None, sometimes, regularly

Table 12.2 Adverse outcomes of treatment

Outcome	Definition
Mortality	Death inhospital
Nerve root injury	Iatrogenic
Vascular injury	Required intervention
Dural tear	With CSF leak
Deep wound infection	Required IV antibiotics
Pulmonary embolus	Proven by imaging study
Readmission after discharge	Within 30 days for any reason
Reoperation	Any time after index surgery for any reason
Other	Wound haematoma, medical complications, etc.

because of industry or government sponsorship, membership of spine societies by data contributors or enrolling only surgical patients, and therefore outcomes are not seen as generalizable to all patients with low back pain [22]. In Australia, a pilot spine care registry has been started by the Spine Society of Australia and Monash University but will enrol only surgical patients initially. At Singapore General Hospital, a spine outcomes registry was established for lumbar cases in 1998 and cervical cases in 2002. At the end of 2017, there were almost 10,000 lumbar and 2,000 cervical patients. The registry receives institutional funding coupled with research grants to support a staff of allied health personnel who assist in the outcomes assessments with the patients. Patient-reported outcomes measures (PROMs) are interpreted for the patients in their local vernacular language. The PROMs used are disease-specific instruments such as the Oswestry Disability Index, North American Spine Society (NASS), Neck Disability Index, AAOS Cervical instrument and Short Form 22 for adolescent idiopathic scoliosis. Quality of life measures used are the Short Form 36 and NASS patient satisfaction scores. These outcome measures are collected preoperatively and post-operatively at weekly intervals of 6, 12 and 24 weeks and at the 2nd and 5th years and up to 10 years post-surgery. Perioperative morbidity and mortality statistics are captured and reported separately from registry data per episode of hospital admission. The vast repository of data from the registry has helped fuel the research into the outcomes of surgical treatments from degenerative spinal disorders, with 22 studies reported in peer-reviewed international journals by the end of 2017.

Appropriateness of Care for Low Back Pain

A study by Williams et al. of usual care by Australian general practitioners (GPs) for patients with low back pain found no improvement in compliance with evidence-based guidelines after the release of the NHMRC guidelines in 2004 [23]. Only 20% of patients received appropriate investigations, medications and advice [24]. As mentioned above, the CareTrack Australia study in 2012 examined the appropriateness of care for 22 common conditions, including low back pain [17]. In a separate analysis of the low back pain subset in the CareTrack study, Ramanathan outlined the indicators used in the study for compliance with the NHMRC guidelines:

- Patients presenting with low back pain have their medical history documented at presentation.
- Patients presenting with low back pain have a physical examination performed and documented at presentation.
- Patients presenting with low back pain have had a neurological examination of the lower limbs performed.
- Patients presenting with low back pain have been asked about/assessed for:
  - Spine fractures (trauma, history of previous fracture, prolonged use of steroids)
  - Cancer (history of cancer, unexplained weight loss, immunosuppression)

  - Infection (fever, IV drug use)
  - Cauda equina syndrome
- Patients with acute low back pain were *not* advised to rest
- Patients with acute low back pain were *not* recommended to have lumbar supports, traction or TENS
- Patients with acute low back pain were *not* prescribed steroids or antidepressants

She identified that barriers to adherence to clinical guidelines include lack of awareness or familiarity, lack of agreement with the guidelines, lack of willingness to change practice or an expectation that patients will not comply. However, in the low back pain group of 164 patients with 6588 encounters, 72% had received appropriate care based on existing guidelines [25]. Unlike the Williams study which only looked at GPs as care providers, in the CareTrack study, the healthcare providers were a mixture of GPs, allied health practitioners and hospital doctors, and this rate correlated with the LBP subset in the US study of 69% [18]. GPs, though, had the lowest compliance rate at 54% of 1557 encounters compared to allied health providers at 83% of 4639 encounters.

In Singapore, a retrospective study of patients referred for physiotherapy treatment at a hospital musculoskeletal clinic for acute low back pain found that 93% of the patients had diagnostic imaging, but there was no difference in functional outcomes after treatment between patients with normal radiology and those with disc protrusions or degeneration [26]. Of the 94 patients referred during a 6-month period, 14 had no radiological abnormality, 42 had a disc protrusion on MRI and 21 had degenerative changes on plain x-ray films. Most of the patients were aged between 30 and 50 years, and 75% had previous low back pain episodes. All patients received manual therapy, back exercises and back pain education with functional improvement in the majority. Of those who improved, there was no significant difference between those with normal radiology and those with abnormalities on plain x-ray or MRI. The authors concluded that their study findings were consistent with international guidelines recommending against radiological investigations in patients presenting with acute low back pain with no sinister symptoms.

Variation in Surgery for Lumbar Degeneration

Variation in the rates of low back surgeries was identified in the first Australian Atlas of Healthcare Variation, and this variation was a focus of analysis in the second Atlas. The average rate of hospitalisations for lumbar spinal decompression between 2013 and 2015 was 81 per 100,000 adults with a range of 30–156. Rates were highest in areas surrounding major cities than in the cities themselves and lowest in remote areas of Australia and areas of low socioeconomic status. Rates were also high in areas of high socioeconomic status and in privately insured patients (81% of all hospitalisations) [20].

Lumbar spinal fusion was, in the past, restricted to the treatment of fractures and deformity, but now the commonest reason for spinal fusion in the USA is degeneration of the spine [27]. The rate of lumbar fusion in Australia is 26 per 100,000 adults with a range from 10 to 69, in other words, 6.9 times as high in the highest area compared with the lowest. Nearly 90% of all fusions are done on private patients. This discrepancy between spinal fusion surgery performed in private versus public hospitals was the subject of a study in 2009 [28]. The authors found that the number of spinal fusion procedures performed in private hospitals in the most populated state in Australia (New South Wales) had increased 166% in the 10 years between 1997 and 2006 from 7.7 per 100,000 population to 20.5 per 100,000. The rate of spinal fusion procedures performed in public hospitals during the same time period had essentially remained unchanged at 2 per 100,000 population. The authors also noted that the figures for the private sector procedures did not include operations performed under worker's compensation insurance and speculated that the true rate is probably much higher as most worker's compensation procedures are performed in private hospitals but are not reported because the payments to hospitals by insurers are outside the national Medicare system.

A similar discrepancy was noted in the UK and prompted the National Institute for Health and Care Excellence to call for lumbar fusions to be permitted only as part of a randomised trial [29].

Summary

In Australasia, healthcare quality reporting is comprehensive but largely unintegrated. This lack of linked data about the quality and safety of care provided to individual patients was identified as a major drawback for effective healthcare improvement by a report from the Grattan Institute [30]. Healthcare providers and funders, both government and private, should share the data they collect with the hospitals and healthcare practitioners who deliver the care so that comparisons can be made and exemplary care shared with all. These data are about process, complications and patient experiences and should be reported in a transparent and accessible way. In turn, providers and hospitals have no access to patient outcomes after discharge from care. These metrics are held in registries or outcome studies and are available only to the contributors or researchers. So, actions to correct deficiencies in the standard of care are limited by the lack of integration of data because the people who can make changes do not have all the information. Integration of data at all levels of reporting should lead to better-quality healthcare for the people that matter the most, the individuals that receive that care.

Acknowledgement The authors acknowledge the contributions of Prof. S.B. Tan *(Director of Spine Service, Dept. of Orthopaedic Surgery, Singapore General Hospital)*, Mr. William Yeo *(Senior Manager of the ODC)* and Ms. Chong Hwei Chi *(Senior Principal Physiotherapist).*

References

1. Australian Bureau of Statistics. Census 2016.
2. Statistics Singapore. Singstat.gov.sg
3. Duckett SJ. The Australian healthcare system. Melbourne.: OUP; 2004.

4. Global Burden of Disease Study 2016. Institute for Health Metrics and Evaluation, University of Washington, Seattle. http://ghdx.healthdata.org/gbd-2016
5. Most efficient healthcare around the world. Bloomberg.com
6. Australian Institute of Health and Welfare 2017. The burden of musculoskeletal conditions in Australia: a detailed analysis of the Australian Burden of Disease Study 2011. Australian Burden of Disease Study series no. 13. BOD 14. Canberra: AIHW.
7. Australian Institute of Health and Welfare 2016. Impacts of chronic back problems. Bulletin 137. Cat. no. AUS 204. Canberra: AIHW.
8. Singapore Burden of Disease Study Group. Epidemiology & Disease Control Division, Ministry of Health, Singapore, 2014.
9. Institute of Medicine. 1990. Medicare: a strategy for quality assurance, vol. 2. Kathleen Lohr, editor. Washington, DC: National Academy Press.
10. Donabedian A. Evaluating the quality of medical care. Milbank Mem Fund Q. 1966;44:166.
11. Agency for Healthcare Research and Quality. The National Healthcare Quality Report; 2003.
12. Wilson RML, Runciman WB, Gibberd RW, Harrison BT, Newby L, Hamilton JD. The quality in Australian health care study. Med J Aust. 1995;163:458–71.
13. Hamilton JD, Gibberd RW, Harrison BT. After the quality in Australian health care study, what happened? Med J Aust. 2014;201(1):23.
14. Jackson T, Michel JL, Roberts RF, Jorm CM, Wakefield JG. A classification of hospital-acquired diagnoses for use with routine hospital data. Med J Aust. 2009;191(10):544–8.
15. The Australian Council on Healthcare Standards. Australasian clinical indicator report: 2009–2016. 18th ed.
16. Chen A, Retegan C, Vinluan J, Beiles CB. Potentially preventable deaths in the Victorian audit of surgical mortality. ANZ J Surg. 2017;87:17–21.
17. Runciman WB, Hunt T, Hannaford NA, Hibbert PD, Westbrook JI, Coiera EW, Day RO, Hindmarsh DM, McGlynn EA, Braithwaite J. CareTrack: assessing the appropriateness of health care delivery in Australia. MJA. 2012;197(2):100–5.
18. McGlynn EA, Asch SM, Adams J, Keesey J, Hicks J, DeCristofaro A, Kerr EA. The quality of health care delivered to adults in the United States. N Engl J Med. 2003;348(26):2636–45.
19. Australian Commission on Safety and Quality in Health care. The First Australian Atlas of Healthcare Variation; 2015.
20. Australian Commission on Safety and Quality in Health Care. The First Australian Atlas of Healthcare Variation; 2017.
21. Clement RC, Welander A, Stowel C, Cha TD, Chen JL, Davies M, Fairbank JC, Foley KT, Gehrchen M, Hagg O, Jacobs WC, Kahler R, Khan SN, Lieberman IH, Morisson B, Ohnmeiss DD, Peul WC, Shonnard NH, Smuck MW, Solberg TK, Stromqvist BH, Van Hoof ML, Wasan AD, Willems PC, Yeo W, Fritzell P. A proposed set of metrics for standardised outcome reporting in the management of low back pain. Acta Orthop. 2015;86(5):523–33.
22. Van Hoof ML, Jacobs WCH, Willems PC, Wouters MWJM, De Kleuver M, Peul WC, Ostelo RWJG, Fritzell P. Evidence and practice in spine registries. Acta Orthop. 2015;86(5):534–44.
23. National Health and Medical Research Council. Evidence-based management of acute musculoskeletal pain. Canberra: NHMRC; 2004.
24. Williams CM, Maher CG, Hancock MJ, McAuley JH, McLachlan AJ, Britt H, Fahridin S, Harrison C, Latimer J. Low back pain and best practice care: a survey of general practice physicians. Arch Intern Med. 2010;170(3):271–7.
25. Ramanathan SAS. Appropriate care for low back pain in Australia: evidence, expert opinion, current practice and patient perspectives. PhD thesis, University of South Australia, 2016.
26. Goh MR, Po IYY, Olafsdottir K. Low back pain in Changi General Hospital: an observational study. Proc Singapore Health Care. 2010;19(3):175–82.
27. Rajaee S, Bae H, Kanim L, Delamarter R. Spinal fusion in the United States: analysis of trends from 1998 to 2008. Spine. 2012;37:67–76.
28. Harris IA, Dao ATT. Trends in spinal fusion surgery in Australia: 1997 to 2006. ANZ J Surg. 2009;79:783–8.

29. National Institute for Health and Care Excellence. Low back pain and sciatica in over 16s: assessment and management. Invasive treatments. NICE guideline NG59. Methods, evidence and recommendations. London: NICE; 2016.
30. Duckett S, Jorm C, Danks L. Strengthening safety statistics: how to make hospital safety data more useful. Melbourne: Grattan Institute; 2017.

Healthcare Systems: India

13

Satish Rudrappa, Deepak Venkatesh Agarkhed, and Sushrut S. Vaidya

General Overview: The Healthcare System of India

Around 5,500 years ago, India's history begins with the Indus-Saraswathi civilization. The Ayurveda, a traditional Indian Medical heritage, was a system of medicine and lifestyle that is practised since ancient Vedic India (> 4000 years). Acharya Charaka, around sixth century BCE, was one of the prime contributors to Ayurveda [1] and was known as "Father of Indian Medicine". Approximately the same time, Acharya Sushruta, the "Father of Indian Surgery", founded the science of Salyatantra (Salya, broken parts of an arrow; tantra, manoeuvers). He was the author of the treatise known as "Sushruta Samhita", which is the foundation of surgery and gives details about surgical instruments, surgical techniques like incisions, probing, extraction of foreign bodies, thermal cauterization, excisions and trocars for draining abscess.

Yoga [1] is part of Vedic philosophy. Maharishi Patanjali, the "Father of Yoga" compiled in his Yoga Sutras (aphorisms). He promoted the Ashtanga Yoga, the eightfolds path of Yoga, Yama (self-restraint), Niyama (self-purification by self-restraint and discipline), Asana (seat or posture), Pranayama (control of breath), Pratyahara (sense withdrawal), Dharana (one-pointed concentration), Dhyana (meditation) and Samadhi (total absorption), for overall development of the human being. These components advocate meditation, breath regulations, physical discipline and restraining the sense organs. The Marjari, Meru Prishthasana, Vyaghrasana, Triyak Bhujangasana, Dhanurasana, Ardha Matsyendrasana and Khatu Pranam

S. Rudrappa (✉)
Neurosciences Department, Sakra World Hospital, Bangalore, Karnataka, India

D. V. Agarkhed
Sakra World Hospital, Bangalore, Karnataka, India

S. S. Vaidya
Economics Department, International College of Liberal Arts (iCLA), Kofu, Yamanashi Prefecture, Japan

J. Ratliff et al. (eds.), *Quality Spine Care*,
https://doi.org/10.1007/978-3-319-97990-8_13

asana are believed to have positive effects on human spine. Yoga has gained popularity in the Western world for its physical, mental and spiritual benefits, resulted in the declaration of June 21 each year as International Day of Yoga by United Nations General Assembly (UNGA).

The progress of India in all sectors including healthcare took backstage due to the policies of colonial British Raj [2]. A major contributor to the current burden of disease and disability in India may be due to lack of scientific or health research systems development during the British regime.

Presently, India is a country with a population of 1.2 billion, spread over 3-lakh sq. km. India is well known for its diversity and widespread cultural influence throughout the world. At present the total median age is 27.9 years despite a population growth rate of 1.17%. Modern population pattern shifts have indicated that over 33.5% of the population resides in urban areas. One of the challenges faced by Indian healthcare delivery systems is that one-quarter of the Indian population lies below the poverty line.

Public health is a state subject. The chief responsibility to provide quality healthcare services to the people of India lies with state governments. Post-independence there was gradual progress in the healthcare sector (Table 13.1). Many national programmes were started to control communicable diseases like malaria, polio and leprosy. Maternal and child health services like prenatal and postnatal care, immunization and oral rehydration therapy were initiated. The first National Health Policy of India (NHP) [3] was formulated in 1983. It focused on the provision of primary healthcare to all by 2000. A National Rural Health Mission (NRHM) [3] was launched in 2005.

Many factors led to growth of allopathic medical practice in India. The rapid development of allopathic medical practice in the Western world, coupled with developments in medical technology, and the breakdown of traditional education system under British colonial rule all contributed to a steady drift toward allopathic medicine. The practice of alternative medicine is still very popular in rural and semiurban areas. Considering this trend, India undertook the AYUSH [1] (Ayurveda, Yoga and Naturopathy, Unani, Siddha and Homoeopathy) programme in 2014. The goal of this effort is optimal development and propagation of Ayurveda, Yoga, Siddha and other alternative medicine elements. A total of 3,598 hospitals and 25,723 dispensaries across the country offer AYUSH treatment, thus ensuring availability of alternative medicine and treatments. In 2017, the Government of India has

Table 13.1 Development of health service in India

S. No.	Health infrastructure	1950–1951	1999–2000
1.	Registered medical practitioners (per 10,000 population)	1.7	5.5
2.	No. of medical colleges	0.28	167
3.	Hospital beds of all types (per 10,000 population)	3.2	9.3
4.	No. of doctors (in ‘000)	61.8	535.2
5.	Hospitals and dispensaries	9209	70,000
6.	No. of nurses	16,550	5,65,696

provided grant-in-aid for setting up of AYUSH educational institutions in states and union territories. India at present has 476 medical schools [4] training 61,390 students for a bachelor course in medicine and surgery.

The WHO report summarized in Table 13.2 provides many insights about the Indian healthcare system in comparison with 35 OECD countries (the Organization for Economic Co-operation and Development including Australia, Japan, the USA, France, and Israel) [5]. The health sector growth trend in India including forecast is shown in Fig. 13.1. With the huge Indian population, the Indian healthcare sector has huge growth potential.

Table 13.2 Comparison of health indicators of India and OECD countries

Health status indicator for 2015 year	Unit of measurement	India	OECD countries
Life expectancy at birth – male	Years	66.9	77.9
Life expectancy at birth – female	Years	69.9	83.3
Infant mortality	Infant deaths per 1000 live births	38	4
Under age 5 mortality	Under age 5 deaths per 1000 live births	48	5
Mortality from all causes	Proportions of all cause deaths, 2012 – %	Injury: 25 Non-communicable diseases: 63 Rest: 12	Injury: 8 Non-communicable diseases: 82 Rest: 10
Mortality from injuries in 2012	Deaths per 100,000 population	112	35
Proportions of injury deaths, 2012	%	Road traffic accidents: 20 Due to fall: 25 Rest: 55	Road traffic accidents: 18 Due to fall: 18 Rest: 64
Maternal mortality	Deaths per 100,000 live births	174	7
Tuberculosis – incidence rate	100,000 population	167	12
Diabetes among adults aged 20–79 years, crude estimates, 2014: male	Percent of population	7.9	9.1
Diabetes among adults aged 20–79 years, crude estimates, 2014: female	Percent of population	7.5	7.6
Ageing: population aged 65 years and over	%	5.6	16.8
Road traffic deaths due to alcohol	%	4.7	
Doctors per 1000 population, 2014		0.7	3.3

(continued)

Table 13.2 (continued)

Health status indicator for 2015 year	Unit of measurement	India	OECD countries
Nurses per 1000 population		1.4	9.1
Radiation therapy units, 2013	Per million population	0.4	7.2
Hospital beds per 1000 population, 2005	Per 1000 population	0.9	4.7
Total expenditure on health per capita, public and private, international dollars, 2016	USD PPP	267 (25% on public, 75% private)	3453 (78% on public, 22% on private)
Change in out-of-pocket spending as a share of total expenditure on health, 2010–2014	% of total expenditure on health	62.4	
Pharmaceutical expenditure per capita, international dollars (USD PPP) 2014	USD PPP	100	
Vaccination rates for hepatitis B (Hep3) children aged around 1, 2014	%	70	91

Source: Health at a Glance Asia/Pacific 2016 OEDC, WHO

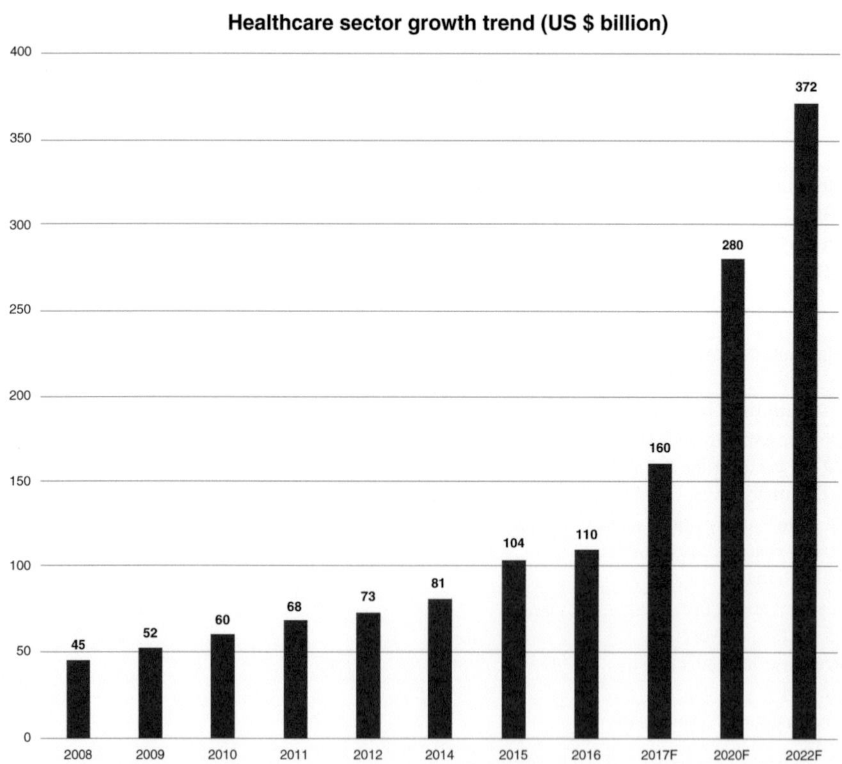

Fig. 13.1 Healthcare sector growth trend (Source: *Frost and Sullivan, LSI Financial Services, Deloitte, Aranca Research*)

Healthcare Delivery System of India

The current healthcare system of India comprises a set of public and private institutions, controlled by the state government, the central government and private organizations. While government spending is reserved for only those institutions owned and run by the central and state governments, India's dynamic medical structure is dominated by those controlled by private organizations. The healthcare system in India is improving, with increased partnerships between the government and private organizations to provide affordable healthcare to all. The Indian healthcare delivery system is classified into two major groups – public and private. The public healthcare system (owned by the government) includes limited secondary and tertiary care institutions in key cities and focuses on providing basic healthcare facilities in the form of primary healthcare centres (PHCs) in rural areas. The private sector delivers the majority of secondary, tertiary and quaternary care institutions with a major concentration in larger cities.

While the global average patient-bed ratio remains to be at 2.5 beds for 1000 individuals, India finds it challenging to provide even 0.9 beds for every 1000 individuals, perhaps suggesting doubts on India's healthcare structure. A contributing factor may be the budget allocation towards the health sector has been deficient in meeting the population's health demands. The gross domestic product (GDP) in India was 2263.79 billion US dollars in 2016. The GDP value of India represents 3.65% of the world economy. Only 1.3% of GDP was spent on healthcare in 2015–2016 by the centre and states. Most developed countries spend from 8% to 15% of GPD on healthcare. With only 4.7% of the gross domestic product (GDP) [6] being allocated towards healthcare in India, out of which 1.3% of the contribution coming from the public sector (government health spent) and 3.4% from the private sector, India's contribution of healthcare as a percent of GDP is one of the lowest in the world. Recent government budgets acknowledge the healthcare plight of India and promise certain goals for improvement in the near future.

Both allopathy and AYUSH are accessible to Indian patients. Figure 13.2 shows the overview of the current health system. However, as per NSSO [7] surveys, 90% of Indians prefer allopathy over AYUSH both in rural and urban India.

The *Lancet* analysed access to and quality of healthcare among and within countries using a new metric, the healthcare access and quality (HAQ) index based on

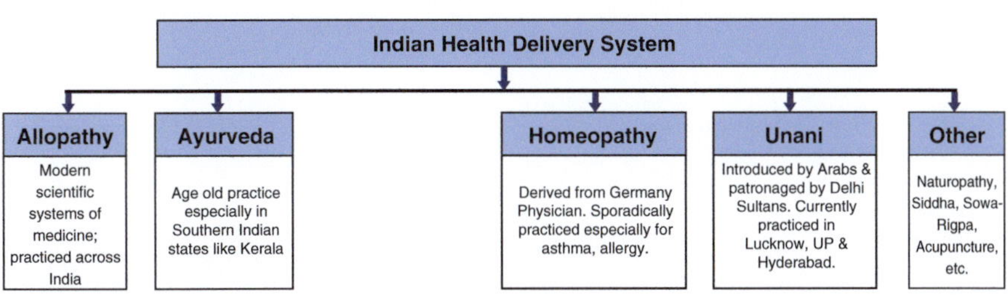

Fig. 13.2 Indian healthcare delivery system

mortality from causes amenable to personal healthcare. Even though India's HAQ index increased from 31 in 1990 to 45 in 2015, India still ranked 154th among 195 countries. In another *Lancet* study, which analysed progress towards universal health coverage (UHC) as one of the Sustainable Development Goal Indicators, India again underperformed relative to other countries, many of which were far less developed.

Public Healthcare System of India

The public healthcare system was originally developed to provide healthcare access regardless of socioeconomic status (Fig. 13.3). The report by the Bhore Committee [3] in 1946 is the foundation of current health policy and healthcare systems. It had recommendations for a three-tiered healthcare system to provide preventive and curative healthcare in rural and urban areas based on the population norms.

A sub-centre (SC) is established in each population of 3000 to 5000 people and serves as the first contact point between the primary healthcare system and the community. Each SC is required to be staffed by at least one auxiliary nurse midwife (ANM)/female health worker and one male health worker.

A primary health centre (PHC) is established in a population of 20,000 to 30,000 people and is the first contact point between the village community and the medical officer. PHCs were envisaged to provide integrated curative and preventive

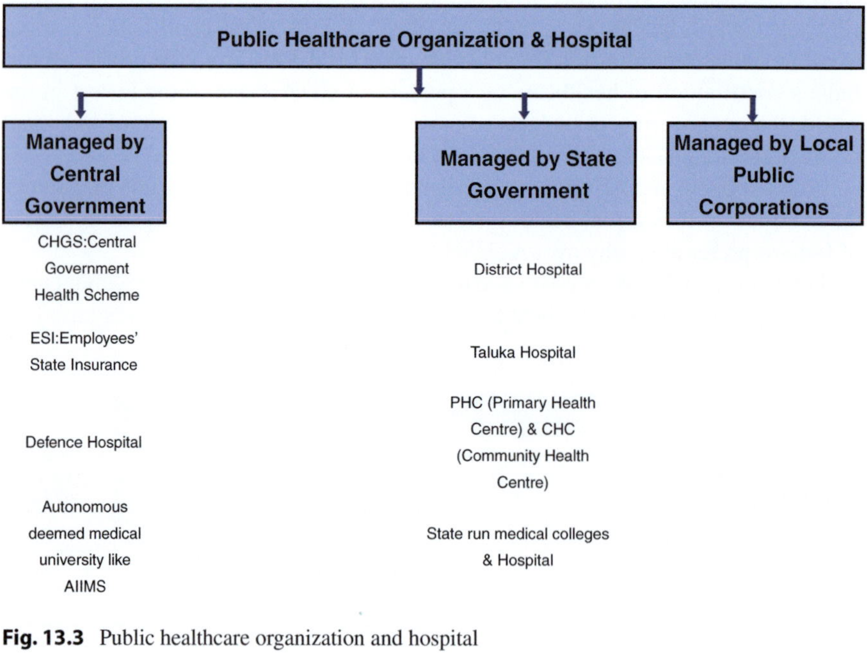

Fig. 13.3 Public healthcare organization and hospital

healthcare to the rural population. The PHCs which are established and maintained by the state governments are to be staffed by a medical officer supported by 14 paramedical and other staff.

Community health centres (CHCs) are established and maintained by the state government for populations of 80,000 to 120,000 people. A CHC is required to be staffed by four medical specialists, a surgeon, a general physician, a gynaecologist/obstetrician and a paediatrician. These physicians are supported by 21 paramedical and other staff. Facilities are mandated to have 30 beds with an operating theatre, X-ray, labour room and laboratory facilities.

In cases of an existing facility such as a district hospital or a subdivisional hospital, a CHC can be declared a fully operational first referral unit (FRU) provided it is equipped to provide round-the-clock services for emergency obstetric and newborn care, in addition to all emergencies that any hospital is required to provide.

Currently there are more than 700 district hospitals, 4,500 CHCs, 24,000 PHCs and 15,000 SCs in India.

Different factors related to public healthcare are divided between the state and national/central government systems in terms of decision-making. The central government addresses broadly applicable healthcare issues such as overall family welfare and prevention of major diseases, while state governments handle aspects such as local hospitals, public health and sanitation. These areas of focus may differ from state to state based on the particular communities involved.

To achieve Universal Healthcare (UHC), in 2017, the government of India proposed multiple new initiatives, including the National Health Policy (NHP), aimed at achieving universal health coverage and delivering quality healthcare services to all at an affordable cost. Pradhan Mantri Surakshit Matritva Abhiyan [8] (PMSMA) was taken up by the central government to provide quality antenatal care (ANC) to every pregnant woman in their second or third trimester, with the goal of reducing the maternal mortality rates.

Health insurance has not made significant penetration in the Indian market; less than 20% of the population has insurance coverage. Among these, 67% are covered under public insurance companies like New India Assurance, United India Insurance or National Insurance. There are multiple private insurance players within the country with variable penetrance. The various National Health Insurance Schemes are presented below.

National Health Insurance Schemes from Government

- Rashtriya Swasthya Bima Yojana (RSBY)
- Employment State Insurance Scheme (ESIS)
- Central Government Health Scheme (CGHS)
- Aam Aadmi Bima Yojana (AABY)
- Janashree Bima Yojana (JBY)
- Universal Health Insurance Scheme (UHIS)

Table 13.3 Government initiatives on healthcare

Government initiatives	Type of benefits	Government spending in US $
National Health Mission	To address the health needs of the underserved rural areas	13.16 billion
Intensified Mission Indradhanush (IMI)	The aim of improving coverage of immunization in the country and reaching every child under 2 years of age and all the pregnant women who have not been part of the routine immunization programme	
National Nutrition Mission (NNM)	To monitor, supervise, fix targets and guide the nutrition-related interventions across the ministries	Three-year budget of US$ 1.40 billion
LaQshya, for Labour Room Quality Improvement	The mobile application for safe delivery and operational guidelines for obstetric high-dependency units (HDUs) and intensive care units (ICUs)	
Ministry of Health and Family Welfare	To tackle lifestyle diseases such as cardiovascular disease (CVD), hypertension, obesity and diabetes in India	Planning to spend US$ 148.22 million

Source: Ministry of Commerce and Industry, Government of India

Around 155 million individuals are covered under the three central government-funded health programmes – Central Government Health Scheme (CGHS), Employees' State Insurance Scheme (ESIS) and Rashtriya Swasthya Bima Yojana (RSBY). Some of the recent major initiatives taken by the Government of India to promote Indian healthcare industry [9] are reviewed in Table 13.3.

Owing to the perceived poor quality of healthcare received at government/public institutions, studies have shown that over 57% of Indians prefer to receive medical care from private institutions compared to those owned and run by the government. Dependency on public and private healthcare systems varies across various states in India.

Private Healthcare System of India

When India became independent in 1947, the private health sector provided only 5–10% of total patient care. In 2005 it accounted for 82% of outpatient visits, 58% of inpatient expenditure and 40% of births in institutions [10].

India's challenges with the healthcare system remain skewed to rural areas as compared to the urban areas. This may be due to the focus on rapid development and the increase in the investments that take place on private healthcare development, catering to the evolving shift in incomes across urban settlers. While the public healthcare system struggles with managing its resources, the same may not be accurate in the private sector. Augmented by government initiatives, private organizations have slowly begun setting up their centres in Tier 2 and 3 sectors. Investments from local parties and through foreign multinational companies foster a systematic integration with the potential for competing with the larger international market. Studies have shown that due to the absence of universal health coverage in India, the out-of-pocket expenditure of the average individual contributes approximately 86% of the private healthcare expenditure.

One positive aspect of healthcare in India is that it is the largest sector in terms of revenue and providing employment. Via the Ministry of Commerce and Industry, the government of India has pointed out several important financial indicators about Indian healthcare. The hospital and diagnostic centres attracted foreign direct investment (FDI) worth US$ 4.99 billion between April 2000 and December 2017, according to data released by the Department of Industrial Policy and Promotion (DIPP). The hospital industry in India stood at US$ 61.79 billion in 2017 and is expected to increase at a compound annual growth rate (CAGR) of 16–17 per cent to reach US$ 132.84 billion by 2023. India is experiencing 22–25 per cent growth in medical tourism, and the industry is expected to double its size from the present (April 2017) US$ 3 billion to US$ 6 billion by 2018. Medical tourist arrivals in India increased more than 50 per cent to 200,000 in 2016 from 130,000 in 2015.

Private healthcare competition has been growing at an exponential rate, with hospitals now competing with one another in terms of the infrastructure for clinical and non-clinical services. India's competitive advantage lies in its large pool of well-trained medical professionals and competitive cost compared to its peers in Asia and Western countries.

Standardization of Indian Healthcare System

With the increase in the public awareness in health, there is a growing demand in India to have quality healthcare. NABH and NABL are accreditation bodies under the Quality Council of India set up by the Ministry of Commerce and Industry and the Department of Science and Technology, respectively. NABH and NABL have prescribed certain conditions for hospitals and diagnostic centres to be fulfilled before they are given accreditation certificates. NABH was set up with the cooperation of Ministry of Health and Family Welfare, Government of India and Indian Health Industry. The board was structured to accommodate the needs of the consumers and setting standards for the progress of the healthcare industry and to provide a boost to medical tourism (Fig. 13.4).

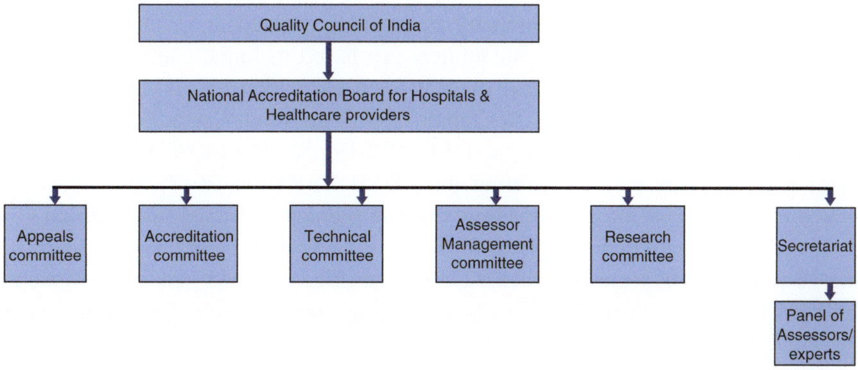

Fig. 13.4 NABH organization composition

Table 13.4 Key performance index of hospital

Name of key performance index	Name of key performance index
Bed occupancy rate & Bed turnover rate	Neonatal mortality (less than 28 days) & Infant mortality (less than 1 year)
Average length of stay	Percentage of demand met by blood bank
LAMA rate	Sputum positive rate
Nurse to bed ratio	Cycle Time for Diagnostic Reporting
Number of drugs expired during the month	Waiting time for OPD consultation
Percent of cancelled surgeries	Patient satisfaction index
Total no. of deaths on operation table and postoperative deaths	Down time of critical equipment
Anaesthesia-related mortality	Death audit conducted during the month
Surgical site infection rate	Medical audits conducted during the month
Biomedical waste management	Management review meeting conducted during the month
LSCS rate	Any other major events during the month

Source: District level hospital, Indian Public Health Standards (IPHS) [11]

The government has brought several hospitals under accreditation processes established by NABH. Some facilities have also had an external review of the quality of the healthcare being provided, with focus on high-quality clinical care, patient safety and respecting patient rights. Facilities are graded against a predetermined set of standards. There are international accreditation bodies, like Joint Commission International, who also provides accreditation for hospitals in India. Currently, there are more than 500 NABH accredited facilities in India. NABH is an institutional member of International Society for Quality in Health Care (ISQua), dedicated to promotion and support of continuous improvement in the safety and quality of healthcare worldwide. Table 13.4 reviews key performance indicators (quality measures) are typically measured in hospital having more than 100 beds [11].

Health Device Industries in India

The Indian Medical Devices industry is presently valued at USD $5.2 billion. Around 800 medical device manufacturers are based in India. Currently, India is counted among the top 20 global medical devices market and is the 4th largest medical devices market in Asia after Japan, China and South Korea. Equipment and instruments (surgical and non-surgical) form the largest segment (53% of the Indian medical device industry), constituting about USD 2.7 Billion (2017), while the estimated market size of the consumer and durable segment is USD $1404 million.

India's healthcare industry is one of the fastest-growing sectors, and in the coming 10 years, it is expected to reach $275 billion (Fig. 13.1). As part of the Make in India initiative, medical device parks are being commissioned to foster greater growth of this sector (Figs. 13.5 and 13.6) [12].

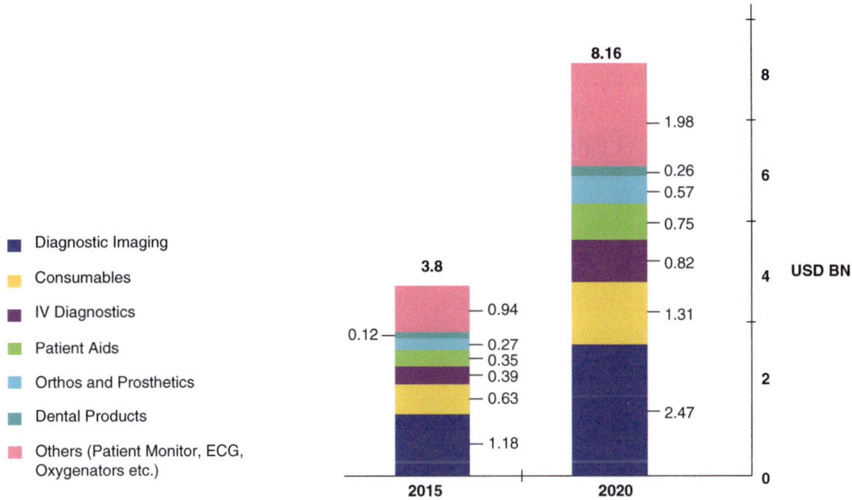

Fig. 13.5 Segment-wise market share of medical devices. (Source: Make in India)

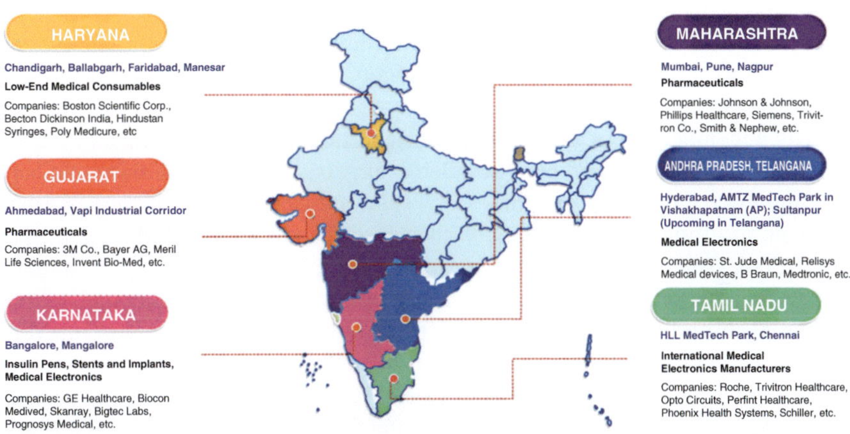

Fig. 13.6 Proposed medical device parks across India

Challenges in the Indian Healthcare System

Challenges remain for the Indian healthcare system. Even 70% of the population is in rural India, hospital infrastructure is concentrated in urban areas. This produces difficulties for accessing beds for rural patients. Although as many as 12 new All India Institute of Medical Sciences (AIIMS) facilities will be developed in different parts of India, there remains long way to go to make bed capabilities match the population. High-end medical devices are mostly imported from abroad, adding the cost of treatment, as India does not have proper R&D facilities and technology for manufacture. As part of the Make in India project, India is developing medical device technology park for research, development, manufacturing and training.

A substantial cost of patient treatment is consumed by drugs and other consumables; optimal price control may require regulatory bodies to insure patient affordability. Growth in healthcare education requires both quality and quantity, as huge numbers of medical staff go abroad. Although the government has made initiatives to private entities to engage in public-private partnership (PPP), with multiple windows for obtaining regulatory clearance, lack of concessions on land, power costs and customs duties on imported equipment remain impediments.

Spine Surgery in India

Until the late 1980s, spine surgery was practised sporadically in India, with spine surgeons mainly performing basic procedures related to degenerative diseases or trauma. By the early 1990s, many surgeons who had trained specifically in spine surgery in the United Kingdom and the United States returned to India. These local pioneers started spine surgery as sole practice and helped develop it to its present status as a dynamic subspecialty. Spine surgery is practised both by orthopaedic and neurosurgical trained specialists. Both specialties have their own spine societies with a membership of over 400 active spine surgeons in each. Considering the population of India, the number of available surgeons is few, and India would benefit from more training in the spine. Many spine surgeons practice mainly in urban hospitals resulting further deficits, with lack of access for semiurban and rural populations. There is a common fear among the public about the spine surgery, with the perception that surgeries may result in further neurological complications leading to disability. Hence acceptance of spine surgery for some is poor. Most patients, especially in rural regions, resort to traditional manipulative techniques rather than approaching the trained specialists. Scoliosis treatment is usually approached only when there is significant deformity leading to neurological and other complications.

Under the auspices of Medical Council of India, fellowship programmes are available to train in spine surgeries for both orthopaedic surgeons and neurosurgeons after completing their residency in their respective fields. There are about 15 hospitals across the country which offer their own fellowship programmes that are not accredited. Many centres perform surgeries mainly related to degenerative spine disorders; there is a dearth of training in deformity corrections.

With the easy access to MRI and CT scans, there is an increase in the detection and treatment of spinal disorders. Spine surgery as an aspect of the overall Indian healthcare market has grown by 32% in the last decade (Fig. 13.7). There are many international and national manufacturers which provide options for spinal instrumentation. Local manufacturers have a larger share than international brands.

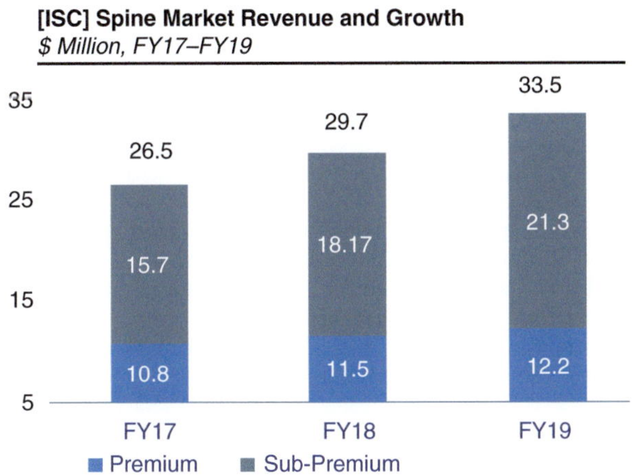

Fig. 13.7 Spine market revenue and growth in India

The cost of the implants manufactured by international companies is usually at an average of 50% more than locally manufactured products, due to multilevel government tax system and absence of local manufacturing from the multinationals within India.

Conclusion

Indian healthcare system is vast and complex. Considering the vast nature of the country with significant disparity in economic status, it will be difficult to have a uniform policy across the country. Malnutrition and communicable diseases are still prevalent which requires urgent intervention. Though universal healthcare is not uniformly distributed due to the participation of alternate medicine, primary healthcare to a certain extent is addressed, but secondary and tertiary care requires significant improvement. With the increase in the population especially in the rural areas, government health policies are not reaching to the predicted extent. Universal health schemes from the government, though required, will have greater economic burden which will result in the loss of quality care. With the increase in the migration to urban areas, there is a progressive participation of public and private health insurers.

As the healthcare sector is emerging as fastest growing sector in India, right direction and initiatives from both government and private players will make healthcare available, affordable, accessible and acceptable. Private participation with uniform policy of participating in health insurance policies from government will have a better future without compromising on patient safety and quality. Considering the vast market and consumption, it is imperative for the governmental organization to invest and also open the market for private participation. In addition, investment in healthcare manufacturing industry and basic science research will add greater value for the future.

References

1. AYUSH. Ministry of Ayush, Government of India, New Delhi. Retrieved May 25, 2008, from Ayush Web site: http://ayush.gov.in/about-the-systems (2018).
2. The Lancet. India-a tale of one country, but stories of many states. Lancet. 2017;390(10111):2413.
3. Chokshi M, Patil B, Khanna R, Neogi S, Sharma J, Paul V, et al. Health systems in India. J Perinatol. 2016;36(S3):S9–S12.
4. MICI. Medical council of India, New Delhi [Internet]. Retrieved May 25, 2008, from: https://mciindia.org/ActivitiWebClient/informationdesk/collegesearch
5. OECD/WHO. Health at a Glance: Asia/Pacific 2016: Measuring progress towards Universal Health Coverage. Paris: OECD Publishing; 2016.
6. KPMG, Union Budget 2017–18 | Healthcare, from KPMG Web site: https://home.kpmg.com/content/dam/kpmg/in/pdf/2017/02/Healthcare.pdf
7. Ministry of Statistics & Programme Implementation, New Delhi, from Web site: http://mospi.nic.in/download-reports?main_cat=NzIy&cat=All&sub_category=All
8. Pradhan Mantri Surakshit Matritva Abhiyan, Ministry for Health and Family Welfare, New Delhi.
9. Health care Industry in India, IBEF publication, Ministry of commerce; 2018.
10. Sengupta A, Nundy S. The private health sector in India. BMJ. 2005 Nov 19;331(7526):1157–8.
11. Indian Public Health Standards. National Health mission publication, IPHS revised guidelines; 2012.
12. Make in India. Retrieved May 20, 2008 [Internet]. Accessed at: http://www.makeinindia.com/article/-/v/sector-survey-medical-devices

Healthcare Systems and Quality Assessment of Spine Care in Japan

14

Motoki Iwasaki and Takahito Fujimori

Outline of the Healthcare System in Japan

The Japanese health insurance system initially started for workers in Japan during the 1920s when the employment-based health insurance plan was established. The universal health insurance system, which is regulated by the Japanese government, has provided comprehensive coverage to all citizens since 1961. There are several plans within the universal health insurance system based on age, employment status, and/or place of residence. Two major plans of health insurance are society-managed, employment-based health insurance and national health insurance. In general, the former covers workers at companies, while the latter covers the self-employed and unemployed.

The health insurance system in Japan covers all permanent residents by public medical insurance. This includes both Japanese and non-Japanese citizens.

Characteristics of Japanese Universal Health Insurance System [1]
- Covering all permanent residents by public medical insurance
- Freedom of choice of medical facilities
  (Free access)
- High-quality medical services with low costs

M. Iwasaki (✉)
Department of Orthopaedic Surgery, Osaka Rosai Hospital, Osaka University Graduate School of Medicine, Sakai, Osaka, Japan

T. Fujimori
Department of Orthopedic Surgery, Japan Community Healthcare Organization, Osaka Hospital, Osaka, Japan

J. Ratliff et al. (eds.), *Quality Spine Care*,
https://doi.org/10.1007/978-3-319-97990-8_14

All health insurance plans provide the same packages of medical care benefits, as determined by the national government. These benefits include hospital fee, outpatient fee, mental healthcare, prescription drugs, home healthcare, and most dental care. Patients are covered by some forms of public insurance system at relatively lower cost, including certain premiums and copayments (10–30%). Home care services are also covered by long-term care insurance. The benefit prices of medical services as well as drugs and approved medical devices are strictly regulated by the government and revised every other year. Private health insurance can provide only a supplementary service in Japan.

The premium rate for public health insurance is based on the individual's income, place of residence, and ability to pay. Cost-sharing varies according to one's age (Fig. 14.1). Patients' copayment for medical expenditure is basically 30%, with the exceptions for children under the age of 6 (20% copayment) and persons over the age of 70 with low incomes (10% copayment) [2]. In addition, there is a high-cost medical care benefit system. It is to avoid copayments made for medical costs becoming too expensive for family budgets (the maximum copayment is set up according to insured persons' income and age).

The Japanese healthcare system is characterized by free access to healthcare facilities and good quality of medical care with comparably low prices [2]. Patients can receive medical services of any physician or at any medical facility of their choice.

This universal health insurance system has been maintained for more than 50 years. Japan has the world's longest life expectancy although the financial management of its health care system has been growing increasingly challenging. Japan

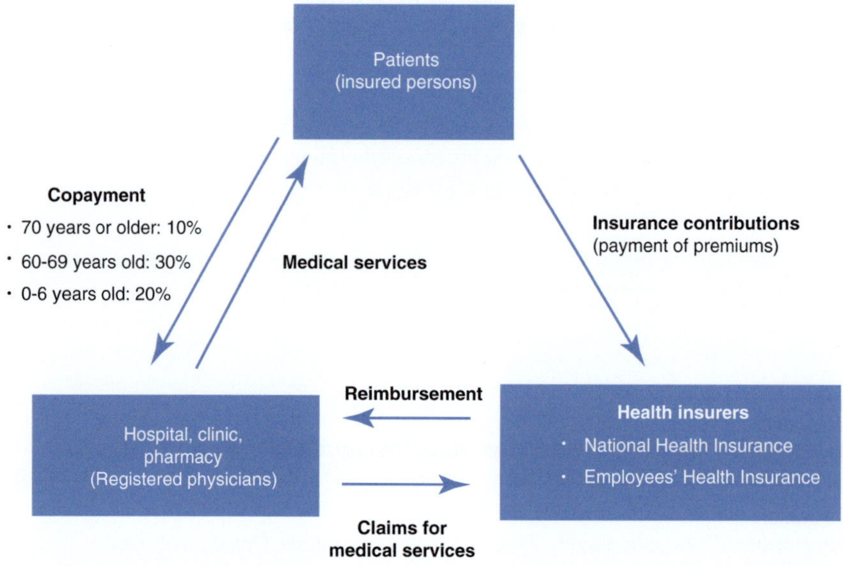

Fig. 14.1 Overview of medical services in Japan

is currently facing problems associated with its rapidly aging society; the number of elderly population is expected to grow from the current 16 million to 20 million by 2020. In contrast, the working population is expected to decline from 109 million to 100 million during the same period [1]. People aged 65 or older reached 27.3% of Japanese population in 2016 and are expected to reach 39.4% by 2055; the population of those over 75 years old will peak by 2025 [1]. The government introduced a medical care system for the elderly in 2008: The late-stage medical care system for the elderly covers those over 75 years old and early-stage medical care for the elderly aimed at 65–74-year-old patients.

Health-Related Outcome Assessments in Japan

The MOS 36-Item Short-Form Health Survey [3] and Euro-QOL 5D are commonly used health-related patient-reported outcome measurements in Japan. These measurements are validated in Japanese population [4, 5]. Users need to apply to the organizations for licensing [6, 7]. There are a variety of disease-specific measures of spine healthcare quality that impact evaluation of Japanese spine patients.

Disease-Specific Types of Health-Related Outcome Assessments: Cervical Spinal Disorders

Nurick Scale

The Nurick scale is physician-based measurement developed in 1972 [8, 9]. The Nurick scale is mainly focused on abilities to walk and to work. Patients are graded from 0 to 5 with higher scores indicating more disabled. The Nurick scale can simply evaluate ambulatory function that is a critical ability for patients. On the other hand, the Nurick score lacks evaluation of the motor function in the upper extremities and sensory function. There is currently no validated Japanese version available.

The Japanese Orthopedic Association (JOA) Scoring System for Cervical Spondylotic Myelopathy

The JOA scoring system for cervical spondylotic myelopathy (CSM) is a disease-specific, physician-reported scoring system developed in 1976 [10]. The scoring system was revised in 1994 [11]. The current JOA scoring system consists of seven domains: motor function in the fingers, motor function in the elbow and shoulder, motor function in the lower extremities, sensory function in the upper extremities, sensory function in the trunk, sensory function in the lower extremities, and bladder function. Calculation of the JOA score is straightforward. Total score can range from −5 to 17, counted by 0.5 point increments, with higher score indicating better function.

Interobserver and intraobserver reliability was tested by the committees of JOA [12]. The JOA scoring system has been widely used in daily clinical practice in

Japan. Nonetheless, there have been some critiques on the JOA scoring system. The domain of the fingers' function includes an ability to use chopsticks. Although chopsticks become spread in western countries, regular use of chopsticks is limited to East Asia. Thus, some authors have developed modified JOA scoring systems that omit the use of chopsticks [13, 14]. These modified JOA scores correlate with the original JOA score; however, the users need to recognize that the modified JOA scoring systems are not identical to the original JOA scoring system [15].

Second, there is not enough evidence of weighting of each score in each domain. It is unknown whether 1 point in motor function in the finger is equivalent for patient's activities of daily life to 1 point in motor function in the lower extremities. Third, statistical power is limited because the score distributes within a narrow range. To improve statistical power, the recovery rate proposed by Hirabayashi is often used [16].

The Japanese Orthopedic Association Cervical Myelopathy Evaluation Questionnaire (JOACMEQ)

The JOACMEQ is a disease-specific, patient-reported outcome measurement developed in 2007 (Table 14.1) [17]. The JOACMEQ was developed to cover the drawbacks of the JOA scoring system. The JOACMEQ consists of five domains: cervical spine function, upper extremity function, lower extremity function, bladder function, and quality of life. Factor loading of the questions is set up so that scores in each domain range from 0 to 100, with higher scores indicating a better condition and higher function. Reliability, internal consistency, criteria validity, and clinically important difference are tested when the JOACMEQ was developed [18–20].

A treatment for a patient is determined to be effective when the score change (the postoperative score-the preoperative score) of the patient is more than 20 points or the postoperative score of the patient is more than 90 points [20].

A drawback of this assessment tool is its complicated calculation of scores. The excel file for calculation can be downloaded from the developer website [21]. As the JOACMEQ is still a new scoring system, there are limited numbers of researchers that use the JOACMEQ as their primary outcome assessment tool.

Disease-Specific Type of Health-Related Outcome Assessments: Lumbar Spinal Disorders

Roland-Morris Disability Questionnaire (RMDQ)

RMDQ is a disease-specific, patient-reported measurement developed in 1983. RMDQ is a common assessment tool for low back pain in Japan. The Japanese version was reported in the literature [22].

Oswestry Disability Index (ODI)

ODI is a disease-specific, patient-reported measurement developed in 1980. ODI is a common assessment tool for lumbar surgery in Japan. Validated Japanese versions were reported in the literatures [23].

Table 14.1 Japanese Orthopaedic Association Cervical Myelopathy Evaluation Questionnaire

Question number	Question	Possible answers				
Q1-1	While in the sitting position, can you look up at the ceiling by tilting your head upward?	Impossible	Possible to some degree (with some efforts)	Possible without difficulty		
Q1-2	Can you drink a glass of water without stopping despite the neck symptoms?	Impossible	Possible to some degree	Possible without difficulty		
Q1-3	While in the sitting position, can you turn your head toward the person who is seated to the side but behind you and speak to that person while looking at his/her face?	Impossible	Possible to some degree	Possible without difficulty		
Q1-4	Can you look at your feet when you go down the stairs?	Impossible	Possible to some degree	Possible without difficulty		
Q2-1	Can you fasten the front buttons of your blouse or shirt with both hands?	Impossible	Possible if I spend time	Possible without difficulty		
Q2-2	Can you eat a meal with your dominant hand using a spoon or a fork?	Impossible	Possible if I spend time	Possible without difficulty		
Q2-3	Can you raise your arm? (Answer for the weaker side)	Impossible	Possible up to shoulder level	Possible though the elbow and/ or wrist is a little flexed	I can raise it straight upward	

(continued)

Table 14.1 (continued)

Question number	Question	Possible answers				
Q3-1	Can you walk on a flat surface?	Impossible	Possible but slowly even with support	Possible only with the support of a handrail, a cane, or a walker	Possible but slowly without any support	Possible without difficulty
Q3-2	Can you stand on either leg without the support of your hand? (The need to support yourself)	Impossible with either leg	Possible on either leg for more than ten seconds	Possible on both legs individually for more than ten seconds		
Q3-3	Do you have difficulty in going up the stairs?	I have great difficulty	I have some difficulty	I have no difficulty		
Q3-4	Do you have difficulty in one of the following motions: bending forward, kneeling, or stooping?	I have great difficulty	I have some difficulty	I have no difficulty		
Q3-5	Do you have difficulty in walking more than 15 minutes?	I have great difficulty	I have some difficulty	I have no difficulty		
Q4-1	Do you have urinary incontinence?	Always	Frequently	When retaining urine over a period of more than 2 hours	When sneezing or straining	No
Q4-2	How often do you go to the bathroom at night?	Three times or more	Once or twice	Rarely		
Q4-3	Do you have a feeling of residual urine in your bladder after voiding?	Most of the time	Sometimes	Rarely		

Table 14.1 (continued)

Question number	Question	Possible answers				
Q4-4	Can you initiate (start) your urine stream immediately when you want to void?	Usually not	Sometimes	Most of the time		
Q5-1	How is your present health condition?	Poor	Fair	Good	Very good	Excellent
Q5-2	Have you been unable to do your work or ordinary activities as well as you would like?	I have not been able to do them at all	I have been unable to do them most of the time	I have sometimes been unable to do them	I have been able to do them most of the time	I have always been able to do them
Q5-3	Has your work routine been hindered because of the pain?	Greatly	Moderately	Slightly (somewhat)	Little (minimally)	Not at all
Q5-4	Have you been discouraged and depressed?	Always	Frequently	Sometimes	Rarely	Never
Q5-5	Do you feel exhausted?	Always	Frequently	Sometimes	Rarely	Never
Q5-6	Have you felt happy?	Never	Rarely	Sometimes	Almost always	Always
Q5-7	Do you think you are in decent health?	Not at all (my health is very poor)	Barely (my health is poor)	Not very much (my health is average health)	Fairly (my health is better than average)	Yes (I am healthy)
Q5-8	Do you feel your health will get worse?	Very much so	A little bit at a time	Sometimes yes and sometimes no	Not very much	Not at all

Calculating formulas:
Cervical spine function: (Q1-1 * 20 + Q1-2 * 10 + Q1-3 * 15 + Q1-4 * 5-50)
Upper extremity function: (Q1-4 * 5 + Q2-1 * 10 + Q2-2 * 15 + Q2-3 * 5 + Q3-1 * 5-40) * 100/95
Lower extremity function: (Q3-1 * 10 + Q3-2 * 10 + Q3-3 * 15 + Q3-4 * 5 + Q3-5 * 5-45) * 100/110
Bladder function: (Q4-1 * 10 + Q4-2 * 5 + Q4-3 * 10+ Q4-4 * 5-30) * 100/80
Quality of life: (Q5-1 * 3 + Q5-2 * 2 + Q5-3 * 2 + Q5-4 * 5 + Q5-5 * 4 + Q5-6 * 3 + Q5-7 * 2 + Q5-8 *3-24) * 100/96)

The Japanese Orthopedic Association (JOA) Scoring System for Low Back Pain

The Japanese Orthopedic Association (JOA) scoring system for low back pain (LBP) is a disease-specific, physician-based scoring system developed in 1986 [24]. Since then, the JOA scoring system for LBP has been a common assessment tool for lumbar surgery in Japan. The JOA scoring system consists of four main domains: subjective symptoms, objective symptoms, activity of daily life, and bladder function, with subscales. Its total score can range from −6 to 29, counted by 1 point, with higher score indicating better function. Interobserver reliability, reproducibility, and validity were reported in the literatures [22, 24, 25]. As similar to the JOA scoring system for CSM, there is no sufficient evidence for weighting of each question.

The Japanese Orthopedic Association Back Pain Evaluation Questionnaire (JOABPEQ)

The JOABPEQ is a disease-specific patient-reported measurement developed in 2007 (Table 14.2) [20, 26, 27]. The JOABMEQ consists of five domains: low back pain, lumbar function, walking ability, social function, and mental health. Each questionnaire was created with reference to the short form health survey with 36 items and the Roland-Morris Disability Questionnaire. As with the JOACMEQ, reliability, internal consistency, criteria validity, and clinically important difference were tested when the JOABPEQ was developed. When the score change is more than 20 points, or the postoperative score is more than 90 points, the treatment is judged as effective [20, 28, 29].

Table 14.2 Japanese Orthopaedic Association Back Pain Evaluation Questionnaire

Question number	Question	Possible answers				
Q1-1	To alleviate low back pain, you often change your posture	Yes	No			
Q1-2	Because of low back pain, you lie down more often than usual	Yes	No			
Q1-3	Your lower back is almost always aching	Yes	No			
Q1-4	Because of low back pain, you cannot sleep well	Yes	No			

Table 14.2 (continued)

Question number	Question	Possible answers				
Q2-1	Because of low back pain, you sometimes ask someone to help you when you do something	Yes	No			
Q2-2	Because of low back pain, you refrain from bending forward or kneeling down	Yes	No			
Q2-3	Because of low back pain, you have difficulty in standing up from a chair	Yes	No			
Q2-4	Because of low back pain, turning over in bed is difficult	Yes	No			
Q2-5	Because of low back pain, you have difficulty putting on socks or stockings	Yes	No			
Q2-6	Do you have difficulty in any one of the following motions: bending forward, kneeling, or stooping?	I have great difficulty	I have some difficulty	I have no difficulty		
Q3-1	Because of low back pain, you walk only short distances	Yes	No			
Q3-2	Because of low back pain, you stay seated most of the day	Yes	No			
Q3-3	Because of low back pain, you go upstairs more slowly than usual	Yes	No			

(continued)

Table 14.2 (continued)

Question number	Question	Possible answers				
Q3-4	Do you have difficulty in going upstairs?	I have great difficulty	I have some difficulty	I have no difficulty		
Q3-5	Do you have difficulty in walking more than 15 minutes?	I have great difficulty	I have some difficulty	I have no difficulty		
Q4-1	Because of low back pain, do you avoid any routine housework?	Yes	No			
Q4-2	Have you been unable to do your job or ordinary activities as well as you would like?	I have not been able to do them at all	I have been unable to do them most of the time	I have sometimes been unable to do them	I have been able to do them most of the time	I have always been able to do them
Q4-3	Has your work routine been hindered because of pain?	Greatly	Moderately	Slightly	Very little	Not at all
Q5-1	Because of low back pain, do you get irritated or get angry at other people more often than usual?	Yes	No			
Q5-2	How is your present health condition?	Poor	Fair	Good	Very good	Excellent
Q5-3	Have you been discouraged and depressed?	Always	Frequently	Sometimes	Rarely	Never
Q5-4	Do you feel exhausted?	Always	Frequently	Sometimes	Rarely	Never
Q5-5	Have you felt happy?	Never	Rarely	Sometimes	Almost always	Always
Q5-6	Do you think you are in decent health?	Not at all (my health is very poor)	Barely (my health is poor)	Not very much (my health is average health)	Fairly (my health is better than average)	Yes (I am healthy)

Table 14.2 (continued)

Question number	Question	Possible answers				
Q5-7	Do you feel your health will get worse?	Very much so	A little bit	Sometimes	Not very much	Not at all

Calculating formulas:
Low back pain: (Q1-1 * 20 + Q1-2 * 20 + Q1-3 * 20 + Q1-4 * 10-70) * 100/70
Lumbar function: (Q2-1 * 10 + Q2-2 * 10 + Q2-3 * 20 + Q2-4 * 10 + Q2-5 * 30 + Q2-6 * 20-100) * 100/120
Walking ability: (Q3-1 * 30 + Q3-2 * 20 + Q3-3 * 10 + Q3-4 * 10 + Q3-5 * 30-100) * 100/140
Social function: (Q3-5 * 4 + Q4-1 * 2 + Q4-2 * 6 + Q4-3 * 10-22) * 100/74
Mental health: (Q5-1 * 3 + Q5-2 * 4 + Q5-3 * 6 + Q5-4 * 6 + Q5-5 * 3 + Q5-6 * 3 + Q5-7 * 3-28) * 100/103

Acknowledgment The authors thank Rena Iwasaki for English correction of this manuscript.

References

1. World Health Organization, Regional Office for South-East Asia. Japan health system review. Health Syst Transit. 2018;8(1):189–92.
2. Ministry of Health, Labour and Welfare. Health and Medical Services. http://www.mhlw.go.jp/bunya/iryouhoken/iryouhoken01/dl/01_eng.pdf
3. Fukuhara S, Bito S, Green J, Hsiao A, Kurokawa K. Translation, adaptation, and validation of the SF-36 health survey for use in Japan. J Clin Epidemiol. 1998;51(11):1037–44.
4. Fukuhara S, Ware JE Jr, Kosinski M, Wada S, Gandek B. Psychometric and clinical tests of validity of the Japanese SF-36 health survey. J Clin Epidemiol. 1998;51(11):1045–53.
5. Ikeda S, Shiroiwa T, Igarashi A, et al. Developing a Japanese version of the EQ-5D-5L value set. J Natl Inst Public Health. 2015;64(1):47–55.
6. EQ 5D. How to obtain EQ-5D. 2018.; Available from: https://euroqol.org/support/how-to-obtain-eq-5d/
7. iHopeQOL. MOS 36-Item Short-Form Health Survey. 2012.; Available from: https://www.sf-36.jp/index.html.
8. Nurick S. The natural history and the results of surgical treatment of the spinal cord disorder associated with cervical spondylosis. Brain. 1972;95(1):101–8.
9. Nurick S. The pathogenesis of the spinal cord disorder associated with cervical spondylosis. Brain. 1972;95(1):87–100.
10. Tsuyama N. The Japanese orthopedic association scoring system for cervical spondylotic myelopathy. J Jpn Orthop Assoc. 1976;50(5):11–2.
11. Hirabayashi K. The Japanese orthopedic association scoring system for cervical spondylotic myelopathy. J Jpn Orthop Assoc. 1994;68(5):134–47.
12. Yonenobu K, Abumi K, Nagata K, Taketomi E, Ueyama K. Interobserver and intraobserver reliability of the Japanese Orthopaedic Association scoring system for evaluation of cervical compression myelopathy. Spine (Phila Pa 1976). 2001;26(17):1890–4. discussion 5
13. Hamburger C, Buttner A, Uhl E. The cross-sectional area of the cervical spinal canal in patients with cervical spondylotic myelopathy. Correlation of preoperative and postoperative area with clinical symptoms. Spine (Phila Pa 1976). 1997;22(17):1990–4. discussion 5
14. Benzel EC, Lancon J, Kesterson L, Hadden T. Cervical laminectomy and dentate ligament section for cervical spondylotic myelopathy. J Spinal Disord. 1991;4(3):286–95.
15. Kato S, Oshima Y, Oka H, et al. Comparison of the Japanese Orthopaedic association (JOA) score and modified JOA (mJOA) score for the assessment of cervical myelopathy: a multi-center observational study. PLoS One. 2015;10(4):e0123022.

16. Hirabayashi K, Miyakawa J, Satomi K, Maruyama T, Wakano K. Operative results and postoperative progression of ossification among patients with ossification of cervical posterior longitudinal ligament. Spine (Phila Pa 1976). 1981;6(4):354–64.
17. Fukui M, Chiba K, Kawakami M, et al. An outcome measure for patients with cervical myelopathy: Japanese Orthopaedic Association Cervical Myelopathy Evaluation Questionnaire (JOACMEQ): part 1. J Orthop Sci. 2007;12(3):227–40.
18. Fukui M, Chiba K, Kawakami M, et al. Japanese Orthopaedic Association Cervical Myelopathy Evaluation Questionnaire (JOACMEQ): part 2. Endorsement of the alternative item. J Orthop Sci. 2007;12(3):241–8.
19. Fukui M, Chiba K, Kawakami M, et al. Japanese Orthopaedic Association Cervical Myelopathy Evaluation Questionnaire (JOACMEQ): part 4. Establishment of equations for severity scores. Subcommittee on low back pain and cervical myelopathy, evaluation of the clinical outcome committee of the Japanese Orthopaedic association. J Orthop Sci. 2008;13(1):25–31.
20. Fukui M, Chiba K, Kawakami M, et al. JOA Back Pain Evaluation Questionnaire (JOABPEQ)/JOA Cervical Myelopathy Evaluation Questionnaire (JOACMEQ). The report on the development of revised versions. April 16, 2007. The Subcommittee of the Clinical Outcome Committee of the Japanese Orthopaedic Association on Low Back Pain and Cervical Myelopathy Evaluation. J Orthop Sci. 2009;14(3):348–65.
21. The Japanese Society for Spine Surgery and Related Research. Outcome Assessment Tools. [cited 2018]; Available from: hottp://www.jssr.gr.jp/english/tool/index.html.
22. Fujiwara A, Kobayashi N, Saiki K, Kitagawa T, Tamai K, Saotome K. Association of the Japanese Orthopaedic Association score with the Oswestry disability index, Roland-Morris disability questionnaire, and short-form 36. Spine (Phila Pa 1976). 2003;28(14):1601–7.
23. Hashimoto H, Komagata M, Nakai O, et al. Discriminative validity and responsiveness of the Oswestry disability index among Japanese outpatients with lumbar conditions. Eur Spine J. 2006;15(11):1645–50.
24. Izumida S, Inoue S. The Japanese Orthopedic Association scoring system for low back pain. J Jpn Orthop Ass. 1985;60(3):4.
25. Fujimori T, Okuda S, Iwasaki M, et al. Validity of the Japanese Orthopaedic association scoring system based on patient-reported improvement after posterior lumbar interbody fusion. Spine J. 2016;16(6):728–36.
26. Fukui M, Chiba K, Kawakami M, et al. Japanese Orthopaedic Association Back Pain Evaluation Questionnaire. Part 3. Validity study and establishment of the measurement scale: subcommittee on low back pain and cervical myelopathy evaluation of the clinical outcome Committee of the Japanese Orthopaedic Association, Japan. J Orthop Sci. 2008;13(3):173–9.
27. Fukui M, Chiba K, Kawakami M, et al. Japanese Orthopaedic Association Back Pain Evaluation Questionnaire. Part 2. Verification of its reliability: the subcommittee on low back pain and cervical myelopathy evaluation of the clinical outcome committee of the Japanese Orthopaedic association. J Orthop Sci. 2007;12(6):526–32.
28. Kasai Y, Fukui M, Takahashi K, et al. Verification of the sensitivity of functional scores for treatment results – Substantial clinical benefit thresholds for the Japanese Orthopaedic Association Back Pain Evaluation Questionnaire (JOABPEQ). J Orthop Sci. 2017;22(4):665–9.
29. Fujimori T, Miwa T, Oda T. Responsiveness of the Japanese Orthopaedic Association Back Pain Evaluation Questionnaire in lumbar surgery and its threshold for indicating clinically important differences. Spine J. 2018. [Epub ahead of print].

Overview of Healthcare System in China

15

Xiongying Chen and Xiang Qian

Introduction

China, officially named the People's Republic of China (PRC), is the world's most populous country, with a population of around 1.382 billion in 2016 [1, 2] according to the Sixth National Population Census of the PRC in 2010. Since the "reform and opening up policy" initiated in 1979, China's gross domestic product (GDP) has grown rapidly for the past several decades with an annual growth rate around 8% and has now officially become the second largest economy in the whole world in 2017 [1, 2]. In 2017, China's GDP was 12.8 trillion USD, while China's healthcare spending was estimated only around 6.2 percent of GDP in 2016 [2], much lower as compared to that of the USA (17.9% in 2017) or other developed countries.

Healthcare in China Before 1949

After the end of imperial Qing dynasty, which lasted from 1644 until 1912, the Republic of China was established on January 1, 1912. In the following years, China was involved in unstable social and economic conditions with multiple wars, including the later Second Sino-Japanese War (1937–1945), ending with the civil war from 1945 to 1949. The civil war concluded with the Chinese Communist Party in control of mainland China [1]. Healthcare for those years before 1949 was very poor. According to the statistics of the government of the Republic of China in the 1930s, the death rate of 13 infectious diseases in China reached as high as 23%. The average life expectancy in China was 31 years before 1949 [3].

X. Chen (✉)
Jackson Hospitalist Program, Jackson Hospital, Montgomery, AL, USA

X. Qian
Anesthesiology, Preoperative and Pain Medicine, Stanford University School of Medicine, Stanford, CA, USA

J. Ratliff et al. (eds.), *Quality Spine Care*,
https://doi.org/10.1007/978-3-319-97990-8_15

During this period, traditional Chinese medicine had played major role, serving the country as the major source of medical services. Traditional Chinese medicine has an ancient history and has been practiced in China for thousands of years; it remains popular to the present.

The first Western medicine effort in China was the founding of a public dispensary for the Chinese at Macau in 1820 [4]. Medical missions in China by protestant Christian physicians and surgeons of the nineteenth and early twentieth centuries laid the foundations for modern medicine in China. Western medical missionaries established the first modern clinics and hospitals, provided the first training for nurses, and opened the first medical schools in China.

In the early twentieth century, missionaries from the USA and European countries started to build more hospitals and clinics in some major cities in China. They also established several Western hospitals. One of the hospitals located in Beijing called Xiehe Hospital (Peking Union Medical College Hospital, PUMCH) was founded in 1906 [5]. PUMCH not only served many sick Chinese patients and represented the highest medical level at that time in China but even after more than 100 years remains one of the top hospitals in China, according to recent best hospital rankings [5]. PUMCH was later affiliated to Peking Union Medical College (PUMC) which was founded in 1917 with support from the Rockefeller Foundation. PUMC is widely considered to be the best medical school in China.

Overview of PRC Healthcare System (1949–Now)

After the establishment of PRC in 1949, the Chinese Ministry of Health (CMH) supervised and controlled China's healthcare system and policies [6]. CMH, together with its counterparts in local provinces or cities, oversees the health needs of the Chinese people. An emphasis on public health and preventive medicine has characterized China's health policy since the early 1950s. At that time, the Chinese government started the "Patriotic Health Campaign," aimed at improving sanitation and hygiene, as well as treating and preventing infectious disease. Diseases such as cholera, typhoid, and scarlet fever, which were rife in China, were nearly eradicated by the campaign [1]. Before 1979, China was a planned economy system, and its healthcare payer system mainly composed of three major parts: the state medical insurance for government employees and military personnel, labor insurance and government insurance for urban people, and Rural Co-operative Medical Scheme (RCMS) for rural residents. All the hospitals and healthcare institutions were public, and healthcare services were largely free.

China's healthcare spending, accounting for about 3% of GDP at that time, had largely met the basic medical and health service needs of most members of society, and the national health level had rapidly improved [7]. Between 1952 and 1982, China's infant mortality rate fell from 200 to 34 per 1000 live births [8]. After the "reform and opening up policy" started in 1979, the public health condition of the Chinese people improved rapidly because of better living conditions, better nutrition, and better healthcare quality overall. However, many of the free public health services provided in the countryside shrank drastically along with the disappearance of people's communes.

After the economic reform and opening up policy, the national healthcare system has also followed the trend of reforms of other industries. The Chinese government gradually eased the direct economic control of the healthcare industry and allowed individual practitioners to enter the government management system [7]. Direct management of public hospitals by the government was reduced. Urban medical health insurance system reform was explored. In the middle of the 1980s, healthcare spending by the Chinese government reduced year by year, and the traditional social health insurance collapsed [9]. As a consequence, the low-income population, especially rural residents, was unfortunately exposed to significant out-of-pocket costs. Further, the Ministry of Health in 1992 put forward a slogan "the construction depends on the country, eat and live on your own," which led to hospitals beginning to focus more on profit and efficiency in patient care, while ordinary people started to pay more out of pocket for healthcare services.

From 1992 to the outbreak of SARS (severe acute respiratory syndrome) in 2003, government expenditure in healthcare as a whole showed a downward trend [10]. Medical service pricing reform started with the government abolishing direct pricing and allowing for-profit medical institutions to implement independent pricing and not-for-profit medical institutions to implement government-guided pricing [7]. "Pharmacy supporting medicine" and "Department contracting" were born under this background. After the 1990s, medical devices and equipment purchases became new venues for hospitals to generate income.

The cost of hospital visits for both urban and rural residents soared, and the phenomenon of "returning to poverty due to illness" increased significantly. By the year 2000, the proportion of personal out-of-pocket payments as a proportion of total medical expenses actually approached the level of 53% [10]. With many hospitals becoming more profit driven when practicing medicine, Chinese residents developed significant dissatisfaction with the Chinese healthcare system.

In 1997, with further economic development and increasing demand from the general public for better healthcare, the Chinese government started a healthcare reform initiative. The Ministry of Health played a leading role in the reform, with main focus on establishing a broader public insurance coverage and increasing the number of public healthcare providers, two main components in China's public healthcare system. In 1999, 49% of urban Chinese had health insurance, as compared with 7% of rural residents and 3% in China's poorest rural western provinces [8]. Three types of government-sponsored medical insurance systems (Urban Residents Basic Medical Insurance, Urban Employee Basic Medical Insurance, and New Rural Co-operative Medical Scheme) were piloted with the goal of covering more of the population [7]. A medical aid system was established in 2005, new in China at the time. The autonomy of healthcare providers was further expanded with a market-driven competition model gradually introduced into hospital management.

Another round of healthcare regulatory reform was started in 2006 due to the fact of "difficult to see a doctor and expensive to see a doctor" becoming a more prominent problem for the general public. Various departments started to strengthen the supervision of medical institutions and issued frequent guidelines to rectify the pricing of drugs, medical devices, lab tests and medical services. To ease the burden on the public healthcare system, the Chinese government also increased its funding to hospitals, rural clinics, and public health insurance agencies during those years, achieving some positive effects with the subsidies increasing annually. From 2000 to 2011, total healthcare expenditures in China increased from USD $51 to $305 per person, with average annual increase of 17.4%. The share of out-of-pocket payments in total health expenditure for the urban population declined from 53% in 2005 to 36% in 2011, with a smaller decrease for the rural population from 53% to 50% [11]. In 2009, the government began a 3-year large-scale healthcare provision initiative worth USD $124 billion [1]. The chief of the Ministry of Health declared the pursuit of a Healthy China 2020, a program to provide universal healthcare access and treatment for all of Chinese by 2020. This goal would be realized by revised policies in nutrition, agriculture, food, and social marketing [11]. Much of the program centered on chronic disease prevention and promoting better lifestyle choices and eating habits. It focused most on urban, populous areas that are heavily influenced by globalization and modernity. By 2011, the campaign resulted in 95% of China's population having basic health insurance coverage [1]. The Chinese central government has also been very supportive of improving China's public health literacy. In 2014, it allocated more than USD $40 million to fund local government programs in this field. There is also other funding, at $5.6 per head, for improving the basic public healthcare services, including health education [1]. Despite the hardship of medical care reform, great success was achieved over this period.

Healthcare in China recently became more privatized and experienced a significant rise in quality. The mortality rate for children under age five in China has dropped by more than two-thirds since 1990, while the maternal mortality rate has been cut by 70 percent [11]. As of 2015, the average life expectancy at birth in China was 76.34 years, and the infant mortality rate was less than 12 per thousand [2]. Both have improved significantly since the 1950s.

In spite of significant improvements in health and the construction of advanced medical facilities, China has several emerging public health problems, such as respiratory illnesses caused by widespread air pollution, hundreds of millions of cigarette smokers, and an epidemic increase in obesity among urban youths, among other public health concerns [1]. The "2020 Health Care Forecast Report" published by Deloitte Consulting predicated that by the year 2020, there will be 160 to 170 million people with high blood pressure in China, more than 100 million people with high cholesterol, 92.4 million with diabetes, and 70 million to 200 million people with overweight or obesity. There is one person suffering from cancer every 30 s in China, one person suffering from diabetes every 30 s, and at least one person dying of cardiovascular and cerebrovascular diseases every 30 s [12].

In October 2016, China National Health and Family Planning Commission (formally the Ministry of Health) issued the "Healthy China 2030 Planning outline," with the strategic theme of "co-building, sharing and Health for all" [11]. The goal of this project is to continuously improve people's health conditions; raise life expectancy to 79; control main health-endangering factors; improve health service, along with expansion in the health industry; and establish inclusive health-improving regulatory systems.

On March 27, 2018, China's National Health Commission replaced China's National Health and Family Planning Commission (NHFPC) as the ministry responsible for health and healthcare in the nation. Restructuring the government bodies sends a strong signal for healthcare system to work on transition from treatment-centered culture to prevention-focused strategy for health [13].

China's Healthcare Structure

The structure of China's healthcare system is complicated. Before 1980, healthcare in China was provided mainly by the government. The Chinese central government had overall responsibility for national health legislation, policy making, and administration. From year 1950 to 1980, the Chinese Ministry of Health was the highest authority for healthcare in China and controlled China's healthcare system and policies. Under the Chinese government, the country's officials rather than local governments largely determined access to healthcare. At those times, healthcare was essentially free to everyone in China. The government operated all clinics and hospitals, and it employed all doctors, nurses, and healthcare workers [8].

Since 1980, China has been experimenting with different systems of healthcare delivery. Free market healthcare reforms were tried, although the Ministry of Health still controls the overall healthcare system in China. In 2013, the Ministry of Health and the National Population and Family Planning Commission (NPFPC) were merged into the National Health and Family Planning Commission (NHFPC) as the main agency for health, under the supervision by the State Council. NHFPC and the local Health and Family Planning Commissions were the health authorities with primary responsibility for organizing and delivering healthcare and supervising hospitals and healthcare providers. The State Administration of traditional Chinese medicine is also affiliated with the NHFPC agency. The China Food and Drug Administration is responsible for drug approvals and licenses. Centers for Disease Control and Prevention exist in local provinces and cities and are administered by the local bureaus or departments of health. Both the National and local Health and Family Planning Commissions have comprehensive responsibilities for health quality and safety, cost control, provider fee schedules, health information technology, and clinical guidelines [6].

The Chinese government has also collaborated with the US Centers for Disease Control and Prevention (CDC) on public health priorities that affect China, the USA, and the global community for more than 30 years. The CDC focuses its China-based work on HIV/AIDS, emerging and re-emerging infectious diseases, immunizations, workforce development, influenza, communicable diseases, laboratory quality and safety, and global health security. The China-CDC partnership is increasingly dedicated to supporting China's role in the international public health community through dissemination of scientific information and support to other developing countries [14].

Various medical schools and hospitals in the USA have established collaboration agreements with Chinese counterparts to develop formal relationships for educational exchanges, joint research projects, patient care collaborations, as well as joint participation in international meetings.

China has increased its healthcare reform rhetoric, touting greater access for foreign investors to healthcare services in recent years.

China's health delivery system is fragmented and hospital-centered. From the perspective of delivery, there are four major categories of providers: hospitals, primary healthcare institutions, professional public health organizations, and others (physician clinics). There are two broad categories of business structure: public and private. With regard to management, there are government-run, social-run, and private-run facilities. China's hospitals divide into five categories: general hospitals, traditional Chinese medicine hospitals, integrated Chinese and Western hospitals, specialty hospitals, and national hospitals.

For primary healthcare institutions, since they are grassroots, the hierarchy is much more complicated. In the past, there were health centers (streets, townships), community health stations/health centers, village clinics/outpatient clinics, etc. For professional health institutions, they are mainly disease prevention/epidemic control centers, blood collection and supply stations, and professional organizations supervised by the Family Planning Commission. Of note, some maternity and child care institutions are not hospitals.

The three-tiered medical systems used in China must serve diverse needs of a large population. The tiers presently include township or village health centers, community health centers, and county or city hospitals. As of the end of October 2016, according to China's National Bureau of Statistics, there were 983,394 medical and health institutions nationwide, including 29,140 hospitals, 926,388 primary healthcare institutions, 24,866 professional public health institutions, and 3000 other health institutions (including family planning technical services) [15]. Among those hospitals, 12,708 are public hospitals and 16,432 are private hospitals. Although there are more private hospitals than public hospitals, 90% of major medical services in China are rendered by public hospitals [16]. Private hospitals have traditionally been viewed by many Chinese as having limited resources, with less qualified doctors than public hospitals, and potentially having profit-seeking motives. Among basic medical and health institutions, there are 34, 000 community health service centers (stations), 37, 000 township health centers, 642,000 village clinics, and 201,000 clinics (Clinical Offices) [17]. The Chinese Government hopes that those community health clinics can play a greater role in the future with the current ongoing new round of healthcare reform.

Hospitals in China are organized according to a three-tiered grade system that recognizes a hospital's ability to provide medical care and medical education and to conduct medical research. Based on this, hospitals are designated as primary, secondary, or tertiary institutions [18]. A primary hospital is typically a township hospital that contains less than 100 beds. They are tasked with providing preventive care, minimal healthcare, and rehabilitation services.

Secondary hospitals tend to be affiliated with a medium-sized city, county, or district and to contain more than 100 beds but less than 500 beds. They are responsible for providing comprehensive health services, as well as medical education, and for conducting research on a regional basis.

Tertiary hospitals complete the list as comprehensive or general hospitals at the city, provincial or national level with a bed capacity exceeding 500. They are responsible for providing specialist health services, perform a greater role with regard to medical education and scientific research, and serve as medical hubs providing care to multiple regions [18].

Based on the level of service provision, size, medical technology, medical equipment, and management and medical quality, the above grades of hospital systems are further subdivided into three subsidiary levels: A, B, and C. This results in a total of nine levels. In addition, one special level –3AAA is reserved for the most specialized hospitals [19]. This hospital system is hence referred to in Chinese as 3 grades and 10 levels.

At the end of 2016, there are 2232 tertiary hospitals (including 1308 tertiary grade A hospitals), 7944 secondary hospitals, 9282 primary hospitals, and 9682 unclassified hospitals in China. Among those large hospitals, there are 1602 hospitals with more than 800 beds [17].

Due to the lack of primary medical doctor and freestanding doctor's clinics in China, residents living in large cities usually go to the hospital for both basic and emergency medical care. Most patients in China can just walk into a hospital and pay for either a "special specialist care" appointment ticket or a "regular care" appointment ticket, based on different listing prices. High-quality medical resources are usually concentrated in China's largest cities. Private hospitals usually serve cash-paying patients, and most of private hospitals are specialty hospitals. Basic healthcare in China is quite affordable when compared with the options in Western countries.

Although most hospitals in China are public hospitals, financially they are independent, meaning that government only provides some basic expenditure with most other costs being the hospital's own responsibility to be generated through various medical services. Therefore more hospitals in large cities are starting to expand their facilities and increase bed numbers in order to admit more patients and attract more referrals from smaller hospitals. One of the largest hospitals in Henan province has more than 10, 000 beds (the most in the world) and is still expanding.

Medical Insurance System in China

Before 1978, urban residents who were mostly government employees were covered by labor insurance and government insurance. This insurance demanded minor out-of-pocket payment but was largely free. After major economic reforms, costs of healthcare rose rapidly. Many government employees lost their healthcare insurance due to reforms in state-owned enterprises [11, 20]. In 1984, the government started implementing free market reforms. People started to lose their free medical care, except those government employees. In 1997, China State Council issued a universal healthcare reform guidelines, an important part of which was to establish medical coverage in urban areas [7]. Urban Employee Basic Medical Insurance (UEBMI) and Urban Residents Basic Medical Insurance (URBMI) were created to cover healthcare expenses for urban-working residents and non-working residents, respectively. Both insurances were run by the Ministry of Human Resources and Social Security [19].

In 1998, UEBMI was introduced to provide healthcare access to urban-working and retired employees in public and private sectors. UEBMI is administrated at municipal level and is mandatory. It is the most generous public health insurance plan and has the highest average premiums and the highest reimbursement rate. The funds of UEBMI came from 8% of the employee's wage: 6% are paid by employers and 2% by employee contribution [11]; these rates vary by time and by municipality. In 2014, roughly 283 million were enrolled in UEBMI, contributing $12.97 billion USD in total and $45.83 USD per capita with expenditure of $10.8 billion USD in total and $38.19 USD per capita [16].

Urban Residents Basic Medical Insurance (URBMI) was piloted in 2007 and was implemented nationwide in 2010. URBMI provides healthcare access to urban residents that are not covered by UEBMI, including children; students in schools, colleges, and universities; and non-working urban residents [21]. It is a government-subsidized, household-level-voluntary medical insurance, administrated at municipal level. Funds of URBMI mainly rely on individual contributions ($39.5 USD for adults, and partly government contributions at least $12.9 USD per capita). Additional government contributions are given to undeveloped central and western regions and poor or disabled individuals [20].

For rural residents, Rural Co-operative Medical Scheme (RCMS) was established as a three-tiered system for rural healthcare access from 1950 to 1980. The RCMS functioned on a prepayment plan that consisted of individual income contribution, a village collective welfare fund, and subsidies from central government [11]. The first tier consisted of barefoot doctors, who were trained in basic hygiene and traditional Chinese medicine. These doctors lived in the village and provide easy access to the rural residents. Township health centers were the second tier of the RCMS, consisting of small, outpatient clinics that primarily hired medical professionals that were subsidized by the Chinese government. Together with barefoot doctors, township health centers were utilized for most common illnesses and disease prevention and vaccination [17]. The third tier of the RCMS, county hospitals, was for the most serious ill or complicated patients. They were primarily funded by the government but also collaborated with local systems for resources (equipment, physicians, etc.).

For those 30 years, although the health insurance system was not perfect, the RCMS focused on disease prevention and early intervention and significantly improved the health condition and life expectancy for rural area residents and decreased simultaneously the prevalence of certain infectious diseases. The malaria rate had dropped from 5.55% of the entire Chinese population to 0.3% of the population during that time. Life expectancy had almost doubled from 35 to 69 years;

infant mortality had been reduced from 250 deaths to 40 deaths for every 1000 live births [11]. In 1976, RCMS reached its peak and covered 85% of the total rural population. However, as a result of agricultural sector reform and the end of people's commune in the 1980s, the RCMS lost its economic and organizational basis and collapsed, with only 9.6% coverage in 1984. By 1999, only 7 percent of those living in rural regions had health insurance.

The New Rural Co-operative Medical Care Scheme (NRCMS) [11] was piloted in 2003 in response to the urgent need for affordable healthcare in rural China. By 2008, more than 90% of the total rural population was enrolled in NRCMS [22]. In 2016, Chinese government decided to merge NRCMS with URBMS to create a universal basic medical scheme [23]. NRCMS is a voluntary insurance scheme subsidized by local and central government. NRCMS differs from RCMS in the following perspectives: administration and risk-pooling are set at county level, much higher than RCMS's village level, and funds of NRCMS are provided by local and central government (for poorer regions) together, which contrasts with the old RCMS that was almost completely funded by the Chinese government and extended universally across all parts of rural China [22]. NRCMS covers expense in all level of public healthcare facilities, though the rate varies by regions and by type of facilities. It provided better access to higher-quality medical service and partly controlled medical costs. NRCMS is appropriate and convenient for China's enormous number of migrant workers who used to have limited access to healthcare [24]. In 2015, NRCMS spent 45 billion USD on 670 million participants and 1.653 billion instances of medical service, with the average of 67.25 USD per capita [15].

However, there are some difficulties that undermine the scheme's effectiveness in reducing out-of-pocket medical costs. Firstly, the benefit package of NRCMS is mostly limited to catastrophic and inpatient care. While these costs are covered, most outpatient visits require substantial individual payment [20]. Secondly, the reimbursement rate varies across level of healthcare facilities, increasing the cost of high-level hospital visit. The details of the NRCMS analysis report show that patients benefit most from the NRCMS at a local level. If patients go to a small hospital or clinic in their local town, the scheme will cover from 70 to 80% of their bill, but if they go to a county one, the percentage of the cost being covered falls to about 60%, and if they need specialist help in a large modern city hospital, they have to bear most of the cost themselves, as the scheme would cover only about 30% of the bill [25]. Due to the inequality of the skill and knowledge of lower-level healthcare physicians and providers, rural residents often do not trust their local doctors even in the county level and would prefer going to large modern city to seek medical care, especially those cancer patients or those patients with heart or lung diseases. This has significantly increased their medical cost out of their own pocket. Furthermore, fee-for-service reimbursement model in the current healthcare system provides incentives for healthcare providers to overprescribe medicine and perform unnecessary procedures or treatments, further adding to the cost [26]. In addition, despite NRCMS reduced actual cost of medical service, patients tend to purchase more medical service (often at their own cost) when under the service of NRCMS, offsetting its effects [27].

Although China now has world's largest health insurance network, China is simply too big and currently still has more than 30 million people living in poverty. A major illness can still lead a family to poverty. The government understands the task of poverty alleviation and has made a commitment to the entire society by winning this tough battle. Among the poor, many are destitute due to major illness and lost capability to work or return to poverty after self-paying for treatment of serious illness under insufficient health insurance coverage. In 2018 and beyond, the Chinese government will continue to intensify its efforts in this regard. The government will use half of the subsidized funds for basic medical insurance while increasing public finances to support major illness insurance, making it possible for more than 20 million people to have access to this type of insurance that cover for major illness, with effort on expanding disease coverage in coming years [28]. At the same time, the government aims to make high-quality medical resources available to broader coverage through the support of "internet plus medical care" and "telemedicine" programs, so that more patients with medical needs can access quality medical resources both offline and online. The Chinese government has also recently encouraged the development of private health insurance sector as a valuable supplement to the public scheme.

Traditional Chinese Medicine

One of the major differences in healthcare systems between China and other countries is the implementation of traditional Chinese medicine (TCM) along with Western medicine, which plays a big role in healthcare in China. China is the only country in the world where Western medicine and traditional Chinese medicine are practiced alongside each other at every level of the healthcare system. Although Western medicine dominates the medical practice, TMC has not been considered as supplementary with the fact that there are a lot of large and tertiary TCM hospitals located all over in China. TCM includes herbal remedies, acupuncture, acupressure, medical massage, moxibustion, and others, including nutritional therapy, which has a unique theoretical and practical approach to the treatment of disease and has developed over thousands of years. TCM-based practice accounts for about 40% of all healthcare services delivered in China in 1997 [29] with somewhat less percentage of healthcare expenditure nowadays.

As with most forms of traditional medicine, the theoretical and diagnostic basis of TCM cannot be fully explained through the standard Western medicine anatomy and pathophysiology perspective. TCM has gathered more acclaim in the last several decades in the West. The Chinese government strongly encourages and promotes TCM through government subsidies to this date. Part of the reason is the belief and trust toward TCM by the general public in China, as well as due to the fact that there are not enough Western medicine-trained physicians in China, especially in the countryside. In spite of the popularity of TCM in China, Chinese patients in general still consider Western medicine superior and being the first choice for medical care.

Challenges of China's Healthcare System

Since the new round of healthcare reform started in 2009, the Chinese government struggles to figure out an effective way to deliver better healthcare service to its 1.3 billion people.

Currently, many minority groups are facing challenges in gaining equality in healthcare access. Due to the 1980s health reform, there has been a general increase in government health subsidies, but, even still, individual spending on healthcare has significantly increased. Inequality between urban and rural areas persists, since much of recent government reform is focused on urban areas [30]. Despite efforts by the NCRMS to combat this inequality, it is still difficult to provide high coverage universal healthcare to rural areas. The unbalanced nature of China's economic development has made China's medical development unbalanced. To add further to this rural inequality challenge, much of the elderly population lives in rural areas are largely remain underinsured while that have been facing even more difficulties in accessing quality healthcare [30].

China's healthcare system in general keeps basic wages low, leading doctors to an incentive-driven practice model including overdiagnosis and procedures and possibly unnecessary surgeries [31]. Second, as in many other countries, to develop a universal coverage for country of this size (1.3 billion people) is an unprecedented challenge, not to mention China's population is getting older faster than anywhere else in the world [30]. Several different healthcare models have been developed across the country to attempt to address those challenges, including the reintroduction of community-based primary care programs, but its effect remains to be seen.

Overdiagnosis, overutilization of medical equipment, and overtreatment are very common in China. Patients stayed in the hospital much longer due to the fact that hospital expenses are more likely to be covered by health insurance while outpatient care expenses are not.

Independent physician clinics or primary care clinics are rare in China and most outpatient clinic services are rendered inside the hospital. Patient medical costs may be offset for evaluation and treatment done in the hospital. Otherwise patients unfortunately will have to pay by their own for outpatient-based diagnosis and treatments. For instance, an uncontrolled diabetes patient will be advised to stay in the hospital for 10 days until the blood glucose is under control, rather than managed as an outpatient. Although the individual patient may pay less, overall healthcare costs are much higher.

Overcharging and overprescribing by physicians is a common theme in many underfunded public hospitals. Physician's low salaries raise the appeal of accepting kickbacks offered by pharmaceutical or medical device companies, although government strongly opposes this behavior and ban this practice with harsh punishments including suspension and even criminal charges in some case. In 2013, 48% of outpatient revenues and 39% of inpatient revenues at tertiary hospitals were from drug prescriptions, according to data from National Health and Family Planning Commission [32].

China is aging fast. The Chinese population is getting older faster than anywhere else in the world. The Chinese government is not fully prepared for this aging problem, and China only has a weak safety net to provide coverage for the elderly. By 2050, the proportion of the population over 65 years old in China is projected to reach around 34%, roughly 500 million people. China's dependency ratio for retirees could rise as high as 44% by 2050.

With population structure changes and with growing numbers of elderly people in China needing a variety of outpatient and chronic care-based medical services, such as primary care, rehabilitation, long-term care facilities, and others, this will become a significant challenge for China's hospital-centered healthcare system, especially as those services are still in their infancy.

China began introducing EHRs to their hospitals and clinics in 2005. Since then, they have been working hard to expand EHR use to as many facilities as possible, under the specific standards and guidelines laid out by the Health Information Standards Professional Committee (HISPC) of the Ministry of Health (MOH). As of 2014, half of all tertiary hospitals in China use their own EHR system, as do 30% of urban health centers and 20% of rural hospitals. This growth is only expected to continue. Unfortunately, those many hundreds of EHR and EMR systems are developed or are operating in different regions with limited or very little cross-region data sharing. There is currently no central governance over regional development and unified planning for a national system. There is in general lack of willingness to share information as well, and there is no general guidance, and it is usually an individual doctors' decision to share medical or health information between different medical and health institutions.

Finally, primary care is still a relatively new term in China. Many Chinese patients who seek medical help in China typically bypass primary care physicians and go straight to hospital-based specialists. In a country once well known for its readily accessible "barefoot doctors," primary care is now in poor condition. As discussed in previous sections, PR China established a three-tiered healthcare system after its foundation in 1949. Primary-level facilities (including community health facilities in urban areas, township health centers, and village clinics in the rural areas) mainly help provide preventive and basic medical services, whereas secondary and tertiary hospitals provide specialized care. Nevertheless, the government was less financially supportive of healthcare industry and has held less accountability since the economic reform in the 1980s. The barefoot doctor model was gradually dismantled when a shift in funding from primary healthcare to hospital-based care occurred; this led to the proliferation of specialized care in hospitals with substantial loss of primary care.

In recent years, China has shifted toward strengthening the primary care system and promoting utilization of primary care. All levels of government have devoted resources into primary care infrastructure construction, personnel training, and other supporting programs, including salary reforms, a zero-profit drug policy, and insurance schemes at the primary care level, in order to reach the major targets of China's ambitious health reforms to meet its people's escalating healthcare needs [33].

Promoting primary care is a major target of the latest health reforms initiated in China in 2009. However, the underutilization of primary care is a prominent problem all over the country, and in general it has not improved with previous health reforms. Underlying causes are multifactorial but can include the following factors: unequal distribution of quality medical providers and medical resources, low training quality of PCPs, the public's lack of trust in the quality of primary care, lack of a gatekeeping function by PCPs, and the detrimental elements of health reform policies focusing on specialty care. One of the efforts to combat this is the development of a grading diagnosis and treatment system, which has been proposed for some time with its purpose to effectively utilize a two-way semi-mandatory referral system to direct patients from a primary care physician to different levels of the specialty hospitals according to patient's condition and severity. Hospitals are asked to give priority access to those patients who are referred by primary care physicians.

Quality Control of China's Healthcare System

Quality is the lifeline of all industries. For the medical industry, quality and safety are directly related to human life and thus are the core part of China's medical reforms.

The Chinese government has taken measures to implement the better quality control measures and the entire health industry has made joint efforts to constantly strengthen the management of medical quality and safety and upgrade systems to be more scientific, more standardized, and more refined [34].

The Department of Health Care Quality, which is within the Bureau of Health Politics and Hospital Administration and is overseen by the National Health and Family Planning Commission (now the National Health Commission), is responsible at the national level for the quality of medical care. The National Health Service Survey is conducted every 5 years (the latest was done in 2013), and a report is published after each survey highlighting data on selected quality indicators [6]. Hospitals and various health institutions use this data to improve their quality stands in the nation.

To be accredited in China, hospitals must obtain a license from the local health authority. Physicians get their practice licenses through hospitals; licenses are subject to renewal. Several national rankings of hospitals are published by third parties, although there are no financial incentives for hospitals to meet quality targets currently. No public quality information about individual doctors is made available [6].

China has a large population. In 2016, the total patient visits nationwide reached 7.93 billion, an increase of 3.1% (240 additional million patient visits) from 2015, and hospital admission nationwide reached 227 million, an increase of 16 million or 8% from 2015 [34].

Previously, the management of medical quality in many hospitals in China continued the traditional method of "statistical data reporting," with facilities regularly reporting data on various medical indicators, such as the average length of stay, mortality rate, and hospitalization cost for various disease treatments. These reports were shared in the internal hospital quality meetings. These reports were generally department based. Medical societies and the Chinese authorities realized there were opportunities to improve this system.

As early as 2004, realizing that clinical drug administration, especially antimicrobial drug management, was an important part of developing a scientific system for delivery of quality medical care and that bacterial resistance had become a very important public health problem in the world, the Ministry of Health promulgated antibacterial drug usage principle and a national antibiotic treatment guideline was issued.

Some technical monitoring systems on the rational use of antimicrobial drugs and the control of drug resistance were established and achieved success over the years. The proportion of antibiotics usage among all medications in medical institutions was 19.7% in 2010, and it has dropped to 11.2% in 2016 [34]. With the more standardized and rational use of antimicrobial drugs, the trend of drug resistance in recent years has been contained. The incidence of MRSA in 2011 in China was about 50% and was less than 30% in 2017, with some hospitals seeing their MRSA occurrence rate to be slightly above 20% [34]. At present, China has established a bacterial resistance surveillance network in more than 1400 hospitals. At the same time, the country vigorously promotes rational clinical drug use and standardizes diagnosis and treatment behaviors in order to control cost and improve quality.

Following release of the "Temporary Directing Principles of Clinical Pathway Management" by the former Ministry of Health in 2009, clinical pathways are now regulated nationally and used in a similar manner as clinical guidelines in Western countries [6]. Established clinical pathways cover more than 1212 disease categories in more than 30 clinical disciplines, and clinical pathway management has been implemented in nearly 7000 hospitals in China [34]. Previously, pathways were created at the individual hospital, rather than the national level [6].

In order to promote the management of medical quality, to strengthen medical quality management, to standardize medical service behavior, and to ensure medical safety, in 2016 the China National Health and Family Planning Commission issued the "Measures for the Management of Medical Quality." The measures gave detailed instructions regarding quality control indicators covering medical institutions, various clinical specialties, and medical technology. It clarified 18 core systems for quality and safety of medical care, including the patient first visit-physician responsibility system, the three-level hospital rounding system, the complicated case discussion system, and the surgical safety checking system, and required all medical institutions to establish internal medical quality control policy. The program also established a Medical Quality (Safety) Information system for adverse events data collecting, recording and reporting. In August 2017, China has established 36 state-level quality control centers that cover the major clinical specialties [34]. Each individual province (region, city) had also established its own quality control centers, and there are a total of more than 1200 quality control centers nationwide. The quality control centers at all levels assist the health and family planning administrative departments to carry out daily quality control work, strengthen vertical and horizontal linkages, and form a network to become a continuous improvement in the quality of medical care in China.

Finally, China's health administration is pursuing the standardization of medical quality and safety supervision. The Chinese government has gradually built and improved national, provincial, and regional medical quality and safety management information reporting, monitoring, and sharing mechanisms to improve medical quality and safety management. They have selected representative and critical quality control indicators and adopted the method of multicenter data source system assessment to organize the preparation of the "National Medical Service and Quality and Safety Report" [34].

With these efforts, the efficiency of medical services and medical service capabilities in China has continuously improved. The in-hospital mortality rate in the secondary and tertiary public hospitals has gradually decreased and stabilized at a relatively low level. In 2015, the total mortality rate of hospitalized patients in tertiary public general hospitals and secondary public general hospitals was 0.71% and 0.48%, respectively, which was 0.03 and 0.06 percentage points lower than in 2014; the hospitalized deaths of surgical patients were 0.38% and 0.21%, respectively. Grade 3 general hospitals fell 0.03 percentage points from 2014, and grade 2 general hospitals remained basically the same as 2014. This data is the result of statistical analysis of 64 million inpatients in nearly 3000 hospitals in China [34].

According to the China Health Statistics Yearbook 2016, the efficiency of medical services in China continues to increase. The average length of stay in hospitals in 2016 was 9.4 days, which was a decrease of 0.2 days compared to 2015; the average length of stay in third- and second-level public general hospitals was 10.1 days and 8.8 days respectively, which was 0.3 days and 0.1 days lower than 2015 respectively [15]. In the past 5 years, the efficiency of China's medical services has been analyzed through the average hospitalization day index and the trend has been declining year by year, which shows that the efficiency of medical services is continuously improving in China.

In May, 2017, Lancet published the global ranking of medical quality and accessibility in 195 countries around the world [35]. The ranking of the global medical quality shows that China has been one of the countries with the largest improvement in the quality of medical care from 1990 to 2015. China's ranking has increased from 110th at the time in 1990 to the 60th in 2015, ranking the third in the world in terms of progress for those 15-year period. The gap index in the quality of interregional medical services in China also narrowed. Such a gap index reduction indicates that while the quality of medical care in China continues to increase, so does the degree of homogeneity.

Quality Control of Spine Care in China

Due to the recent rapid economic development in China, there has been rapid development in the biomedical fields [36]. Spine care in China is also developing rapidly. According to 2010 statistical data, there were more than 50,000 Chinese orthopedic surgeons. Due to its vast population and emerging status, China is becoming a leading force in medical research, including in the field of orthopedics and spine care.

This increase has been paralleled by an increase in contributions to the scientific literature by Chinese spine surgeons [37].

In China, spine care is generally part of orthopedic departments, usually affiliated with a major hospital. Outpatient orthopedic surgical centers or independent groups of orthopedic surgeons are rare in China.

Various guidelines have been developed and published by experts in the orthopedic field as the guiding medical care of spine conditions, with topics such as "consensus of Chinese orthopaedic experts on diagnosis and treatment of ankylosing spondylitis" and "Prevention of venous thromboembolism after major orthopaedic surgery" [38–41]. There is no universal metrics or spine care quality control measures accepted nationwide. The quality control of spinal surgery relies on the individual hospital policy and especially individual orthopedic departments' policies. For instances, in one of the grade 3 hospitals in a large city in the southern part of China, the orthopedic department has detailed quality management policies regarding the operating room, nursing care, and rates of non-planned reoperations. For spinal surgery, the orthopedic department has a detailed guideline for various spinal surgery perioperative nursing care protocols.

Nationally, the mortality rate or surgical adverse event rates are not available publicly, although internally individual departments have statistics available for risk control and for internal quality improvement activities.

Most quality measures consist of process and structural measures rather than capturing patient outcomes. Patients in China choose their operating hospital based on health insurance arrangement, although they can choose whichever hospital they want to go to within a given system. There is no public information regarding individual hospital's quality performance available, so individual "word of mouth" and patient opinions may impact choice of a facility.

References

1. China. [Internet] [Accessed 2018 Apr 2]. Available from: http://en.wikipedia.org/wiki/China.
2. China Statistics year book 2017., www.stats.gov.cn/tjsj/ndsj/yearbook2017.
3. Life expectancy increases by 44 years from 1949 in China's economic powerhouse Guangdong. http://www.en.people.cn/90001/90776/90882/6776688.html.
4. Medical Missions in China. [Internet] [Accessed 2018 Apr 2]. Available from: http://en.wikipedia.org/wiki/China.
5. Peking Union Medical College. [Internet] [Accessed 2018 Apr 2]. Available from: http://en.wikipedia.org/wiki/China.
6. Fang H. China: International Health Care System Profiles. [Accessed 2018 Apr 2]. Available from: http://international commonwealthfund.org/countries/china. 2015.
7. Wang Xl. The historical evolution and institutional reflection of government regulation in Chinese Medical Market. [Accessed 2018 Apr 2]. Available from: http://www.hprc.org.cn/gsyj/jjs/hyyxs/201211/t20121130_205403.html.
8. Blumenthal CD, Hsiao W. Privatization and its discontents – the evolving Chinese health care system. N Engl J Med. 2005;353:1165–70.
9. Chen M, Zhao Y, Si L. Who pays for health care in China? The case of Heilongjiang province. PLoS One. 2014;9(10):e108867.

10. Long Q, Xu L, Bekedam H, Tang S. Changes in health expenditures in China in 2000s: has the health system reform improved affordability. Int J Equity Health. 2013 June 13;12:40.
11. Healthcare reform in China. [Internet] [Accessed 2018 Apr 2]. Available from: https://en.wikipedia.org/wiki/Healthcare_reform_in_China.
12. Deloitte Center for Health Solutions. Healthcare and Life Sciences Predictions 2020. A bold future? [Internet] [Accessed May 16, 2018] Available at: https://www2.deloitte.com/content/dam/Deloitte/global/Documents/Life-Sciences-Health-Care/gx-lshc-healthcare-and-life-sciences-predictions-2020.pdf.
13. Editorial, Health-care system transition in China. Lancet. 2018;391(10128):1332.
14. Centers for Disease Control and Prevention. Global Health – China. Page last updated: April 2, 2018. Accessed at: www.cdc.gov/globalhealth/countries/china.
15. China Statistics Yearbook 2016. www.stats.gov.cn/tjsj/ndsj/2016/indexch.htm.
16. China's hyped healthcare reform is stuck. [Accessed 2018 Apr 2]. Available from: wwwbusinessinsidercom, Aug 9, 2015.
17. State Council. Health and Family Planning Committee. China Health and Family Planning Statistical Yearbook 2016: Beijing Peking Union Medical College Press; 2017. isbn:9787567906433.
18. Classification of Chinese Hospitals. [Internet] [Accessed 2018 Apr 2]. Available at: https://en.wikipedia.org/wiki/Classification of Chinese Hospitals.
19. State Council, China. "Guidelines on Urban Residents Basic Medical Insurance Pilots" 2007., http://www.gov.cn/zhuanti/2015-06/13/content_2878973.htm.
20. Barber SL, Yao L. Development and status of health insurance systems in China. Int J Health Plann Manag. 2011 Oct 1;26(4):339–56.
21. Ministry of Health, China State Council. China Health Statistic Yearbook 2008. Beijing: Peking Union Medical College Press; 2008. ISBN 9787811360578. OCLC 276710548
22. Wagstaff A, Magnus J, Gao LX, Junchen Q. Extending health insurance to the rural population: an impact evaluation of China's new cooperative medical scheme. J Health Econ. 2009;1:1–19.
23. Pan XF, Xu J, Meng QY. Integrating social health insurance systems in China. Lancet. 2016;387(10025):1274–5.
24. Meng QY, Xu K. Progress and challenges of the rural cooperative medical scheme in China. Bull World Health Organ. 2014;92(6):447–51.
25. Liu YL, Hu SL, Fu W, Hsiao W. Is community financing necessary and feasible for rural China? Health Policy. 1996;3:155–71.
26. Sun XY, Jackson S, Carmichael G, Sleigh AC. Prescribing behavior of village doctors under China's new cooperative medical scheme. Soc Sci Med. 2009;68(10):1775–9.
27. Cheng LG. NRCMS: Economic Effects or Health Effects? Economic Research Journal. 2012; 01:120–133-via CNKI.
28. Li KQ. At least 20 million people should be able to enjoy major illness insurance this year. Economy Daily March 2018;13:11.
29. Hesketh T, Zhu WX. Health in China. Traditional Chinese medicine: one country, two systems. BMJ. 1997 Jul 12;315(7100):115–7.
30. Chen LY, Standing H. Gender equity in transitional China's healthcare policy reforms. Fem Econ. 2008;13(3–4):189–212.
31. Liu YL, Hsiao WC, Eggleston K. Equality in health and health care: the Chinese experience. Soc Sci Med. 1999;10:1349–56.
32. Statistical Communique on the Development of Health and Family Planning in China in 2013. [Internet] [Accessed May 16, 2018] Available at: http://www.nhfpc.gov.cn/guihuaxxs/s10742/201405/886f82dafa344c3097f1d16581a1bea2.shtml.
33. Shanxi Health and Family Planning Yearbook 2016. Northwest University Press, ISBN: 978-7-5604-3800-9.
34. Health and Family Planning Commission held medical quality publicity media meeting. August 15, 2017. [Internet] [Accessed 2018 Apr 2]. Available from: http://www.nhfpc.gov.cn/zhuz/xwfb/201708/18dd11c70ea74e6595a64fab49a0b73f.shtml.

35. GBD 2015 Healthcare Access and Quality Collaborators, and others. Healthcare Access and Quality Index based on mortality from causes amenable to personal health care in 195 countries and territories, 1990–2015: a novel analysis from the Global Burden of Disease Study 2015. Lancet. 2015;390(10091):231–66.
36. Zou YM, Li Q, Xu WD. Scientific research output in orthopaedics from China and other top-ranking countries: a 10-year survey of the literature. BMJ Open. 2016;6(9):e011605.
37. Jia ZW, Ding F, Wu YH, He Q, Ruan D. The 50 most-cited articles in orthopaedic surgery from mainland China. Clin Orthop Relat Res. 2015 Jul;473(7):2423–30.
38. Qiu GX, Dai KR. Operative orthopaedics. 1st ed. Beijing: People's Medical publishing House; 1982.
39. Qiu GX, Dai KR. Operative orthopaedics. 3rd ed. Beijing: People's Medical publishing House; 2005. p. 1061.
40. Chinese Orthopaedics Association. Chinese specialist consensus on treatment of customary pain in orthopaedics. Orthop Surg. 2010;2:169–74.
41. Chinese Orthopaedic Association. Prevention of venous thromboembolism after major orthopaedic surgery. Orthop Surg. 2010;2:81–5.

Part IV

Implementation of Quality Reporting

16 Conditions of Care and Episode Groups

Mohamad Bydon, Mohamed Elminawy, and Mohammed Ali Alvi

Increased Spending on Healthcare in the USA

For several decades, administrators and policy advisors have made efforts to curb healthcare costs. The USA has been ranked as the highest spending nation in percent GDP expenditure on healthcare for the last decade, with annual healthcare expenditure reaching $3.1 trillion in 2014, approximating one-fifth of the entire economy [1]. Moreover, despite high spending on healthcare, the USA has low rankings on certain health performance indicators among its peers [2, 3]. Efforts to control increasing costs have been made by all fronts of healthcare including provider organizations, insurance companies, and government payers. Policy reforms introduced by the Affordable Care Act (ACA) predominantly focused on the reimbursement and incentive structure of the current system.

Transition to Value-Based Care

The predominant fee-for-service (FFS) system focuses solely on the services provided and does not account for patient outcomes or for service costs. This led to increased costs by rewarding providers for the volume and complexity of services they provide on a per capita basis [4, 5]. Toward the end of last decade, several investigators found that higher intensity of care does not necessarily result in higher quality of care. Moreover, studies found that significant cost savings may be readily achievable by focusing on ways to reduce unnecessary and preventable hospital

M. Bydon (✉) · M. Elminawy · M. A. Alvi
Mayo Clinic Neuro-Informatics Laboratory, Mayo Clinic, Rochester, MN, USA

Department of Neurologic Surgery, Mayo Clinic, Rochester, MN, USA
e-mail: Bydon.Mohamad@mayo.edu

J. Ratliff et al. (eds.), *Quality Spine Care*,
https://doi.org/10.1007/978-3-319-97990-8_16

inpatient admissions and readmissions, emergency department (ER) visits, unnecessary inpatient lengths of stay, preventable conditions and hospital-acquired conditions, unnecessary invasive procedures, and high-end diagnostic tests [6–10]. The concept of "value" in healthcare was further defined, focusing upon the quality of healthcare provided to patients through the attributes of accessibility, patient experience, and quality of service relative to cost-effectiveness. The aim of "value"-based care is to provide optimal healthcare to the population using the least amount of resources necessary, thereby lowering the cost.

With the advent of the ACA, this value-based care model was adapted and a task force was developed to design innovative payment models. This task force was led by the Center for Medicare and Medicaid Services (CMS) Innovation Center. Its guiding principle was to "test innovative payment and service delivery models to reduce program expenditures…while preserving or enhancing the quality of care furnished to individuals under such titles." Several value-based purchasing (VBP) initiatives were introduced including but not limited to accountable care organizations (ACO) [11], Comprehensive Care for Joint Replacement model, a cardiac payment model [12], Hospital Inpatient Quality Reporting Program [13], and Bundled Payments for Care Improvement Initiative (BPCI) (Table 16.1).

Table 16.1 Human Health Services (HHS) framework categorizing healthcare payment according to how providers receive payment

Payment framework				
	Category 1	Category 2	Category 3	Category 4
Shifting from volume to value	Fee-for-service with no link to quality	Fee-for-service with link to quality	Alternative payment model built on fee-for-service architecture	Population-based payment
Description	Payments are based on volume of services and not linked to quality or efficiency	At least a portion of payment vary based on the quality or efficiency of healthcare delivery	Some payment is linked to effective management of a population or an episode of care.[a] Payments are still triggered by delivery of services, but opportunities for shared savings or 2-sided risk	Payment is not directly triggered by service delivery so volume is not linked to payment. Clinicians and organizations are paid and responsible for the care of a beneficiary for a long period of time (e.g., >1 year)
Examples of some currently innovative programs undertaken by CMS	Limited in Medicare fee-for-service as majority of payments now are linked to quality	Hospital value-based purchasing program, Physician Value-Based Modifier (VM) program,[b] Readmission/Hospital-Acquired Condition Reduction Program	Accountable care organizations, medical homes, Bundled Payments for Care Improvement, ESRD Quality Incentive Program, Medicare-Medicaid financial alignment initiative fee-for-service model	Advanced payment programs for eligible organizations

Courtesy of cms.gov

[a]Episode groups are established for Category 2, 3, 4 to help the shift toward value-based purchasing programs

[b]The resource portion of MIPS will replace the current VM program

Bundled Payments for Care Improvement Initiative (BPCI)

BPCI was launched in January 2013 by the US Center for Medicare and Medicaid Services (CMS) through its innovation center authority. This payment system was envisioned to account for all costs associated with patient care for a single visit or "episode." In the context of surgical care, this translates into a single payment for the hospital, the operating physician, instrument and equipment cost (examples include biologics, bone graft, spinal instrumentation, etc.), and providers of post-acute care. The goal of bundled payment systems is to transition the risk of cost management from the payer to healthcare providers so that unnecessary procedures, diagnostic testing, and long postoperative lengths of stay could be discouraged [14, 15]. Under this model, decisions regarding apportionment of care and resources within an episode are shifted from the payer to individual providers and hospitals. This was launched as a 3-year program, endorsed by the US Secretary of Human and Health Services [16], as part of a broader effort to test the feasibility of *episode-based payment models* which could help transition from the current FFS payment system to a pay-for-performance (P4P) payment system while maintaining focus on health outcomes [17]. Soon after the announcement, a pilot study was initiated by CMS in collaboration with selected providers to test the efficacy of episode-based bundling in ten acute care conditions.

In this pilot study, for a patient undergoing a surgery, an episode was defined as the period from 3 days before surgery to 30 days following discharge from the hospital. A *bundle* is initiated when a patient is admitted to the hospital. CMS has taken 179 diagnosis-related groups (DRGs) and rolled them into 48 different *episode groups*, capturing many of the high volume and high cost of care conditions including stroke, spinal fusion, major joint procedures, congestive heart failure (CHF), pneumonia, etc. [18].

BPCI defined four models in which patients were evaluated as either A) all Medicare Severity Diagnosis-Related Groups (MS-DRGs) (model 1) or B) 48 *episode groups* (models 2–4). Models 1 and 4 focus on an inpatient setting, whereas models 2 and 3 create opportunities for providers to manage patients while they are on the continuum of care. Healthcare providers including hospitals, physician group practices, and skilled nursing facilities constitute the "entities at risk." Third-party organizations that help to facilitate providers to participate in these programs are referred to as "conveners," while providers working under a convener are termed "episode initiators" (Table 16.2).

Table 16.2 Bundled payment care initiative models

	Model 1	Model 2	Model 3	Model 4
Episode	All DRGs; all acute patients	Selected DRGs; hospital plus post-acute period	Selected DRGs; post-acute period only	Selected DRGs; hospital plus readmissions
Services included in the bundle	All part A services paid as part of the MS-DRG payment	All non-hospice part A and B services during the initial inpatient stay, post-acute period and readmissions	All non-hospice part A and B services during the post-acute period and readmissions	All non-hospice part A and B services (including the hospital and physician) during initial inpatient stay and readmissions
Payment	Retrospective	Retrospective	Retrospective	Prospective

Courtesy of cms.gov

Differentiating Bundled Payment from Other Payment Models

There are nuances within bundled payment mechanisms that distinguish them from previous payment models. Payment of a fixed amount of money to a hospital is not new; DRG-based payments have been in use since the advent of Prospective Payment System (PPS) in 1983 [19]. This system does not incentivize hospitals to improve their outcomes and cost-efficiency nor does it incentivize them to ration care away from sicker patients, one of the potential adverse consequences of a move to bundled payments [20].

There have been other examples of bundled cost payments in the USA. The Texas Heart Institute over 30 years ago initiated a single lump payment system for all coronary artery bypass grafting (CABG) procedures [21]. The Geisinger Health System in 2007 also tried a similar payment system [22]. "Case-rate" payment systems are another example of bundled cost models that have been used for organ transplants.

Episode Groups

Episodes are defined as the set of services provided to diagnose, manage, and follow up on a clinical condition or treatment. Claims are structured based on episodes of care as they address a specific condition bounded by a time frame; for its pilot study, CMS set the timeline for surgical patients as 3 days preoperatively to 30 days post-discharge [23]. Episode groups are based on specific conditions or procedures, for example, the care provided during a hospital admission for spinal fusion surgery including the preoperative assessment, the procedure itself, the use of bone graft and other pertinent material, perioperative care provided by nurses and hospital staff, postoperative care while still inpatient, as well as postoperative care after discharge, such as a skilled nursing or rehabilitation facility. All services provided during the episode time frame are included in the episode groups. Trigger codes are diagnoses that define the episode, such as the ICD code for a lumbar fusion. The episodes also include "sequelae" codes for clinically plausible subsequent events, such as postoperative infections or deep venous thrombosis.

Terms Used in Episode Groups

Resource use: Resource use are the expenses spent during patient care. Currently programs like value-based payment modifier (VBPM) are being used by CMS to calculate resource use. With episodes of care, all related services provided over a defined period of time will be captured and evaluated.

Trigger codes: Diagnostic or procedure codes like ICD 9, ICD 10, CPT, HCPCS, or MS-DRG that initiate an episode group.

Relevant services: Procedure or service codes included in an episode group.

Look back period: The time before the trigger code occurs for services such as pre-operative evaluation.

Closing rule: The period following the trigger code.

Parts A and B Medicare claims data: Include the seven claim types: inpatient hospital facility, outpatient (OP) hospital facility, physician/supplier part B (PB), skilled nursing facility (SNF), home health (HH), hospice (HS), and durable medical equipment (DME).

Cost is defined by allowed amounts on Medicare claims data, which includes both Medicare trust fund payments and beneficiary deductible and coinsurance.

Types of Episode Groups Established

These are three types of episode groups on which cost measures can be based:

1. *Chronic Conditions Episode Groups*:
   These episode groups account for the patient's clinical history at the time of a medical visit and their current health status.
2. *Acute Inpatient Medical Condition Episode Groups*:
   These episode groups represent treatment for self-limited acute illness or treatment for flares or an exacerbation of a condition that requires a hospital stay.
3. *Procedural Episode Groups (Using CPT/HCPCS Codes)*:
   These episode groups focus on procedures of a defined purpose or type, e.g., axial decompression (including laminectomy), spinal fusion, treatment of spinal fracture, deformity, etc.

Episode of Care Conceptual Model

Episodes are made of three consecutive steps defining an episode using a combination of logic rules and medical billing codes specific to each episode type, namely, (a) opening, (b) grouping, and (c) closing [24] (Fig. 16.1).

(a) Opening (Triggering Codes)

A specific trigger code is identified by Current Procedural Terminology CPT codes, ICD procedure codes, or Healthcare Common Procedure Coding System (HCPCS) codes, and conditions are identified through specific Medicare Severity Diagnosis-Related Group (MS-DRG) codes or by using the International Classification of Diseases ICD-10 diagnosis code on a claim. Specific billing codes indicate the presence of the episode condition/procedure.

In some episodes, two separate occurrences are required to improve the likelihood that the patient has the medical condition [24]. Once a trigger event is identified, grouping algorithms begins, and either grouping, method A or B, is applied [24].

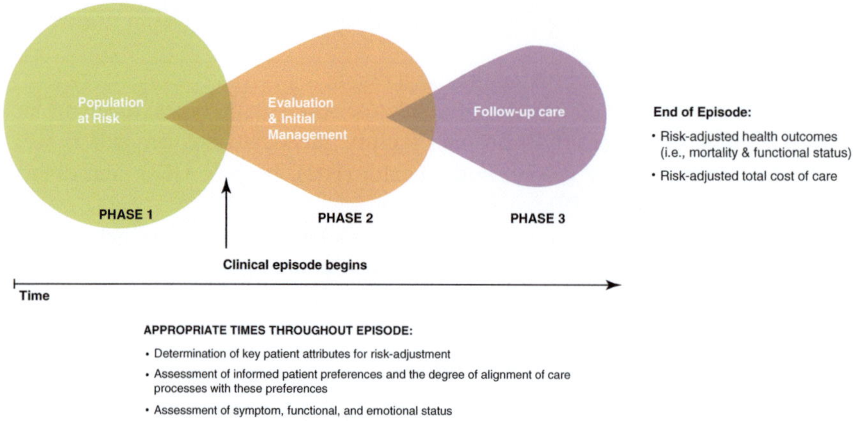

Fig. 16.1 Episode group construction. (Courtesy of cms.gov)

(b) Grouping Services

Once a trigger event is identified, a grouping algorithm pursues which utilizes clinical rationale to define associated services on the claims during the episode window. There are two main grouping methods. Method A was developed by the Center for Medicare and Medicaid Innovation to fulfill requirements of the ACA. Method B was developed by CMS based on supplemental QRURs. There are some commonalities and differences between both algorithms discussed below.

Method A

Method A uses a set of codes to identify an episode and stack them together. The first sets of codes are the trigger codes that determine which episode a diagnosis is most likely associated with. If more than one episode is opened at a time, method A will use a hierarchical set of rules to identify relatedness to each other. Additionally, codes for "relevant services" such as diagnostics testing and imaging are added. These codes are more general and could be relevant to more than one episode. Finally, the third set of codes is called "relevant diagnoses," which are signs, symptoms, and other diagnoses related to the episode condition or procedure.

Method A only scrutinizes the principal diagnosis on a given claim to determine if it is relevant. For each episode type, codes are specified based on their probable clinical relevance to an episode. An episode can be associated with another episode for two reasons: (i) when a procedure is performed for the treatment of a condition and (ii) when a procedure or condition episode is considered as aftereffects or secondary results of a condition.

Method B

Method B distinguishes two categories of care:

Treatment Services:

There are services explicitly related to the healthcare provider managing the patient's condition as well as ancillary services. For condition episodes, two types of services are considered treatment: (i) all services occurring during the trigger inpatient stay and (ii) physician services provided by the managing provider in the 3 days prior to the episode trigger event.

For procedural episodes, two types of services are considered treatment: (i) all services occurring on the day of the procedure (or all services during the inpatient stay if the trigger procedure is performed in the inpatient setting) and (ii) all services in a fixed period before and after the trigger event on days the patient is treated by the managing provider.

Clinically Associated Services:

This includes services that are not considered as treatment but clinically related to the episode (e.g., routine follow-up as well as services linked to the occurrence of adverse outcomes fully or partially influenced by care delivered during treatment).

Method B examines services in the context of each episode independently. A service is either clinically associated with a given episode or not, regardless of other episodes the patient may be experiencing. Episodes also do not interact with each other. If a service is associated with more than one episode type, the full cost of the service will be assigned to all associated episodes.

(c) Closure

Episodes are closed in the final step after a specified length of time based on the typical course of care provided for a given episode type or as a result of patient death.

Depending on the condition to which it is applied and the clinical course of that condition, an individual may move bidirectionally between phases, for example, from follow-up care back into the evaluation and treatment phase.

Calculating Episode Cost Measures

The following steps calculate the cost for all episodes in an episode group:

1. Observed costs for each episode are determined by aggregating standardized amounts for services related to a given condition or procedure that occur within the episode window.
2. Expected costs for each episode are determined through risk adjustment.
3. The ratio of observed to expected payment-standardized cost is summed for all episodes attributed to a provider and that sum is then divided by the total number of episodes attributed to the provider.
4. The result from step 3 is then multiplied by the national average observed episode cost to generate the risk-adjusted average episode cost, which represent the cost measure score.

For an underlying chronic condition which clinically does not end, a specified period (e.g., a 12-month window) is generally defined to capture the healthcare services related to the treatment of that condition.

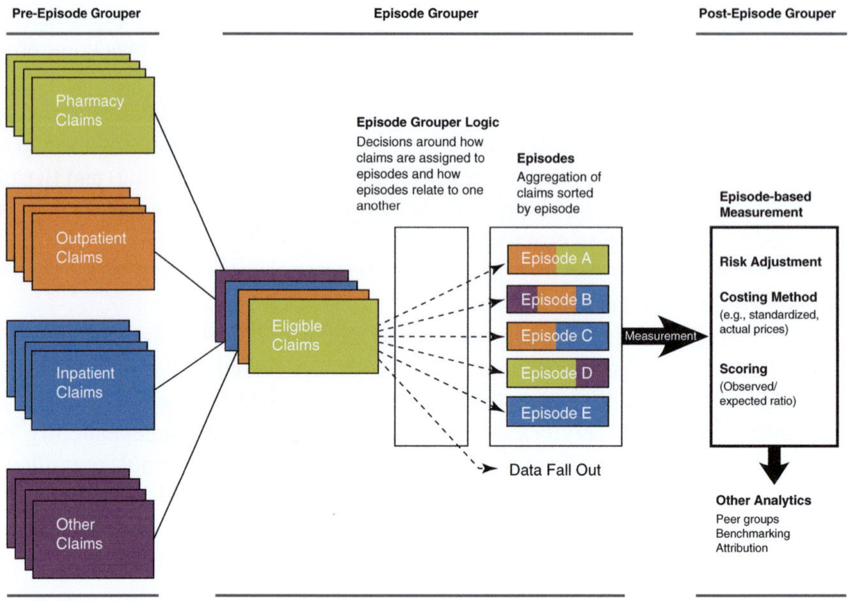

Fig. 16.2 Evaluating episode groupers. (Courtesy of cms.gov)

Payment Standardization and Risk Adjustment

Payment standardization adjusts the allowed amount for a service to facilitate cost comparisons and limit observed differences in costs to those that may result from healthcare delivery choices. Payment-standardized costs remove any payment differences due to adjustments for geographic differences in wage levels or policy-driven payment adjustments such as those for teaching hospitals. Risk adjustment accounts for patient characteristics that can influence spending and are outside of clinician control like illness severity, age, and patient comorbidities.

Attribution of Episodes to a Clinician

Since there are several providers involved in the care of each patient, it was imperative to formulate a way to identify each provider and their respective episode services. After an episode opening, each attributed clinician is identified using the relevant Taxpayer Identification Number/National Provider Identifier (TIN-NPI):

- For procedural episode groups, episodes are attributed to the clinician(s) rendering the trigger services (HCPCS/CPT procedure codes).
- For acute inpatient medical condition episode groups, episodes are attributed to the clinician(s) rendering at least 30 percent of inpatient evaluation and management (E&M) services during an inpatient hospitalization with the medical Medicare Severity Diagnosis-Related Groups (MS-DRGs) for the episode group (Fig. 16.2).

Bundled Payment in Other Surgical Areas

There have been several studies in different surgical specialties focusing upon bundled payment structures. Birkmeyer et al. studied Medicare beneficiaries undergoing CABG, hip fracture repair, colectomy, and spine surgery from 2005 to 2007 [20]. The results for spine surgery from this study are presented in subsequent sections. They found the average total payment to be the highest for CABG, amounting to $45,358, followed by $28,352 for colectomy and $27,570 for hip fracture repair. They found that hospital payments accounted for the largest portion of the total payment for all procedures, including 79.5% for CABG, 59.7% for hip fracture repair, and 77.3% for colectomy. Within hospital payments, DRG payment for the hospitalization constituted the highest portion across all surgeries. Thirty-day readmissions also formed a substantial portion of overall hospital costs, with an average of $3000/episode and accounting for 6.1% of average total payment in colectomy, 7% in CABG, and 16.2% for hip fracture repair. Surgeon payment portion varied from 4.4% for hip fracture repair to 5.3% for colectomy and 6% for CABG. Post-acute care payment portion was also found to be variable for these procedures ranging from 6.9% for CABG to 8.6% for colectomy and 27.5% for hip fracture repair. The authors concluded that hospital payments currently vary significantly and can be reduced by incentivizing hospitals to improve quality and efficiency.

Total hip replacement (THR) and total knee replacement (TKR) have been extensively studied in the context of the Comprehensive Care for Joint Replacement (CCJR) initiative, a 90-day bundled payment model for episode of care for Medicare beneficiaries undergoing these procedures [25]. Preliminary studies showed that the initiative resulted in increased patient satisfaction as well as 22% reduction in associated costs [26]. Another study presented results from the first 21 months of the BPCI initiative which showed that Medicare payments declined significantly for those hospitals participating in the initiative, from $30,551 before the program to $27,265 after 21 months. The decrease in payment was attributed primarily to decreased use of post-acute care [27].

Bundled and Episode-Based Payment Models in Spine Care

The Need for Cost-Efficiency in Back Pain and Spine Care

Spine care is frequently cited as an area in dire need of quality and value improvement [28]. One of the primary reasons is the prevalence of back pain and the cost associated with its care. Back pain is the number one cause of disability and also the most common reason of seeing a doctor in the USA. The 2010 Global Burden of Disease Study showed that back pain was associated with 83 million adjusted life years lost [29]. Moreover, costs associated with back pain are high. Back pain has been referred to as a billion dollar industry [30], with one study showing that medical costs associated with back or neck pain were almost twice as that of most other complaints [31, 32]. According to a recent estimate, the cost of care for conditions related to back and neck pain among Medicare patients increased by 15 times just in the last decade and is now expected to approximate care for chronic conditions such as diabetes [33]. Another study reported that almost $290 billion were spent between 2000 and 2010 on almost four million spinal fusion episodes [34].

Variations in Payments Between Different Spine Surgeries

The total average payment for all spine procedure as per the bundled episode-based payment model ranges from $23,877 to $32,467 in the reported literature [15, 20, 35]. Post-discharge care including rehabilitation has been found to account for 3–9.8% of the bundled amount [15, 20]. Ugiliweneza et al. used MarketScan to study patient costs associated with cervical and lumbar surgery and found significant variation in costs even within the same DRGs [15]. They found that total bundled payment ranged from $12,518 for DRG 491 (back and neck procedures except spinal fusion) to $116,096 for DRG 456 (spinal fusion except cervical with spinal curvature/malignancy/infection or extended fusion with major comorbidity and complication) in 30-day bundle, from $13,188 for DRG 491 to $119,779 for DRG 456 in 60-day bundle, and from $13,188 for DRG 491 to $123,691 for DRG 456 in 90-day bundle. Even within the same DRG, significant variations were noticed. The lowest variation in 30-day and 60-day bundles that authors found was in DRG 491 where the difference between the minimum and maximum bundled cost was $159,436 for 30-day and $87,793 for 60-day bundle. In the 90-day bundle, the DRG with minimum variation was 472 (cervical fusion with major comorbidity and complication) where the difference between the minimum and maximum bundled cost was found to be $207,367. The highest variation across 30-day, 60-day, and 90-day bundles was found to be in DRG 456, where the differences between the minimum and maximum bundled cost were found to be $221,927, $252,961, and $253,893, respectively. Utilization of post-discharge facilities also varied across DRGs with a minimum of 0.6% for DRG 473 and a maximum of 28% for DRG 456. Similarly, portion of bundled costs for readmission also varied across DRGs ranging from 1% for DRGs 455, 472, and 473 to 7% for DRG 456. These results illustrate the heterogeneous nature of spine care and the impact of procedure type and patient conditions in spine surgery.

Another study utilized the Medicare Provider Analysis and Review (MedPAR) files to assess variations of bundled payment distributions across hospitals for surgical intervention for three common spinal disorders (disc herniation, spinal stenosis, and spondylolisthesis) [35]. The authors found that most of the variation in bundled payment cost between the highest paid and lowest paid hospitals was attributed to the difference in cost for index hospitalizations and post-acute care. They found that physician services cost accounted for only 12%. After adjustment for frequency of fusion-based procedures between highest and lowest paid hospitals, the variation was eliminated with the residual variation being attributed for post-acute care and readmissions, especially in the setting of spondylolisthesis and disc herniation [35]. Thus, in terms of cost, spinal surgeries are not only heterogeneous within treatment groups but may also depend heavily on the institutional practices.

Advantages of Episode-Based Payment Models in Spine Care

The overarching goal of bundled episode-based payment is a step toward optimum and cost-efficient delivery of care. Although some of the cost savings may be realized by optimization of care, an unanticipated consequence that may produce cost savings may be rationing care away from sicker patients. Payers including CMS realize this potential outcome; payers must ward off this potential adverse effect upon patient access. It should be noted that the hypothesized cost savings through this model will depend on several factors among which regional differences and hospital/provider variations are the two most important factors [15]. The profound variation of costs for a given DRG across different hospitals also represents an opportunity for savings using a bundled care model. For instance, one study estimated that reducing costs by the hospitals in the most expensive quintile to national average would generate savings of $162 million [15]. The length of a bundle also has cost implications. According to a study, increasing bundle length captures proportionately more costs and hospitalizations without reducing costs for the providers [36].

Such incentivized payment models also stimulate more efforts to benchmark quality outcomes to external organizations and institutions. The benefits of benchmarking and evaluating practices against local and national peer institutions include cost-effectiveness and patient satisfaction [20, 37, 38]. In the context of spine surgery, institutions with high fusion rates may choose to participate in a registry and then compare its rates with other institutes of similar characteristics to assess its practices [15]. Another motivation of adapting a bundled payment model is the leverage in negotiating with vendors for graft material, implants, and other items. One study stated that by mandating vendors to comply with average national prices in order to keep them on an "approved devices" list, institutions were able to save $950 per single-level ACDF [39].

Several prominent healthcare institutions have adapted episode-based bundled models for spine surgery. A recent study surveyed such institutions to find the reasons for adapting these payment models. The authors found that the most common motivation behind adapting a bundled payment model was facilitation in recruiting third-party administrators and corporations [40]. Other major reasons included motivation to prescreen patients to identify patients requiring surgery and shared profit increases for physicians and hospitals [40]. Adapting such models is also expected to promote further research into surgical techniques that have the potential to decrease morbidity and readmissions, thereby reducing costs [41].

Disadvantages and Challenges in Using Bundled Care for Spine Care

Though BPCI is geared toward optimizing patient care with the incentive to drive down costs, some experts have expressed valid concerns in adapting this model. There are several challenges in designing an appropriate bundling model for spine-related procedures and care. One such concern is the potential danger of physicians selecting low-risk healthier patients to treat, patients that may have lower spending for hospitals and physicians. One anecdotal example was presented by Schoenfeld et al., who showed that bundled cost for DRG 459 representing a patient undergoing a spinal fusion with complications or comorbidities was $65,124 compared to $43,363 for DRG 460 representing a patient undergoing a spinal fusion without any complication or comorbidity [35]. Additional evidence of this potential unintended consequence is that some spine centers have already started denying surgery to patients who have significant comorbid condition burden [40]. Rather than "heal the sick," hospitals and providers are encouraged to "treat the healthy." Another challenge is defining a balance of financial risk that would be divided between payers and physicians/providers. In this approach, spine surgeons may be disincentivized from elective spine procedures in some patients, although the impact of this conflict of interest has not been studied [35]. There is a profound variation in surgical techniques and nuances applied for a particular pathology. For instance, a grade 1 lumbar spondylolisthesis may be surgically managed by lumbar decompression or by decompression combined with lumbar fusion, which is known to elevate the cost of care [31, 33, 42, 43]. Similarly, for a patient with cervical myelopathy, surgeons may choose to employ cervical arthroplasty (30-day bundle cost, $19,425) over anterior cervical discectomy and fusion or ACDF (30-day bundle cost, $26,095) [35]. Rather than decide on surgical approach based on individual patient characteristics, providers may make decisions based on cost first and appropriate selection or patient need later. Moreover, under this model, a minor change in the number of patients with major comorbidities or complications is expected to drastically impact long-term sustainability and reimbursements for a provider [35].

A reputable institution recently published its results after transitioning to a BPCI program from a FFS model, for total joint replacement, cardiac valve replacement, and lumbar spinal fusion [44]. The overarching objective across all procedures is to demonstrate cost savings by decreasing the length of stay, decreasing 90-day readmissions, and facility-based post-acute care. While the program was able to demonstrate cost savings in total joint replacement and cardiac valve procedures, the effect in spine surgery was the opposite. The results showed that on average, the episode per cost increased by $8291 compared to previous FFS model. This rise in cost was attributed to a changing case mix owing to increased referral in the study period and increased surgical costs. Another reason that the authors stated was the increased use of transforaminal lumbar interbody fusion (TLIF), which is associated with higher surgical costs compared to posterior lumbar interbody fusion (PLIF) albeit with better clinical outcomes [45].

Conclusion

While bundled and episode-based payment models represent promising methods to curb healthcare costs in the USA, it is necessary that physicians and hospitals adapt to this changing landscape and set policies to respond to these new payment systems. Although this change in payment models has yielded positive results in several surgical fields, the results in spine surgery have been less impressive. The impact of the new payment models on patient access is not well understood. Although some savings are likely to be realized from care optimization, a fear remains the savings may be realized from rationing care away from the sickest patients who are often the most in need of care.

References

1. NHE-Fact-Sheet. 2017.; Available: https://www.cms.gov/Research-Statistics-Data-and-Systems/Statistics-Trends-and-Reports/NationalHealthExpendData/NHE-Fact-Sheet.html
2. Davis K, Stremikis K, Schoen C, Squires D. Mirror, mirror on the wall, 2014 update: how the US health care system compares internationally. The Commonwealth Fund. 2014;16:1–31.
3. Squires DA. The U.S. health system in perspective: a comparison of twelve industrialized nations. Issue Brief. 2011;16:1–14.
4. Bundled Payments for Care Improvement (BPCI) Initiative: General Information | Center for Medicare & Medicaid Innovation [Internet]. [cited 9 Feb 2018]. Available: https://innovation.cms.gov/initiatives/bundled-payments/
5. Protection P, Act AC. Patient protection and affordable care act. Public Law. 2010;111:759–62.
6. McIlvennan CK, Eapen ZJ, Allen LA. Hospital readmissions reduction program. Circulation. 2015;131:1796–803.
7. Jencks SF, Williams MV, Coleman EA. Rehospitalizations among patients in the Medicare fee-for-service program. N Engl J Med. 2009;360:1418–28.
8. Zhang W, Watanabe-Galloway S. Ten-year secular trends for congestive heart failure hospitalizations: an analysis of regional differences in the United States. Congest Heart Fail. 2008;14:266–71.
9. Krumholz HM, Merrill AR, Schone EM, Schreiner GC, Chen J, Bradley EH, et al. Patterns of hospital performance in acute myocardial infarction and heart failure 30-day mortality and readmission. Circ Cardiovasc Qual Outcomes. 2009;2:407–13.
10. Bueno H, Ross JS, Wang Y, Chen J, Vidán MT, Normand S-LT, et al. Trends in length of stay and short-term outcomes among Medicare patients hospitalized for heart failure, 1993–2006. JAMA. 2010;303:2141–7.
11. Marcoux RM, Larrat EP, Vogenberg FR. Accountable care organizations: an improvement over HMOs? P T. 2012;37:629–50.
12. Centers for Medicare & Medicaid Services (CMS), HHS. Medicare Program; Advancing Care Coordination Through Episode Payment Models (EPMs); Cardiac Rehabilitation Incentive Payment Model; and Changes to the Comprehensive Care for Joint Replacement Model (CJR). Final rule. Fed Regist. 2017;82:180–651.
13. Averill RF, Hughes JS, Goldfield NI. Paying for outcomes, not performance: lessons from the Medicare inpatient prospective payment system. Jt Comm J Qual Patient Saf. 2011;37:184–92. 145
14. Mok JM, Martinez M, Smith HE, Sciubba DM, Passias PG, Schoenfeld A, et al. Impact of a bundled payment system on resource utilization during spine surgery. Int J Spine Surg. 2016;10:19.
15. Ugiliweneza B, Kong M, Nosova K, Huang KT, Babu R, Lad SP, et al. Spinal surgery: variations in health care costs and implications for episode-based bundled payments. Spine. 2014;39:1235–42.
16. U.S. Department of Health USD, Services H, Others. Better, smarter, healthier: in historic announcement, HHS sets clear goals and timeline for shifting Medicare reimbursements from volume to value. Washington, DC. 2015
17. Centers for Medicare & Medicaid Services CFM, Others. Bundled Payments for Care Improvement (BPCI) initiative: general information. Available at https://innovation.cms.gov/initiatives/bundled-payments/View in Article. Accessed July 13, 2017, 2015.

18. Bundled Payments for Care Improvement (BPCI) Initiative: General Information | Center for Medicare & Medicaid Innovation [Internet]. [cited 9 Feb 2018]. Available: https://innovation.cms.gov/initiatives/bundled-payments/
19. Mistichelli J. Diagnosis related groups (DRGs). Bioethics Research Library, Kennedy Institute of Ethics, Georgetown University; 1984.; Available: https://repository.library.georgetown.edu/handle/10822/556896
20. Birkmeyer JD, Gust C, Baser O, Dimick JB, Sutherland JM, Skinner JS. Medicare payments for common inpatient procedures: implications for episode-based payment bundling. Health Serv Res. 2010;45:1783–95.
21. Miller HD. From volume to value: better ways to pay for health care. Health Aff. 2009;28:1418–28.
22. Abelson R. In bid for better care, surgery with a warranty. NY Times. 2007;17: 531–533.
23. MACRA: MIPS & APMs. 2017.; Available: https://www.cms.gov/Medicare/Quality-Initiatives-Patient-Assessment-Instruments/Value-Based-Programs/MACRA-MIPS-and-APMs/MACRA-MIPS-and-APMs.html
24. Home. 2017.; Available: https://www.cms.gov
25. Ibrahim SA, Kim H, McConnell KJ. The CMS Comprehensive care model and racial disparity in joint replacement. JAMA. 2016;316:1258–9.
26. Blue Cross Blue Shield. Media Center | Blue Cross Blue Shield North Carolina [Internet]. [cited 14 Feb 2018]. Available: http://mediacenter.bcbsnc.com
27. Dummit LA, Kahvecioglu D, Marrufo G, Rajkumar R, Marshall J, Tan E, et al. Association between hospital participation in a Medicare bundled payment initiative and payments and quality outcomes for lower extremity joint replacement episodes. JAMA. 2016;316:1267–78.
28. Resnick DK, Tosteson ANA, Groman RF, Ghogawala Z. Setting the equation: establishing value in spine care. Spine. 2014;39:S43–50.
29. Hoy D, March L, Brooks P, Blyth F, Woolf A, Bain C, et al. The global burden of low back pain: estimates from the global burden of disease 2010 study. Ann Rheum Dis. 2014;73:968–74.
30. MacLellan L. The $100 billion per year back pain industry is mostly a hoax. In: Quartz [Internet]. Quartz; 26 Jun 2017 [cited 9 Feb 2018]. Available: https://qz.com/1010259/the-100-billion-per-year-back-pain-industry-is-mostly-a-hoax/
31. Martin BI, Deyo RA, Mirza SK, Turner JA, Comstock BA, Hollingworth W, et al. Expenditures and health status among adults with back and neck problems. JAMA. 2008;299:656–64.
32. Davis MA, Onega T, Weeks WB, Lurie JD. Where the United States spends its spine dollars: expenditures on different ambulatory services for the management of back and neck conditions. Spine. 2012;37:1693–701.
33. Chen E, Tong KB, Laouri M. Surgical treatment patterns among medicare beneficiaries newly diagnosed with lumbar spinal stenosis. Spine J. 2010;10:588–94.
34. Goz V, Weinreb JH, McCarthy I, Schwab F, Lafage V, Errico TJ. Perioperative complications and mortality after spinal fusions: analysis of trends and risk factors. Spine. 2013;38:1970–6.
35. Schoenfeld AJ, Harris MB, Liu H, Birkmeyer JD. Variations in Medicare payments for episodes of spine surgery. Spine J. 2014;14:2793–8.
36. Sood N, Huckfeldt PJ, Escarce JJ, Grabowski DC, Newhouse JP. Medicare's bundled payment pilot for acute and postacute care: analysis and recommendations on where to begin. Health Aff. 2011;30:1708–17.
37. Miller DC, Gust C, Dimick JB, Birkmeyer N, Skinner J, Birkmeyer JD. Large variations in Medicare payments for surgery highlight savings potential from bundled payment programs. Health Aff. 2011;30:2107–15.
38. Cutler DM, Ghosh K. The potential for cost savings through bundled episode payments. N Engl J Med. 2012;366:1075–7.
39. Oren J, Hutzler LH, Hunter T, Errico T, Zuckerman J, Bosco J. Decreasing spine implant costs and inter-physician cost variation: the impact of programme of cost containment on implant expenditure in spinal surgery. Bone Joint J. 2015;97-B:1102–5.
40. Kazberouk A, McGuire K, Landon BE. A survey of innovative reimbursement models in spine care. Spine. 2016;41:344–52.

41. Sullivan R, Jarvis LD, O'Gara T, Langfitt M, Emory C. Bundled payments in total joint arthroplasty and spine surgery. Curr Rev Musculoskelet Med. 2017;10:218–23.
42. Deyo RA, Mirza SK, Martin BI, Kreuter W, Goodman DC, Jarvik JG. Trends, major medical complications, and charges associated with surgery for lumbar spinal stenosis in older adults. JAMA. 2010;303:1259–65.
43. Schoenfeld AJ, Weiner BK, Smith HE. Regional variation and spine care: an historical perspective. Spine. 2011;36:1512–7.
44. Bundled Care Program Failed to Reduce Fusion Surgery Costs. The Back Letter; 2018;33. https://doi.org/10.1097/01.BACK.0000529682.00072.aa, 33.
45. Jubelt LE, Goldfeld KS, Blecker SB, Chung W-Y, Bendo JA, Bosco JA, et al. Early lessons on bundled payment at an Academic Medical Center. J Am Acad Orthop Surg. 2017;25:654–63.

Aligning Healthcare Systems

17

Gabriel S. Makar, Michael Gutman, Mayan Lendner, David A. Janiec, Christina Vannello, Michael E. West, and Alexander R. Vaccaro

Abbreviations

ACO	Accountable Care Organization
CIN	Clinical Integrated Networks
CMS	Centers for Medicare and Medicaid Services
CVA	Cerebrovascular accident
DVT	Deep venous thrombosis
MACRA	Medicare Access and CHIP Reauthorization Act of 2015
MIPS	Merit-Based Incentive Payment System
NDI	Neck Disability Index
ODI	Oswestry Disability Index
PCMH	Patient-Centered Medical Homes
PCSP	Patient-Centered Specialty Practices
PE	Pulmonary embolism
SF12	12-item Short Form Health Survey
SSI	Surgical site infection
VAS	Visual analog scale

G. S. Makar · M. Gutman · M. Lendner · D. A. Janiec · C. Vannello
M. E. West · A. R. Vaccaro (✉)
Rothman Institute, Philadelphia, PA, USA
e-mail: Alex.Vaccaro@rothmaninstitute.com

J. Ratliff et al. (eds.), *Quality Spine Care*,
https://doi.org/10.1007/978-3-319-97990-8_17

Where We Are Today

Healthcare has not changed drastically since the inception of Medicare and Medicaid in the 1960s: the patient sought care, the provider gave care, and the insurer managed payments. As simple as the basic concept of health insurance may seem, each participant in the transaction has divergent goals in mind – patients desire the most benefits for premiums paid, providers seek maximum compensation for care, and insurers focus on cost control and profitability. Each stakeholder is working continuously to further their individual interests; the focus of care, the patient's health, may become lost due to goal misalignment.

It is not difficult to understand how the healthcare industry and its participants have reached to this point. Insurance is traditionally organized around indemnifying parties against loss. Health insurance must go beyond merely paying the transactional costs of care; it must coexist with support and not impede the acquisition of optimal health, all of which make it far more challenging than other types of insurance. Health insurance, despite its nomenclature, has never been about health but rather about cost coverage and profitability.

It is no surprise that the primary interests of the patient, the provider, and the insurance payer are at time divergent. Patients want services, as it is their perception that they have already paid for them. Providers want maximum compensation for work performed. Payers are focused on lowering cost. Although there has been significant legislation over the past 10 years with a focus on "value" (quality/cost), insurance companies continue to reward/penalize providers/healthcare systems on cost vs. value, and a disconnect between the actual cost of care and the portion of that cost that the patient is responsible for still exists. No party in the interaction, not even the patient, has at all times the primary focus of health.

Every patient should get exactly what he or she needs at the time of treatment, understanding that anything more is wasteful and that anything less is clinically inappropriate, potentially resulting in additional future care and cost.

Value optimization should be the natural by-product of an efficient care process, not the driver. There are many inefficient processes, systems, strategies, and attitudes which require adjustment if the healthcare industry is to operate effectively. Effective patient care needs oversight and direction from the physician accompanied by mutual decision-making with the patient as well as a consistent set of standards or "best practices." By including patients in shared clinical decision-making, providers will improve patient engagement to create a better understanding of and adherence to care pathways [1, 2]. Interestingly, our system has seen a historical shift with traditional fee for service insurance products toward "patient entitlement features" which at times are a significant hindrance for optimal care [1, 3]. With traditional insurance products, patients at times have been far too aggressive in the decision process regarding their care, focusing on benefit structure as opposed to care and what is clinically necessary and not wasteful [4].

Concurrent with technology increasing the number of interventions available is an aging patient demographic with increasing healthcare demands. Alone, these two factors risk significant increase in healthcare expenditures and illustrate the need for quality of care and assessment of clinical effectiveness. There is universal change in healthcare focus from volume to value, requiring a significant change in how all stakeholders realign in the care of patients.

Care Coordination

Creating a care paradigm to minimize fragmentation of care is not a simple task. Patients have historically been passed back and forth between providers without optimal coordination of information and, hence, without optimal coordination of care. Such fragmentation is a symptom of a volume-driven healthcare system which favors redundant procedures and the potential for wasteful care. A shift to a value-based system requires an alignment of incentives where the patient benefits due to expedited, meaningful care. In this approach, the physician is rewarded for coordinating proper care, improving outcomes and avoiding wasteful care [5]. Studies assessing adverse events in primary care physicians found that almost 50% of adverse events were due to communication-associated errors [6]. Communication and care coordination redesign is a collaborative effort that includes all parties involved in the patient's health.

Payers must also eliminate barriers that can impinge on the patient and provider working collaboratively to achieve optimal outcomes. Plan designs may include incentivizing plan members (patients) to seek out clinically appropriate, cost-efficient options for their healthcare. Reimbursement redesign would have to include simplifying administrative procedures (e.g., supplying reasonable, clear, and uniformly applied authorization guidelines) and reward quality of service over quantity of service. Most of the current administrative processes that inhibit proper care are a response to the overutilization of services, which is encouraged in a fee-for-service system. In a value-based system, plan design should incentivize members and providers to choose efficient care pathways, reducing both overutilization and related administrative excesses created to control them [6]. Incentives such as reducing patient co-payments for using preferred providers or utilizing preventive services have been shown to increase patients' use of high-value resources. Ultimately, these types of incentives drive patient behaviors toward high-value resources, leading to higher-value care [7]. From a practitioner perspective, the transition to a value-based system will take time, but earlier adopters that are attentive to both care and cost will benefit as adjustments are made to legislation and within the industry [8, 9].

Because the value-based care equation addresses both quality and cost efficiency, physicians are not only placed at the center of patient care but now have greater financial responsibilities and accountability related to the patient's care in the form of incentives and penalties aligned with performance. Although still cost focused in some markets, insurers are now leveraging quality measures and outcome assessments to adjust reimbursements for physicians [10, 11]. These measures are playing a more vital role in monitoring healthcare system efficacy than ever before. Establishing universal quality measures and accurately interpreting those measures continue to be an area of research and debate. The current movement toward bringing quality, outcomes, and patient health to the forefront of the value proposition discussion is essential in aligning healthcare systems.

Transparency

One of the tools being used in the movement to value-based care is information. As basic as this may sound, healthcare as an industry has had a dearth of information available to its consumers: patients, payers, and other providers. Legislation, such as the Medicare Access and CHIP Reauthorization Act of 2015 (MACRA) passed by the federal government, calls for more transparency in regard to healthcare costs and activities [12]. Public reporting of costs, readmissions, and adverse events increases transparency in healthcare; when provided to patients, payers, and providers, proper information can potentially reduce harm and cost resulting from miscommunication, especially when that data is delivered in a timely fashion so that behavior and decision-making may be adjusted as needed [13]. Quality reporting, if used to alter compensation models, will increase a healthy competition in the industry by forcing clinicians to optimize clinical care protocols. Optimization of protocols should improve the standard-of-care and ultimately increase value by both improving quality and reducing cost [14]. The introduction of quality into the payment matrix has fueled much debate in regard to payment methodology and the use of uniform instruments for measurement, including which elements providers will be held accountable. Initially, the value attached to "quality" must be significant enough to get attention and modify behavior rather than cost, with quality being defined as "quality of life and functional capacity."

There is great potential value that transparency may add. It may be assumed that commercial payers will follow this lead and also focus upon transparency in reporting of clinical outcomes. It is quite difficult to implement standards in areas of healthcare where substantial variation still exists. Spine surgery is one area challenged by objective measurement when the very same procedure can be executed in many different ways: timing of intervention, instrumentation, and grafting, among other components of the same procedure, can all vary from surgeon to surgeon. The development of best practices, grounded in evidenced-based medicine, becomes imperative.

Practice Standards

Practice standards have greatly improved with the evolution of patient-centered care initiatives. Patient-Centered Medical Homes (PCMH), Accountable Care Organizations (ACOs), Patient-Centered Specialty Practices (PCSP), and Clinical

Integrated Networks (CIN) are all value-based care initiatives that highlight care coordination and risk sharing to improve outcomes and minimize wasteful care. These care models strive to optimize care for the individual patient, as opposed to generically applying uniform care pathways based on condition; the latter is supported, and possibly encouraged, under a system which does not rely on value as a part of the measurement of clinical success. Coordinating this level of care requires the provider to engage in the patient's care before, during, and after any type of intervention, otherwise known as episodic care. The specialist therefore becomes the primary caregiver in the window of time defined by the patient condition and is accountable for tailoring the treatment plan to the specific and individual need of the patient.

Care Navigator

In order to provide this level of attention and ensure continuity of treatment to a patient throughout an entire episode of care, a patient navigation system should be established, led by a Navigator [15]. The Care (Nurse) Navigator has the singular goal of providing a tailored level of care to each patient, ensuring the most efficient outcome, hence creating value. All patients should be risk stratified/assessed in order to determine the preliminary care pathway. The Navigator is responsible for following the pathway unless conditions of the patient or environment change. The Care Navigator's role ensures that patients are closely monitored over their entire course of care. They address the specific needs of the patient and are able to confirm clinical information, educate the patient, assist with post-acute setup in the home, and act as patient guides through the post-acute care period. A Care Navigator helps reduce communication mishaps by coordinating care between healthcare providers as well as confirming the proper location for any type of intervention and postoperative care, ultimately reducing readmission rates and complications. When a Care Navigator is engaged, the patient receives effective and efficient care: providers are freed up to be resources for other patients, and insurance payers ultimately pay less for equal or higher-quality care [16].

The patient-centered approach becomes integral to any treatment process, starting with the care providers' collection of medical and social information. This information is collected via a standardized survey and subsequently used to produce a standardized risk assessment which will serve as a template for the customization of future care. At the start of care, the risk assessment model produces a score that categorizes the patient as low, moderate, or high-risk, for both medical and social risks. These scores help determine the likelihood of the patient being readmitted to the hospital or experiencing a complication and allow for the determination of the type of facility in which the intervention can safely be conducted, the latter of which may include a surgical center, specialty hospital, community hospital, or tertiary medical center. Risk assessment also helps determine the type of post-intervention care a patient may need. Following the implementation of patient risk assessment

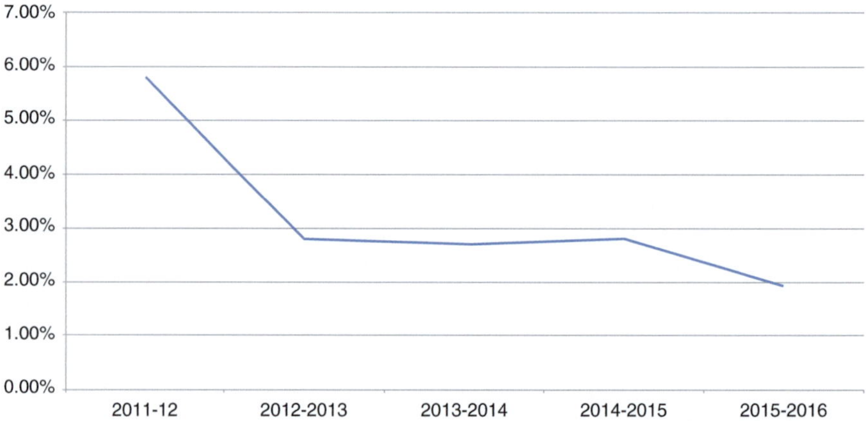

Fig. 17.1 30-day readmission rate of total joint arthroplasty at Thomas Jefferson University Hospital. Rothman Institute was successful in dropping their readmission rate for from 6% in 2011 to 2% in 2016 in part due to the implementation of a Nurse Navigator to their practices

and nurse navigation, Rothman Institute was successful in dropping readmission rates of the total joint arthroplasty population at Thomas Jefferson University Hospital from 6% in 2011 to 2% by 2016 (Fig. 17.1). Similar success may be achieved in other areas of treatment as well.

Quality Assessment

The quality of healthcare delivered is not universal across physicians, departments, or hospitals, despite advancements in medical technology and patient care [17]. It is necessary to measure quality by implementing evidence-based quality assessment metrics, holding all measured entities to the same standards. CMS defines quality measures as "tools that help us measure or quantify healthcare processes, outcomes, patient perceptions, and organizational structure and/or systems that are associated with the ability to provide high-quality health care and/or that relate to one or more quality goals for health care" [18]. Quality assessment measures should provide useful information on care delivered. One hurdle, however, is determining when in the care process to best collect and analyze quality measures. Some procedures may have more potential long-term complications than others. Similar measurement periods for analysis of readmission rates comparing two procedures for the same diagnosis may not be an optimal measure of quality. In this example, the choice of procedure will depend on the patient, their comorbidities, risk assessment, and physician's discretion. Evidence-based quality metrics used at Rothman Institute to assess care include readmissions, complications, infection rate, ODI, NDI, VAS scores, SF12 survey scores, and re-operative rate [19, 20].

Readmission rates have always been a key indicator for quality assessment and patient outcomes across various departments and hospitals [21]. Readmissions are extremely costly to hospitals, and even a marginal decrease in readmission rates can produce substantial savings [22]. An analysis of both the rate of readmissions and primary reason for readmissions within 30 and 90 days postoperatively provides an avenue for improvement in reduced cost and improved quality [23–26]. Assessing the patient's risk of readmission preoperatively provides a better understanding of which patients might require intensive medical optimization prior to surgery. Interpreting the cost metric in terms of patient risk and outcome is where value is created.

The development of a tool that not only risk assesses the patient but also directly correlates the risk score to the likelihood of readmission allows for improved outcomes and reduced cost (Fig. 17.2). Different care pathways can be developed for high-, moderate-, and low-risk patients. If these pathways can result in better management of risk and therefore a higher likelihood of a good outcome for the patient – as measured by instance, severity, and cost of readmissions over time – value is optimized.

Minimizing perioperative complications has taken a higher priority with healthcare payers as they become interested in potential areas of care improvement relative to cost savings as a part of the value-based model [27–30]. Common orthopedic complications, ranging from periprosthetic fracture, pulmonary embolus (PE), and deep vein thrombosis (DVT) to less common complications such as respiratory failure due to

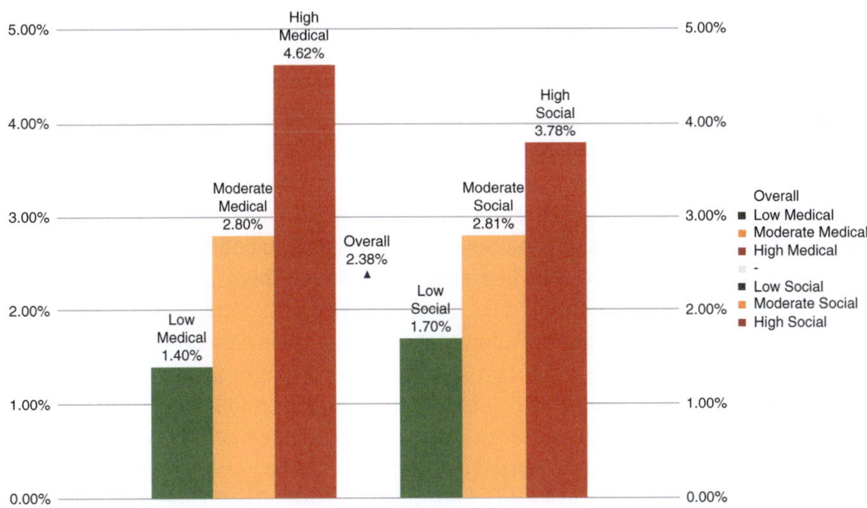

Fig. 17.2 Readmission rates by risk level in patients at Thomas Jefferson University Hospital (2016). Risk stratification according to a number of criteria was able to successfully predict which patients were more likely to be readmitted to the hospital

intubation, vascular injury, or cerebrovascular accident (CVA), create a platform for optimizing pre-, peri-, and postoperative management of patients. Although many complications are not avoidable, optimizing patients will decrease the susceptibility for preventable patient complications. Similar to readmission rates, stratifying patients according to risk level has also proved to be useful for understanding which patient populations have a higher probability of complications [31]. To deliver quality care, it is necessary to understand likely complications most often attributable to each surgery. Further, understanding correlations between patient comorbid conditions and potential complications for each surgery makes tailoring care for patients even more important than before. Improved quality metrics around complications allow providers to move away from the one-size-fits-all standard of care and provide the best possible care. As before, tailored care, resulting in the precise care needed on a patient-to-patient basis, aligns with maximum efficiency and reduces cost.

Minimizing infection rate continues to be an important focus, as most perioperative infections are often seen as preventable, although in practice this view may be inaccurate. Spinal operations complicated by an infection are emotionally difficult for patient and family [32, 33]. Postoperative spinal infections range from an incidence of 0.5% to 20% depending on the procedure and the health of the patient [34]. In an analysis of 3673 spinal procedures, the most common reason for an early readmission was infection, accounting for 32% of all unplanned readmissions [35–37]. The variability in spinal procedure practices and the lack of true quality assessment methodologies make it difficult to translate the impact of surgical site infections (SSIs) on quality outcome measures. Although a substantial amount of research has been done on infection rates across various fields, little has been studied correlating postoperative infection and quality of care delivered [35]. In spine surgery, an infection is one of the most common causes of 30-day readmission and has been documented as costing up to an additional $38,000 in adult deformity cases and $12,600 in posterior cervical cases [36–38]. Smoking history and glycemic control were found to be two significant factors related to SSI and can be viewed as potentially modifiable along with other factors to optimize patients prior to surgery [39].

Adding real value to the care equation also introduces an element than has long been overlooked: actual patient outcomes. It is important to understand if the patient actually received benefit from an intervention. Has there been a reduction in pain? Is the patient higher functioning? Has he or she been able to return to work? Any discussion of quality that does not address the change to the patient's condition after surgery is missing the most important aspect of care. Most insurance payers – and, for that matter, many surgeons – do not collect this information in any organized and consistent manner. Many do not even have a system which can accommodate the data in the first place. Patient-reported outcomes should be collected preoperatively to measure disability, general health, and quality of life. They should be specific, validated instruments used for specific diseases, and the same instruments should again be collected at specific postoperative intervals as a step in documenting patient improvement. The information collected by these instruments is not only useful at the patient level but can also be used to amass data at the surgeon or facility level to understand and compare surgical effectiveness between various individuals and entities. Establishing/developing efficient methods of collecting outcome measures and achieving a high level of post-op compliance/completion will be necessary in order to truly evaluate the care path taken for patients.

Finally, interpretation and use of data are of the utmost importance in value-based care. Value-based care is a major disruption to the healthcare industry. If data are not properly collected, interpreted, and used, there is no value added and likely limited progress. Information must be communicated and actionable to be of relevance to clinicians. After acquiring the appropriate measures, providers need to understand what each outcome measure means to the health of the patient and the quality of care provided.

More general indicators of the value proposition are addressed in the federal government's Merit-Based Incentive Payment System (MIPS), initiated in 2017, which incorporates quality reporting metrics from numerous prior programs under the Centers for Medicare and Medicaid Services (CMS) to assess performance on a more universal platform. MIPS will assess performance across four distinct categories: quality measures, resource use, advancing care (meaningful use of electronic health records), and clinical practice improvement activities [40, 41]. However, these categories are collectively proxies for improvement in the adoption of value-based care, each contributing to quality improvement or cost efficiency. MIPS is intended to provide the government insight in regard to the successes and challenges associated with value-based care. It, as well, provides a platform which can identify and reward achievement in value-based care.

As noted, all of the aforementioned data and reporting must be actionable. Used together, they are important tools which provide information that can be used in the comparison of protocols, pathways, and approaches across physicians. They can expose the pros and cons of various techniques and procedures, forcing discussions in regard to the adoption of best practices and, ultimately, reduction in unnecessary practice variation, which most often results in inefficiencies and higher cost.

Following the implementation of best practices and other clinically appropriate standardization, shared decision-making tools and predictive models can be used to optimize patient selection and manage factors which impact success. These tools and predictive models might include risk stratification for patients so that providers performing a greater number of operations on high-risk populations would not be penalized unfairly [42]. In the high-risk specialty of spine surgery, categorizing patients through predictive modeling or other data correlation tools could be extremely valuable.

Variation in quality measures does exist and is expected when measuring performance across institutions. Although eliminating all variation may not be possible, comparing standardized institutional data could decrease variation and reduce outliers. Quality improvements achieved through value-based care should be scalable because they pertain specifically to patient care, as opposed to provider (facility or surgeon) efficiencies.

Success in value-based care is not something that is achieved by completing any series of tasks but rather something that is an ongoing work. Best practices are not static but instead processes that evolve, as needed, across time following ongoing review and management. Nowhere is this better understood than at Rothman Institute. Surgeons are committed to a best practices environment that begins in research, through which evidence-based medicine can be developed and implemented. Collaborative discussions among subspecialists result in common care pathways that ensure every patient receives proven, best-in-class orthopedic care. Moreover, providing each patient with exactly the care that he or she needs, simultaneously, results in the optimum economic outcome.

It is important to remember, however, that true value-based care is patient facing and does not end within the four walls of any given provider. It was understood early on at Rothman Institute that the industry shift to value meant the investment in and development of new resources could forge relationships with other high-quality, efficient partners in patient care. Rothman Institute has relationships with facility orthopedic service-line management and has additionally initiated numerous service-line co-management agreements, at the facilities in which its surgeons operate. Recognizing the importance of well-managed post-acute care, Rothman Institute also developed a contracted network which it calls its Quality Care Alliance Partners. All care partners are monitored on an ongoing basis to ensure compliance to prescribe care pathways.

Thorough, continual review of quality and financial data has allowed Rothman Institute to understand the components of successful healthcare management in a value-based environment. Information is shared transparently within the practice to encourage healthy competition and innovation; information is shared externally to advance the practice of all providers in the economic chain. Rothman Institute has parlayed the integration of data, best practices, and clear communication into a healthy expansion of its practice.

Conclusion

Value-based care has only recently disrupted the healthcare industry. It conceptually challenges the very underpinnings of what has been accepted healthcare industry practice. Transitioning from a disjointed system that rewards volume in favor of coordinated activity and outcomes is no small task. The perception of each of the operators in the system – patients, providers, and payers – is challenged under value-based care, as each has a separate agenda that often does not synchronize with all stakeholders. The idea of true value-based care connects the patient, provider, and insurer closer together regarding high-quality, cost-effective care with incentive, engagement, and alignment at its core.

New metrics rewarding the correct care and the appropriate level of care have emerged, forcing care to be patient-facing, rather than procedure-driven. This has prompted the introduction of new care team members, such as Nurse Navigators, whose function is to guide patients from the point of diagnosis and establishment of a care pathway through the patient's post-acute care period following any type of intervention.

As a result, aligning healthcare would become a product of care processes tied to efficient patient care. By providing each patient with exactly the care needed, the most efficient care pathway would be established. Individualized care, rooted in best practices and controlled variation, should result in both the highest level and the most efficient care. Care provided at this level across the spectrum, by default, becomes the efficient model for population health.

Still, there are areas of variation that need to be addressed to arrive at the goal of value-based care. Transparency is important, as it permits informed consumer decisions, as well as a way to truly gauge relative performance. Data also allows for improvement through the development of consistent measures (readmissions, complications, infection rates, patient-reported outcomes, etc.) which can then be correlated to health events and used for predictive modeling. This developed data can then be shared with providers in a consistent manner for continuous improvement. All of the component pieces contribute to alignment within an industry which heretofore has been, at best, fractured in its approach in the provision of healthcare.

References

1. Molenaar S, Sprangers MA, Postma-Schuit FC, Rutgers EJ, Noorlander J, Hendriks J, et al. Feasibility and effects of decision aids. Med Decis Making. 2000;20(1):112–27.
2. Finset A. Patient education and counseling in a changing era of health care. Patient Educ Couns. 2007;66(1):2–3.
3. Ullrich PF Jr, Vaccaro AR. Patient education on the internet: opportunities and pitfalls. Spine (Phila Pa 1976). 2002;27(7):E185–8.
4. Martin BI, Deyo RA, Mirza SK, Turner JA, Comstock BA, Hollingworth W, et al. Expenditures and health status among adults with back and neck problems. JAMA. 2008;299(6):656–64.
5. Wilson RM, Runciman WB, Gibberd RW, Harrison BT, Newby L, Hamilton JD. The quality in Australian health care study. Med J Aust. 1995;163(9):458–71.
6. Bhasale AL, Miller GC, Reid SE, Britt HC. Analysing potential harm in Australian general practice: an incident-monitoring study. Med J Aust. 1998;169(2):73–6.
7. Thomson S, Schang L, Chernew ME. Value-based cost sharing in the United States and elsewhere can increase patients' use of high-value goods and services. Health affairs (Project Hope). 2013;32(4):704–12.
8. Ray JC, Kusumoto F. The transition to value-based care. J Interv Card Electrophysiol. 2016;47(1):61–8.
9. Conrad DA. The theory of value-based payment incentives and their application to health care. Health Serv Res. 2015;50(Suppl 2):2057–89.
10. Brunt CS, Jensen GA. Medicare part B reimbursement and the perceived quality of physician care. Int J Health Care Finance Econ. 2010;10(2):149–70.
11. Cheng EM, Sanders AE, Cohen AB, Bever CT Jr. Quality measurement: It's here to stay. Neurol Clin Pract. 2014;4(5):441–6.
12. Casalino LP. The Medicare access and CHIP reauthorization act and the corporate transformation of American medicine. Health Aff (Project Hope). 2017;36(5):865–9.
13. Sharma K, Metzler I, Chen S, Mayer JE Jr, Meara J. Public reporting of healthcare data: a new frontier in quality improvement. Bull Am Coll Surg. 2012;97(6):6–13.
14. Marshall MSP, Brook R, Leatherman S. Dying to know: public release of information about quality of health care. London: Nuffield Trust; 2000.
15. McMullen L, Banman T, DeGroot JM, Scott S, Srdanovic D, Mackey H. Providing novice navigators with a GPS for role development: oncology nurse navigator competency project. Clin J Oncol Nurs. 2016;20(1):33–8.
16. Kocher RP, Adashi EY. Hospital readmissions and the affordable care act: paying for coordinated quality care. JAMA. 2011;306(16):1794–5.

17. McGlynn EA, Asch SM, Adams J, Keesey J, Hicks J, DeCristofaro A, et al. The quality of health care delivered to adults in the United States. N Engl J Med. 2003;348(26):2635–45.
18. Centers for Medicare and Medicaid Services. Centers for Medicare and Medicaid Services: Quality Measures. Available from: https://www.cms.gov/Medicare/Quality-Initiatives-Patient-Assessment-Instruments/QualityMeasures/
19. Patel AA, Donegan D, Albert T. The 36-item short form. J Am Acad Orthop Surg. 2007;15(2):126–34.
20. McCormick JD, Werner BC, Shimer AL. Patient-reported outcome measures in spine surgery. J Am Acad Orthop Surg. 2013;21(2):99–107.
21. Westert GP, Lagoe RJ, Keskimaki I, Leyland A, Murphy M. Health Policy (Amsterdam, Netherlands). An international study of hospital readmissions and related utilization in Europe and the USA, 2002;61(3):269–78.
22. Anderson GF, Steinberg EP. Hospital readmissions in the Medicare population. N Engl J Med. 1984;311(21):1349–53.
23. Jencks SF, Williams MV, Coleman EA. Rehospitalizations among patients in the Medicare fee-for-service program. N Engl J Med. 2009;360(14):1418–28.
24. Pugely AJ, Martin CT, Gao Y, Mendoza-Lattes S. Causes and risk factors for 30-day unplanned readmissions after lumbar spine surgery. Spine (Phila Pa 1976). 2014;39(9):761–8.
25. Sherrod BA, Johnston JM, Rocque BG. Risk factors for unplanned readmission within 30 days after pediatric neurosurgery: a nationwide analysis of 9799 procedures from the American College of Surgeons National Surgical Quality Improvement Program. J Neurosurg Pediatr. 2016;18(3):350–62.
26. Purger DA, Pendharkar AV, Ho AL, Sussman ES, Yang L, Desai M, et al. Outpatient vs inpatient anterior cervical discectomy and fusion: a population-level analysis of outcomes and cost. Neurosurgery. 2018;84(4):454–64.
27. Buerba RA, Fu MC, Grauer JN. Anterior and posterior cervical fusion in patients with high body mass index are not associated with greater complications. Spine J. 2014;14(8):1643–53.
28. Kim BD, Smith TR, Lim S, Cybulski GR, Kim JYS. Predictors of unplanned readmission in patients undergoing lumbar decompression: multi-institutional analysis of 7016 patients. J Neurosurg Spine. 2014;20(6):606–16.
29. Nandyala SV, Marquez-Lara A, Park DK, Hassanzadeh H, Sankaranarayanan S, Noureldin M, et al. Incidence, risk factors, and outcomes of postoperative airway management after cervical spine surgery. Spine (Phila Pa 1976). 2014;39(9):E557–63.
30. Schoenfeld AJ, Carey PA, Cleveland AW 3rd, Bader JO, Bono CM. Patient factors, comorbidities, and surgical characteristics that increase mortality and complication risk after spinal arthrodesis: a prognostic study based on 5,887 patients. Spine J. 2013;13(10):1171–9.
31. Willson MC, Ross JS. Postoperative spine complications. Neuroimaging Clin N Am. 2014;24(2):305–26.
32. Corniola MV, Stienen MN, Tessitore E, Schaller K, Gautschi OP. Minimally invasive spine surgery: past and present. Rev Med Suisse. 2015;11(495):2186–9.
33. Smith ZA, Fessler RG. Paradigm changes in spine surgery: evolution of minimally invasive techniques. Nat Rev Neurol. 2012;8(8):443–50.
34. Gruskay J, Smith J, Kepler CK, Radcliff K, Harrop J, Albert T, et al. The seasonality of postoperative infection in spine surgery. J Neurosurg Spine. 2013;18(1):57–62.
35. Glotzbecker MP, Riedel MD, Vitale MG, Matsumoto H, Roye DP, Erickson M, et al. What's the evidence? Systematic literature review of risk factors and preventive strategies for surgical site infection following pediatric spine surgery. J Pediatr Orthop. 2013;33(5):479–87.
36. Kuhns BD, Lubelski D, Alvin MD, Taub JS, McGirt MJ, Benzel EC, et al. Cost and quality of life outcome analysis of postoperative infections after subaxial dorsal cervical fusions. J Neurosurg Spine. 2015;22(4):381–6.
37. Yeramaneni S, Robinson C, Hostin R. Impact of spine surgery complications on costs associated with management of adult spinal deformity. Curr Rev Muscoskelet Med. 2016;9(3):327–32.
38. Bernatz JT, Anderson PA. Thirty-day readmission rates in spine surgery: systematic review and meta-analysis. Neurosurg Focus. 2015;39(4):E7.

39. Anderson PA, Savage JW, Vaccaro AR, Radcliff K, Arnold PM, Lawrence BD, et al. Prevention of surgical site infection in spine surgery. Neurosurgery. 2017;80(3S):S114–S23.
40. Medicare Program. Merit-Based Incentive Payment System (MIPS) and Alternative Payment Model (APM) Incentive Under the Physician Fee Schedule, and Criteria for Physician-Focused Payment Models. Final rule with comment period. Fed Regist. 2016;81(214):77008–831.
41. NASS. Guide to Navigating CMS Quality Initatives and Avoiding Penalties for CY 2016. National American Spine Society; 2016.
42. McGirt MJ, Bydon M, Archer KR, Devin CJ, Chotai S, Parker SL, et al. An analysis from the quality outcomes database, Part 1. Disability, quality of life, and pain outcomes following lumbar spine surgery:predicting likely individual patient outcomes for shared decision-making. J Neurosurg Spine. 2017;27(4):357–69.

Building Quality Metrics into a Practice

18

Clemens M. Schirmer

Background

The quality aspect of healthcare delivery has been on the forefront of changes seen in the last few decades. The US National Quality Strategy has three overarching aims: to improve the quality of care, to improve the health of the population, and, different but certainly related, to reduce the cost of care [1, 2]. These goals are commonly accepted; more controversial is that the achievement of these aims depends, in part, on the collection and reporting of quality measures.

There are currently more than 400 measures or metrics endorsed by the US National Quality Forum [2]. Supporters of concepts such as quality metrics and physician scorecards posit that better health can be achieved by following guidelines developed for single diseases, and speculate, in line with traditional strategies for process and quality improvement (QI), such as Six Sigma and lean thinking, that a summation of single-disease guidelines accurately describes the quality of care delivered by a physician or physician practice [3, 4].

A metric or measure, used interchangeably in this chapter, is a standard measure for assessing performance in a particular area. Metrics are essential for any program directed at continuous improvement. Using metrics may show how stakeholders are interconnected and may foster compatibility of results.

Scope of the Issue in Spine Care

The reader of this text may know back problems are a common issue in the United States with a profound effect on healthcare costs [5]. Consider the following:

C. M. Schirmer
Comprehensive Stroke Center, Department of Neurosurgery and Neuroscience Institute, Geisinger, Danville, PA, USA
e-mail: cmschirmer@geisinger.edu

J. Ratliff et al. (eds.), *Quality Spine Care*,
https://doi.org/10.1007/978-3-319-97990-8_18

- Low back pain (LBP) is second only to upper respiratory problems for the number of physician visits each year.
- A small percentage of patients who see a doctor for their back pain will develop persistent, disabling LBP—the estimated cost of which approaches $50 billion per year in the United States.
- Spondylosis, intervertebral disc disorders, and other back problems were among the top 20 most expensive inpatient conditions in 2011 across all payers, accounting for approximately $11.2 billion dollars spent on hospital costs for the services and excluding physician fees [1].
- Back pain is the primary cause of disability in people under 50 years of age.

Faced with the high cost of surgical spine care in an industry transitioning to value-based payments, health systems are implementing solutions to analyze the effectiveness of surgical interventions—and improve patient engagement and the quality of spinal care.

In general, measures should be targeted to a specific area and should collect accurate and complete data. A metric also should clearly convey performance in a timely and relevant manner. Medicare via its Better Quality Information (BQI) project, more recently incorporated into subsequent quality improvement initiatives, recommends carefully building consensus around a small number of measures (3 priorities versus 30). Once these measures are put into practice and trust among participants grows, coalitions and governing bodies can expand the number of metrics [6].

Implementing Quality Measurement: A Stepwise Approach

Several steps from data entry to analysis will have to be operationalized for meaningful implementation. Using an outside framework, such as the surgeon-led Neuropoint Alliance Quality Outcome Database Spine module [7], addresses most of the following points but is not necessarily the only way to address these challenges. The following concerns are relevant to consideration of a QI framework:

- Data collection methods must be transparent to the entity being reported on. When there is trust in the credibility of the data and results, practice groups are more likely to support publicly reporting their data. Abstraction is hugely important and should be dedicated to professional staff with limited bias whenever possible.
- Credibility and whole practice mapping require limited selection or sampling. Ideally all patients for a practice group or surgeon should be included, limiting the usability of administrative datasets since this would prevent capturing uninsured or out-of-network payers.
- Data validation is a systematic process for reviewing a body of data against a set of criteria to ensure the data are adequate for their intended use.

Developing a data validation process early is important for participant buy-in and trust in the process to be effective. Data validation is an integral component. Standardized data submission tools to organize the administrative and clinical data files required for calculation of measures should be organized in a consistent format, facilitating the audit of data used to calculate the measures.

- Confidentiality and privacy. A measurement framework protects patient confidentiality by containing any patient-identifiable piece of information remaining with the host organization. This also includes the area of concerns best summed as "who owns the data."
- Audits or checks determine whether the measurement specifications were applied by contributors in a manner that would allow for the same results. Review of the data warehouse construction also ensures that data for inclusion have been pulled from all available and appropriate sources. Each contributor should validate its denominator files for each data submission in regular intervals.
- Feedback and clinician engagement are a necessity; execution should test reports internally and then work with stakeholders on reports for physicians and groups before moving to production.
- Translation of results into practice: Low ratings have the potential to make a participant look bad and results should emphasize that low ratings are opportunities for improvement rather than prompting punitive reactions or viewing them as shameful.
- Defining high and low ratings. If not carefully defined, one group or clinician can end up with three stars and another with two when in fact their performance is not significantly different. Any initiative should work with its stakeholders and national analytic experts to define a methodology that addresses this issue.

Usually using an outcomes registry or database to analyze surgical spine care outcomes is not technical but organizational. It requires a workgroup—a permanent, integrated team of clinicians, technologists, analysts, IT, and quality personnel tasked with turning insights derived from data into better clinical outcomes and a registry. A corresponding surgical spine workgroup consists of a physician, nurse practitioners, a business analyst, data architect, and a representative from patient quality and safety.

Even with a registry in place, most often, there are very little outcomes data to work with. We still lack a single, accepted, standard measure for quantifying spine surgery outcomes. Open questions are:

- Determining the best method for evaluating spine surgery outcomes
- Gathering outcomes data to establish a baseline for outcomes analysis
- Developing a healthcare analytics platform for assessing the effectiveness of surgical procedures

With the ability to consistently measure outcomes, practitioners would be able to reduce variation in care—and improve quality and cost.

Table 18.1 QOD surgical spine non-MIPS measures

Measure ID	Measure title
NPA 3	Functional Outcome Assessment for Spine Intervention
NPA 4	Quality of Life Assessment for Spine Intervention
NPA 5	Patient Satisfaction with Spine Care
NPA 6	Spine-related procedure Site Infection
NPA 11	Unplanned Reoperation Following Spine Procedure Within the 30-day Post-Operative Period
NPA 12	Selection of Prophylactic Antibiotic Prior to Spine Procedure
NPA 14	Medicine Reconciliation Following Spine Related Procedure
NPA 15	Risk–assessment for Elective Spine Procedure
NPA 16	Depression and Anxiety Assessment Prior to Spine-Related Therapies
NPA 17	Narcotic Pain Medicine Management Following Elective Spine Procedure
NPA 18	Smoking Assessment and Cessation Coincident with Spine-related Therapies
NPA 19	Body Mass Assessment and Follow-up Coincident with Spine-related Therapies
NPA 20	Unhealthy Alcohol Use Assessment Coincident With Spine Care
NPA 23	Spine/Extremity Pain Assessment

See [8]

Instruments for Measuring Outcomes

At baseline most health systems data consist primarily of pain scores reported by patients before and after surgery—a very subjective measure of surgical success and data from morbidity and mortality reviews of surgical practice.

The Quality Outcomes Database (QOD) has been approved as a 2018 Centers for Medicare and Medicaid Services (CMS)-Approved Qualified Clinical Data Registry (QCDR) for the Merit-Based Incentive Program (MIPS) 2018 reporting year.

The QOD Surgical Spine QCDR offers 14 unique surgical spine non-MIPS (Merit-Based Incentive Payment System) measures approved by the CMS. A participating registry-eligible professional (EP) can choose from these measures to report for purposes of satisfying the quality portion of MIPS and avoid associated penalties [8]. See Table 18.1 for a list of surgical spine care measures available through the QOD for 2018 MIPS reporting.

Patient-Reported Measures

Patient-reported baseline data and outcomes, preferentially using integrated electronic data-capture solutions, can be immensely helpful to supplement objective measures. Baseline QOL data is gathered by the staff during an office visit approximately 30 days before the surgical procedure. Due to the nature of surgical spine procedures and the time associated with recovery and physical therapy, staff engage the patients to complete the survey again at 3 months, 6 months, 9 months, and 1 year post-procedure.

Table 18.2 Patient-reported outcome measure examples

Measure	Purpose
Patient Health Questionnaire-2 (PHQ-2)	Designed to screen for depression
Patient Health Questionnaire-9 (PHQ-9)	Screening, diagnosing, monitoring and measuring the severity of depression
Oswestry Disability Index (ODI)	Designed to assess limitations of various activities of daily living, primarily targeted for low back pain patients
Neck Disability Index (NDI)	Designed to measure the impact of neck pain on the patient's ability to manage in everyday life
Euro QOL five-dimensional (EQ-5D)	General QOL measurement tool, in contrast to the ODI and NDI, which are targeted to specific spinal conditions

Using an automated, integrated approach for capturing data reduces the inefficiencies and the opportunities for error associated with paper data recording. The digitized information flows directly from the patient portal into the EHR and is available for analysis. This also plays an important role in driving measurable patient engagement. Gathering QOL data digitally has created a meaningful way to engage the health system's patients, sometimes through its patient portal.

A number of tools and surveys are currently used to assess patient-reported surgical spine outcomes throughout the healthcare industry. These various QOL instruments measure the physical, emotional, and social well-being of the patients undergoing treatment for spinal disorders; however, none of the tools alone are sufficient. See Table 18.2 for a list of patient-reported measures.

Systems of Care and Processes in Simple and Complex Nonlinear Environments

Concepts of Complexity

The reductionist approach to scientific inquiry has served mankind well over time and many believe that systems are improved by deconstructing overall system performance and management into component elements [9]. Healthcare may not be appropriately treated by linear approximation and may be better conceptualized as a complex adaptive system—where learning people and institutions (called "agents" in the complex adaptive system vernacular) nonlinearly interact with the environment, resulting in emerging creative behaviors rather than rigidly adhering to a standardized set of linear processes for diagnosing and treating single diseases [10, 11]. Failure to realize this behavior may lead some to erroneously conclude that practices have failed by not implementing standardized interventions [10].

Industrial QI approaches have improved care delivery in mechanical linear domains, such as limited aspects of elective spine surgery [12], ventilator-associated pneumonia bundles [13, 14], and central line bundles [15, 16], where processes do not change appreciably for different patients. These processes commonly have few variables (5 and 8 for the two examples given), and it is reasonable to assume that measurable process steps are causally connected to patient-oriented outcomes. Such is not the case for outcome-based measures and overall care, which is more complex than other specialties with many more inputs and outputs [17, 18]. If more than 20 variables are included in a process control algorithm, the impact of measurement inaccuracies, for instance, results in cumulative noise that makes distinguishing individual variable effects very difficult [19].

Process Standardization

Traditional QI stipulates that optimal quality is achieved when a linear process occurs the same way each time [4]. Real patients do no lend themselves to this simplification due to the wide variety of patient needs. Not all health problems initially encountered at a practice lead to a definitive diagnosis that would trigger a standard care pathway which accounts for each patient's comorbidities, disease severity, medication tolerance, beliefs, desires, and socioeconomic factors [20]. Given the paucity of evidence, surgeons must often rely on creativity, problem-solving, and adaptability to develop a custom care plan.

Process Controls

Input variables in processes, such as hospital central line bundles, are largely controlled by or tagged to specific actions by clinicians (e.g., washing hands, using chlorhexidine antiseptics). In contrast, complex adaptive systems have no single point of control [9], and input variables for care processes and health outcomes are often beyond the control of the physician and patient [21], such as socioeconomic factors [22] and poverty [23]. Identifying hot spots and improving care for disadvantaged populations [24] may be generalizable, but the improved outcomes of these programs were more likely achieved by creating care plans adapted to the unique circumstances of high-risk patients needing changed physician payment models for these approaches to spread more rapidly and consistently to other vulnerable populations [25].

Alignment of Interests

Outcomes may be prioritized differently by independent agents in a complex adaptive system, may vary depending on the external environment of the system, and likely change with time [3, 4], creating challenges for policy makers attempting to measure the outcomes of healthcare practices in different settings.

Well-aligned quality measures for spine care should promote accountable performance and boost clinicians' motivation by rewarding them for managing complexity, solving problems, and thinking creatively when addressing the unique circumstances of each patient [26, 27]. Instead, misaligned QI metrics and directives, e.g., electronic health records (EHRs) [28], have contributed to burnout among physicians, as documented in primary care [29], causing some to advocate for the quadruple aim by adding the goal of enhancing professional satisfaction and well-being to the well-known "Triple Aim" [30]. Notably some primary care physicians believe existing metrics may paradoxically encourage poor quality of care [31, 32].

Outcome Goal Precision

Specialists are more likely than generalists to follow disease-specific guidelines, but this assumes a single unifying correct diagnostic or treatment option based on the organ of interest and does not convey similar uniformity of outcomes [33]. When physicians deviated from single-disease guidelines, it is often for medically appropriate reasons [34, 35].

The translation of traditional QI to the healthcare setting requires rational agents and patients who follow expert advice, whereas in reality patients come with a wide range of priorities that may not be aligned with those of their caregivers.

Traditional QI metrics allow for little variance of the timing of intervention goals. For example, the Centers for Medicare and Medicaid Services (CMS) core quality indicator set includes a hospital metric that aspirin will be prescribed to every patient with an acute myocardial infarction at hospital discharge [36]. The best time frame to attempt to achieve an idealized goal, such as weight loss before spine surgery, can be complex.

Quantitative Aspects of Quality in a Spine Practice

A rigid list of quality metrics, usually process-oriented, purporting to summarize the quality of care discounts the actuality of a complex adaptive system. Learning, adaptability, and self-organization highlight practice aspects most worthy of improvement efforts, while priorities evolve with time [9]. Complex interactions and interdependencies emerge within such a system that cannot be understood or predicted simply by measuring individual elements of the system—one cannot assume that the whole is merely a sum of the measurable parts [11, 37]. These realities imply that measures based on linear models, such as MS-DRG groups and severity indices, are less than optimal summaries of surgical quality [38].

Examples from Other Specialties Associated with Better Outcomes

Other specialties have demonstrated that quality initiatives are associated with better outcomes or lower costs, e.g., the comprehensiveness of services provided by family physicians that is associated with fewer complications or mortality, lower costs, and fewer hospitalizations [39–41], the smaller practice size associated with reduced hospitalizations from preventable conditions [42], and the rate of generic prescription writing [43]. Other measures suggested economies of scales for larger care systems including increased time for office visits for complex patients, 24/7 access to local clinic professionals, and careful selection of referral specialists [44].

Some of these examples, refined over time, also support the notion that better measurement of a practice may be that it regularly undertakes self-reflection and measures its patient care, with regulators worrying less about exactly what each practice is attempting to measure and improve. This approach would focus on the positive features of a complex adaptive system: self-organization, emergence, and coevolution with the environment [45].

Risk Adjustment

Risk adjustment of summative quality scorecards is crucial to guarantee that surgeons and practices are gauged impartially, because the characteristics of the associated patient population have a large effect on the reported results of standard QI metrics. Studies of these quality scorecards conclude that caring for complex patients in a safety-net setting strongly predicts failure to meet common quality goals in hospitals [46, 47] and primary care settings [48–50]. The National Quality Forum highlights that socioeconomic aspects are important factors of patient outcomes, that current measurements do not account for these factors, and that adequate risk adjustments for quality outcomes do not currently exist [51]. Key opinion leaders have proposed risk adjustment for patient panels [52], but currently rigorous methods are lacking, and existing models give different results [53]. As a result, current summative quality scorecards continue to disadvantage surgeons who care for the most vulnerable patient populations. Clinicians who are more attentive to the social and cultural context are more likely to deliver positive patient outcomes [54] when adjusting care plans, though measuring such context takes sizable work [55].

Goal Target Number and Absolute Goals

Quality scorecards are not easy to interpret, and metrics where 0% or 100% are the targets are difficult to manage in practice, even though they are suggested goals in Joint Commission surveys. There is a discrepancy of prospects between the reality of healthcare and traditional notions of industrial QI, e.g., Six Sigma, implying adherence to process measures 99.9997% of the time [56]. Uptake of recommended tests or treatments can never be 100% in the outpatient setting, even in populations with homogenous socioeconomic status. For example, even though many patients may indicate that they are willing to undergo colon cancer screening when asked by their physicians, uptake of recommended screening or adherence to chronic disease management goals is low, often measured at less than 50% of eligible patients [57–60].

Intermountain Healthcare expects variance of 5–15% in some of its quality measures and scrutinizes physicians for complying with a protocol too much [61].

Scorecard Comprehensiveness

The comprehensiveness of services offered by physicians creates a tension between payers who seek to be reassured with numerical data that participating practices provide high-quality care and the practical limits and uncertain validity of data collection and reporting. One may posit that a few well-chosen measures will represent a large fraction of the work delivered in a specialty practice, e.g., hip and knee replacement surgery [62]. For a practice that mostly performs such surgeries, this metric may allow policy makers to determine whether the practice is performing well. Such a two-disease measure would be inappropriate and inadequate for specialties with less narrow disease focus [18].

On the converse, an excess of individual measures may become cumbersome and expensive to collect and report. Even worse, these myriad measures will still be unlikely to capture the richness of the interactions between the primary care practice professionals and patients. Family physicians have been observed to manage nearly 500 different diagnoses in 3,344 recorded patient encounters in a national study [18]; even when diagnoses are clustered into groups (e.g., low back pain syndromes and headaches), 25 of these clusters account for only 60% of the diagnoses [63], making it unrealistic to represent a complex adaptive system with a finite number of dependent and independent variables [11].

The cost to a practice is also burdensome. Just to maintain a patient-centered medical home accreditation has been estimated to cost $120,000 per provider annually [64]. More often than not, scorecards constructed based on EHR data represent an ideal case as envisioned by system designers and differ from the reality experienced by patients and physicians [45].

"All-In" Exceptions and Utilization Reporting

Future quantitative quality scorecards should borrow a concept from the British National Health Service QOF pay-for-performance system currently called exception reporting [65]. As opposed to selecting a group of patients to report on, British practitioners are given a list of reasons that allow them to remove individual patients from quality reports. Examples include patients new to their practice, patients who decline recommended tests or treatments, and patients with comorbidities that render a disease-specific quality metric inappropriate. This concept has also been known as patient choice or shared decision reporting [66].

Surgeons may also be held accountable when they do choose to not subject their patients to interventions. This measure of avoidance is also not well captured by traditional QI which focuses on positive action. The Choosing Wisely campaign provides a thoughtful framework to develop new metrics to reduce unnecessary tests and treatments [67].

Patient Satisfaction Versus Patient-Centric Outcome Measures

Patient satisfaction scores have been linked to rendering inappropriate services, such as prescribing unnecessary antibiotics [68]. Patients' goals and treatment preferences are not the same as patient satisfaction, and there is evidence that greater patient satisfaction scores are associated with worse outcomes, including higher mortality rates [69–71]. This suggests significant gaps in knowledge about the relevance of patient satisfaction scores to quality and stresses caution and the need for further research in this area.

A lofty goal is to measure more patient-centric outcomes at a population level, such as death rates (risk adjusted for age, comorbidities, and socioeconomic factors), disability (absence from work, limitation of activities), ease of access, and some measures of patient experience of care (respect, treatment burden). Measures like these may be more difficult to develop and implement, but they are likely to be more meaningful for achieving societal goals [72, 73].

Care Patterns and Peer Assessment

Perhaps a better approach to reassure payers, regulators, and patients of high-quality care would be to replace most quantitative measures with adequately funded peer-reviewed assessments of patterns of care, as proposed recently in Scotland [74]. Peer-reviewed assessments would also be more consistent with evaluation principles of a complex adaptive system, where qualitative assessments of relationships between agents provide a more meaningful understanding of the quality of care provided than externally mandated numeric targets [37, 75].

Conclusion

Spine practitioners comfort with complexity, ambiguity, and uncertainty—and their ongoing relationships with their patients allow them to negotiate flexible diagnostic and treatment plans based on patient-specific risk factors and probabilities of serious disease [76, 77]. At its core QI assumes the existence of a definitive and measurable right answer in a given situation; in contrast, physicians often deliver high-value care by doing the best but knowing that perfection will never be achieved given that patients are not perfect or idealized.

Adaptability rather than standardization should be the cornerstone of complex care. The national trends of rigid metrics and the current focus on scorecards must be reversed for systems to do a better job of delivering patient care at lower costs.

Specialty-specific measures are a significant advance that spine practitioners may pursue in this area [8]. Helping those who measures us become better at doing so should be an objective; once a metric is in place, it becomes more difficult to contest whether or not it should apply.

References

1. Agency for Healthcare Research and Quality. About the National Quality Strategy (NQS). n.d. http://www.ahrq.gov/workingforquality/about.htm#aims. Accessed 9 Apr 2018.
2. Agency for Healthcare Research and Quality. NQF-endorsed measures. n.d. https://www.qualitymeasures.ahrq.gov/browse/nqf-endorsed.aspx. Accessed 9 Apr 2018.
3. de Brantes F, Galvin RS, Lee TH. Bridges to excellence: building a business case for quality care. JCOM-WAYNE PA. 2003;10:439–46.
4. Institute of Medicine (U.S.), editor. Crossing the quality chasm: a new health system for the 21st century. Washington, D.C: National Academy Press; 2001.
5. Becker's Hospital Review. Top 20 most expensive inpatient conditions. n.d. https://www.beckershospitalreview.com/finance/top-20-most-expensive-inpatient-conditions.html. Accessed 8 Apr 2018.
6. Prachanronarong A. The better quality information to improve care for medicare beneficiaries project: exploring approaches to physician performance measurement. Am Health Drug Benefits. 2008;1:22–6.
7. QOD Spine Registries. n.d. http://www.neuropoint.org/registries/qod-spine/. Accessed 9 Apr 2018.
8. Qualified Clinical Data Registry Reporting. n.d. http://www.neuropoint.org/qcdr-reporting-mips/. Accessed 9 Apr 2018.
9. Rouse WB. Health care as a complex adaptive system: implications for design and management. Bridge-Wash-Natl Acad Eng. 2008;38:17.
10. Sturmberg JP, Martin CM, Katerndahl DA. Systems and complexity thinking in the general practice literature: an integrative, historical narrative review. Ann Fam Med. 2014;12:66–74. https://doi.org/10.1370/afm.1593.
11. Eoyang G, Berkas T. Evaluation in a complex adaptive system. 1998 [Internet] Retrieved from: https://www.researchgate.net/publication/237571019_Evaluation_in_a_Complex_Adaptive_System
12. Meyer H. At UPMC, improving care processes to serve patients better and cut costs. Health Aff (Millwood). 2011;30:400–3. https://doi.org/10.1377/hlthaff.2011.0139.
13. Morris AC, Hay AW, Swann DG, Everingham K, McCulloch C, McNulty J, et al. Reducing ventilator-associated pneumonia in intensive care: impact of implementing a care bundle. Crit Care Med. 2011;39:2218–24. https://doi.org/10.1097/CCM.0b013e3182227d52.
14. Bird D, Zambuto A, O'Donnell C, Silva J, Korn C, Burke R, et al. Adherence to ventilator-associated pneumonia bundle and incidence of ventilator-associated pneumonia in the surgical intensive care unit. Arch Surg Chic Ill 1960. 2010;145:465–70. https://doi.org/10.1001/archsurg.2010.69.
15. Galpern D, Guerrero A, Tu A, Fahoum B, Wise L. Effectiveness of a central line bundle campaign on line-associated infections in the intensive care unit. Surgery. 2008;144:492–5.; discussion 495. https://doi.org/10.1016/j.surg.2008.06.004.
16. Guerin K, Wagner J, Rains K, Bessesen M. Reduction in central line-associated bloodstream infections by implementation of a postinsertion care bundle. Am J Infect Control. 2010;38:430–3. https://doi.org/10.1016/j.ajic.2010.03.007.
17. Katerndahl DA, Wood R, Jaen CR. A method for estimating relative complexity of ambulatory care. Ann Fam Med. 2010;8:341–7. https://doi.org/10.1370/afm.1157.

18. Katerndahl D, Wood R, Jaén CR. Complexity of ambulatory care across disciplines. Healthc Amst Neth. 2015;3:89–96. https://doi.org/10.1016/j.hjdsi.2015.02.002.
19. Young RA, Roberts RG, Holden RJ. The challenges of measuring, improving, and reporting quality in primary care. Ann Fam Med. 2017;15:175–82. https://doi.org/10.1370/afm.2014.
20. Rosendal M, Carlsen AH, Rask MT, Moth G. Symptoms as the main problem in primary care: a cross-sectional study of frequency and characteristics. Scand J Prim Health Care. 2015;33:91–9. https://doi.org/10.3109/02813432.2015.1030166.
21. Hershberger PJ, Bricker DA. Who determines physician effectiveness? JAMA. 2014;312:2613. https://doi.org/10.1001/jama.2014.13304.
22. Stringhini S, Sabia S, Shipley M, Brunner E, Nabi H, Kivimaki M, et al. Association of socioeconomic position with health behaviors and mortality. JAMA. 2010;303:1159–66. https://doi.org/10.1001/jama.2010.297.
23. Foege WH. Social determinants of health and health-care solutions. Public Health Rep Wash DC 1974. 2010;125(Suppl 4):8–10. https://doi.org/10.1177/00333549101250S403.
24. Gawande A. Medical Report: The hot spotters—can we lower medical costs by giving the neediest patients better care. 2011.
25. Phillips RL, Pugno PA, Saultz JW, Tuggy ML, Borkan JM, Hoekzema GS, et al. Health is primary: family medicine for America's health. Ann Fam Med. 2014;12:S1–12. https://doi.org/10.1370/afm.1699.
26. Pink DH. Drive: the surprising truth about what motivates us. London: Penguin; 2011.
27. Cassel CK, Jain SH. Assessing individual physician performance: does measurement suppress motivation? JAMA. 2012;307:2595–6. https://doi.org/10.1001/jama.2012.6382.
28. Rabin RC. A growing number of primary-care doctors are burning out. How does this affect patients? Wash Post. 2014.
29. Linzer M, Levine R, Meltzer D, Poplau S, Warde C, West CP. 10 bold steps to prevent burnout in general internal medicine. J Gen Intern Med. 2014;29:18–20. https://doi.org/10.1007/s11606-013-2597-8.
30. Bodenheimer T, Sinsky C. From triple to quadruple aim: care of the patient requires care of the provider. Ann Fam Med. 2014;12:573–6. https://doi.org/10.1370/afm.1713.
31. Greenhalgh T, Howick J, Maskrey N, for the Evidence Based Medicine Renaissance Group. Evidence based medicine: a movement in crisis? BMJ. 2014;348:g3725. https://doi.org/10.1136/bmj.g3725.
32. Waddimba AC, Burgess JF, Young GJ, Beckman HB, Meterko M. Motivators and hygiene factors among physicians responding to explicit incentives to improve the value of care. Qual Manag Health Care. 2013;22:285–301. https://doi.org/10.1097/QMH.0000000000000006.
33. Harrold LR, Field TS, Gurwitz JH. Knowledge, patterns of care, and outcomes of care for generalists and specialists. J Gen Intern Med. 1999;14:499–511.
34. Persell SD, Dolan NC, Friesema EM, Thompson JA, Kaiser D, Baker DW. Frequency of inappropriate medical exceptions to quality measures. Ann Intern Med. 2010;152:225–31. https://doi.org/10.7326/0003-4819-152-4-201002160-00007.
35. Steinman MA, Dimaano L, Peterson CA, Heidenreich PA, Knight SJ, Fung KZ, et al. Reasons for not prescribing guideline-recommended medications to adults with heart failure. Med Care. 2013;51:901–7. https://doi.org/10.1097/MLR.0b013e3182a3e525.
36. Center for Medicare & Medicaid Services. Clinical quality measures finalized for eligible hospitals and critical access hospitals beginning with FY 2014. n.d. https://www.cms.gov/regulations-and-guidance/legislation/ehrincentiveprograms/downloads/2014_cqm_eh_final-rule.pdf. Accessed 8 Apr 2018.
37. Kordowicz M. Do systems and complexity theories aid our understanding of poor performing general practices? Editor Board. 2012.
38. Green LA. The implications of measuring complexity. Ann Fam Med. 2010;8:291–2. https://doi.org/10.1370/afm.1147.
39. Bazemore A, Petterson S, Peterson LE, Phillips RL. More comprehensive care among family physicians is associated with lower costs and fewer hospitalizations. Ann Fam Med. 2015;13:206–13. https://doi.org/10.1370/afm.1787.

40. Hussey PS, Schneider EC, Rudin RS, Fox DS, Lai J, Pollack CE. Continuity and the costs of care for chronic disease. JAMA Intern Med. 2014;174:742–8. https://doi.org/10.1001/jamainternmed.2014.245.
41. Saultz JW. Interpersonal continuity of care and care outcomes: a critical review. Ann Fam Med. 2005;3:159–66. https://doi.org/10.1370/afm.285.
42. Casalino LP, Pesko MF, Ryan AM, Mendelsohn JL, Copeland KR, Ramsay PP, et al. Small primary care physician practices have low rates of preventable hospital admissions. Health Aff Proj Hope. 2014;33:1680–8. https://doi.org/10.1377/hlthaff.2014.0434.
43. Federman AD, Halm EA, Siu AL. Use of generic cardiovascular medications by elderly Medicare beneficiaries receiving generalist or cardiologist care. Med Care. 2007;45:109–15. https://doi.org/10.1097/01.mlr.0000250293.24939.2e.
44. Milstein A, Gilbertson E. American medical home runs. Health Aff (Millwood). 2009;28:1317–26. https://doi.org/10.1377/hlthaff.28.5.1317.
45. Hollnagel E. The ETTO principle: efficiency-thoroughness trade-off: why things that go right sometimes go wrong. Aldershot: Ashgate Publishing, Ltd; 2009.
46. Rajaram R, Chung JW, Kinnier CV, Barnard C, Mohanty S, Pavey ES, et al. Hospital characteristics associated with penalties in the Centers for Medicare & Medicaid Services hospital-acquired condition reduction program. JAMA. 2015;314:375–83. https://doi.org/10.1001/jama.2015.8609.
47. Skinner J. Mortality after acute myocardial infarction in hospitals that disproportionately treat black patients. Circulation. 2005;112:2634–41. https://doi.org/10.1161/CIRCULATIONAHA.105.543231.
48. Reschovsky JD, O'Malley AS. Do primary care physicians treating minority patients report problems delivering high-quality care? Health Aff (Millwood). 2008;27:w222–31. https://doi.org/10.1377/hlthaff.27.3.w222.
49. Bach PB, Pham HH, Schrag D, Tate RC, Hargraves JL. Primary care physicians who treat blacks and whites. N Engl J Med. 2004;351:575–84. https://doi.org/10.1056/NEJMsa040609.
50. Hong CS, Atlas SJ, Chang Y, Subramanian SV, Ashburner JM, Barry MJ, et al. Relationship between patient panel characteristics and primary care physician clinical performance rankings. JAMA. 2010;304:1107–13. https://doi.org/10.1001/jama.2010.1287.
51. National Quality Forum. Risk adjustment for sociodemographic factors 2014. http://www.qualityforum.org/risk_adjustment_ses.aspx. Accessed 8 Apr 2018.
52. Fiscella K, Burstin HR, Nerenz DR. Quality measures and sociodemographic risk factors: to adjust or not to adjust. JAMA. 2014;312:2615–6. https://doi.org/10.1001/jama.2014.15372.
53. Kent DM, Shah ND. Risk models and patient-centered evidence: should physicians expect one right answer? JAMA. 2012;307:1585–6. https://doi.org/10.1001/jama.2012.469.
54. Weiner SJ, Schwartz A, Sharma G, Binns-Calvey A, Ashley N, Kelly B, et al. Patient-centered decision making and health care outcomes: an observational study. Ann Intern Med. 2013;158:573–9. https://doi.org/10.7326/0003-4819-158-8-201304160-00001.
55. Valdez RS, Holden RJ, Novak LL, Veinot TC. Transforming consumer health informatics through a patient work framework: connecting patients to context. J Am Med Inform Assoc. 2015;22:2–10. https://doi.org/10.1136/amiajnl-2014-002826.
56. Henderson KM, Evans JR. Successful implementation of Six Sigma: benchmarking general electric company. Benchmarking Int J. 2000;7:260–82.
57. Leard LE, Savides TJ, Ganiats TG. Patient preferences for colorectal cancer screening. J Fam Pract. 1997;45:211–8.
58. Anderson WF. Colorectal cancer screening for persons at average risk. Cancer Spectrum Knowl Environ. 2002;94:1126–33. https://doi.org/10.1093/jnci/94.15.1126.
59. Green AR, Peters-Lewis A, Percac-Lima S, Betancourt JR, Richter JM, Janairo M-PR, et al. Barriers to screening colonoscopy for low-income Latino and white patients in an urban community health center. J Gen Intern Med. 2008;23:834–40. https://doi.org/10.1007/s11606-008-0572-6.
60. Sharma AE, Willard-Grace R, Hessler D, Bodenheimer T, Thom DH. What happens after health coaching? Observational study 1 year following a randomized controlled trial. Ann Fam Med. 2016;14:200–7. https://doi.org/10.1370/afm.1924.

61. Goitein L, James B. Standardized best practices and individual craft-based medicine: a conversation about quality. JAMA Intern Med. 2016;176:835. https://doi.org/10.1001/jamainternmed.2016.1641.
62. Damberg CL, Baker DW. Improving the quality of quality measurement. J Gen Intern Med. 2016;31:8–9. https://doi.org/10.1007/s11606-015-3577-y.
63. Stange KC, Zyzanski SJ, Jaén CR, Callahan EJ, Kelly RB, Gillanders WR, et al. Illuminating the "black box". A description of 4454 patient visits to 138 family physicians. J Fam Pract. 1998;46:377–89.
64. Magill MK, Ehrenberger D, Scammon DL, Day J, Allen T, Reall AJ, et al. The cost of sustaining a patient-centered medical home: experience from 2 states. Ann Fam Med. 2015;13:429–35. https://doi.org/10.1370/afm.1851.
65. Doran T, Kontopantelis E, Fullwood C, Lester H, Valderas JM, Campbell S. Exempting dissenting patients from pay for performance schemes: retrospective analysis of exception reporting in the UK Quality and Outcomes Framework. BMJ. 2012;344:e2405. https://doi.org/10.1136/bmj.e2405.
66. McCartney M, Treadwell J, Maskrey N, Lehman R. Making evidence based medicine work for individual patients. BMJ. 2016:i2452. https://doi.org/10.1136/bmj.i2452.
67. ABIM Foundation. Choosing wisely. n.d. http://www.choosingwisely.org/. Accessed 8 Apr 2018.
68. Wexler R. Patient satisfaction as a quality metric promotes bad medicine. JAMA Intern Med. 2014;174:1418. https://doi.org/10.1001/jamainternmed.2014.1624.
69. Kupfer JM, Bond EU. Patient satisfaction and patient-centered care: necessary but not equal. JAMA. 2012;308:139. https://doi.org/10.1001/jama.2012.7381.
70. Fenton JJ. The cost of satisfaction: a national Study of patient satisfaction, health care utilization, expenditures, and mortality. Arch Intern Med. 2012;172:405. https://doi.org/10.1001/archinternmed.2011.1662.
71. Mold JW, Lawler F, Schauf KJ, Aspy CB. Does patient assessment of the quality of the primary care they receive predict subsequent outcomes? An Oklahoma Physicians Resource/Research Network (OKPRN) study. J Am Board Fam Med. 2012;25:e1–12. https://doi.org/10.3122/jabfm.2012.04.120106.
72. Reuben DB, Tinetti ME. Goal-oriented patient care—an alternative health outcomes paradigm. N Engl J Med. 2012;366:777–9. https://doi.org/10.1056/NEJMp1113631.
73. May C, Montori VM, Mair FS. We need minimally disruptive medicine. BMJ. 2009;339:b2803. https://doi.org/10.1136/bmj.b2803.
74. BBC News. 'Outdated' QOF GP payment system scrapped in Scotland 2015. http://www.bbc.com/news/uk-scotland-scotland-politics-34419123. Accessed 8 Apr 2018.
75. Crabtree BF, Nutting PA, Miller WL, McDaniel RR, Stange KC, Jaen CR, et al. Primary care practice transformation is hard work: insights from a 15-year developmental program of research. Med Care. 2011;49:S28–35. https://doi.org/10.1097/MLR.0b013e3181cad65c.
76. Young RA, Bayles B, Benold TB, Hill JH, Kumar KA, Burge S. Family physicians' perceptions on how they deliver cost-effective care: a qualitative study from the Residency Research Network of Texas (RRNeT). Fam Med. 2013;45:311–8.
77. Katerndahl D. Providing complex (rather than complicated) chronic care. J Am Board Fam Med. 2014;27:6–7. https://doi.org/10.3122/jabfm.2014.01.130285.

19 Impact of Quality Assessment on Clinical Practice, Intermountain Healthcare

Mark J. Ott and Griffin H. Olsen

Abbreviations

APCs	Advanced practice clinicians (including physician assistants, nurse practitioners, and nurse midwifes)
DPCs	Doctor procedure cards
EMR	Electronic medical record
PSI 90	Patient safety indicator 90 (a composite of multiple publicly report patient safety outcome metrics
RBC	Red blood cells

Introduction

This chapter shows how value assessment can have dramatic impact on clinical practice, with steadily improving quality while reducing the cost of care for patients and for the healthcare system. The method that has proven repeatedly successful within Intermountain Healthcare is to present to clinicians their specific data in a way that allows them to make choices and to see how their colleagues do the same thing in different ways. To understand how this was accomplished in the Intermountain Healthcare system and how this can be used in other healthcare systems requires understanding of the history and organization of Intermountain Healthcare.

M. J. Ott (✉)
Central Region Administration, Intermountain Healthcare, Murray, UT, USA
e-mail: mark.ott@imail.org

G. H. Olsen
Surgical Services Clinical Program, Intermountain Healthcare, Murray, UT, USA

J. Ratliff et al. (eds.), *Quality Spine Care*,
https://doi.org/10.1007/978-3-319-97990-8_19

Intermountain Healthcare was created as a not-for-profit healthcare organization in 1975 as a gift to the communities of the Intermountain West of the United States by The Church of Jesus Christ of Latter-Day Saints. The leadership of the then newly created Intermountain Healthcare was given 15 independent community hospitals scattered across the states of Utah, Wyoming, and Idaho; but more importantly the leaders of this new organization were given the charge to become "a model healthcare system" and to meet the healthcare needs of the peoples in those communities regardless of their ability to pay for those services. Intermountain Healthcare has since grown to include 23 hospitals; ~200 outpatient clinics, urgent care clinics, and outpatient pharmacies; a health insurance plan (SelectHealth) covering ~850,000 lives; an employed medical group of ~2,000 employed physicians and advanced practice clinicians (APCs) along with twice that many independent clinicians also delivering care in Intermountain Healthcare hospitals; and a workforce of ~40,000 employees who provide exceptional care. From the charge, "to become a model healthcare system," there arose a commitment to collecting data on patient outcomes and continually working to improve those outcomes while simultaneously reducing the cost of care. From its initial inception as an organization, an electronic data warehouse (EDW) was created along with an electronic ordering and data collection system known as Tandem/Help. This transitioned over the years into an updated system, Help2, which eventually transitioned into the current Cerner-based electronic medical record (EMR) called iCentra.

Data collection, data analysis, and the sharing of that data with clinicians and administrators are what make possible the Intermountain Healthcare's vision statement to "Be a model health system by providing extraordinary care and superior service at an affordable cost." To carry out this vision, multiple data sources are integrated and organized for presentation to clinicians of their personal performance data on safety, quality, patient experience, patient access, and cost metrics. These data reports/dashboards need to be shared with them in a way that engages physicians and other care providers to voluntarily improve the care of their patients and to increase the fulfillment of these care providers. They need to be concise and timely and fit into the clinicians' pre-existing workflows. Only healthcare organizations have the resources to gather, analyze, and share these data, and only fully integrated healthcare organizations that have access to hospital data, outpatient data, insurance claim data, and patient and provider satisfaction data are able to comprehensively address the full spectrum of the value equation. Intermountain Healthcare is fortunate to be such a fully integrate healthcare system, and its experience is relevant to the rest of the United States and to the global healthcare market since it also has a mix of physician employment models. Approximately a third of the physicians caring for patients in the

Intermountain Healthcare system are employed by Intermountain Healthcare, and two-thirds are independent practitioners. Regardless of employment models, clinicians respond similarly when they are given their validated outcomes and cost data. The following case studies are examples of how the sharing of specific quality and cost data sets with clinicians is done within Intermountain Healthcare and the clinical impact that has occurred.

Blood Utilization

Red blood cell (RBC) transfusion is the most commonly performed procedure in US hospitals [1]. Blood transfusion can be given in excess of their true benefit to patients and can increase adverse outcomes, mortality, and cost [2–4]. Review of our data demonstrated that our clinicians were over transfusing patients to the detriment of their outcomes and adding cost to their care. As a result, we developed and implemented an automated electronic blood ordering and tracking system to monitor RBC ordering and administration. With the specific goal to reduce both the number of patients receiving RBC transfusion and the amount of RBC they received when a transfusion was indicated, we re-designed how we documented blood orders and administrations in our EMR. We started the reengineering of our EMR for blood ordering and administration in 2010. In 2011 we implemented the new blood program in 3 of our largest facilities, and by July of 2012 we completed the implementation at all 22 facilities. Simultaneously we initiated a system-wide educational effort of thousands of physicians and staff through division and staff meeting presentation, online educational modules, and hands-on practice sessions. These educational efforts were tailored to the specific roles of indications and ordering by physicians and APCs and separately to the delivery roles involving unit clerks, nurses, anesthesiologists, and the blood bank personnel. Referential performance was provided monthly via email to any physician whose inpatients received an RBC transfusion in the previous month (Fig. 19.1). The email contained a hyperlink that would take them to their own transfusion dashboard (Fig. 19.2). Finally, results were also presented regularly at physician meetings by a physician champion. The physician champion also responded to individual physician data concerns by phone and/or email 24/7. Each clinician could then see their own transfusion patterns for the past year and compare their transfusion thresholds to the best evidence guidelines, which we supplied them in the email. We specifically did not tell them if their transfusion of their patients was appropriate or not, since this was ultimately their clinical decision.

The percentage of patients receiving RBC decreased by 30% from 1/1/2012 to 1/31/2015. The number of RBC units transfused decreased from 49.64 units per

a

From: SurgeryClinicalProgram@imail.org
Subject: Transfusion Reduction
Date: Mon, 19 Jan 2015 22:04:02 +0000

Dear Esteemed Colleague:
You are receiving this email as an attending provider of record for a patient discharged in the month of December 2014 who received a blood transfusion during that hospitalization. Intermountain Healthcare has established a Clinical Board Goal for 2014 (listed below) focused on reducing the number of unnecessary PRBC transfusions in the adult population. By clicking on this link Physician Blood Utilization Report from a computer inside the Intermountain Healthcare firewall and using your standard Intermountain user ID/password, you can view your transfusion data.

Goals
Decrease the amount of two unit transfusions **and** transfusion for Hematocrit > 22.9% to 45.0 % or less average for measurement period January 1, 2104- December 31, 2014 for system (excluding bone marrow transplant patients).
Most patients do not need an elective blood transfusion for hematocrits above 21%. When a blood transfusion is appropriate, one unit instead of two units is usually the appropriate dose. Please consider giving your patient one unit of blood and then reevaluating the patient before routinely giving them two units of blood. We know that this is different from what you may have learned in medical school and residency, but is well supported by the best evidence based guidelines below.

Please compare your personal blood transfusion practice to these best evidence based guidelines for transfusion indications based on hematocrit level and medical history:

b

Potential PRBC Transfusion Indication Recommendations	
Indication	**Threshold Hct/Hgb**
o Asymptomatic	21/7
o Tachycardia, shortness of breath, tachypnea, orthostasis, and/or syncope with no explanation other that anemia	24/8
o Marrow suppressive therapy	27/9
o To reduce cardiac stress in severe CHF	30/10
o Shock with global tissue ischemia manifested by hemodynamic instability and/or elevated lactic acid (greater than 4 mmol/L)	
o Local ischemic disease of heart or brain	
o Acute hemorrhage or blood loss not immediately controllable	Based on hemodynamics not hematocrit

If you have any questions please contact your hospital or surgical services medical director, or Mark Ott, MD Surgical Services Medical Director. Mark.Ott@imail.org.

Mark Ott, MD
Medical Director
Surgical Services Clinical Program

Fig. 19.1 (**a**, **b**) Blood utilization automated email sent monthly to any physician who had an inpatient that received an RBC transfusion in the previous month

1000 patient days pre-intervention to 34.55 units per 1000 patient days post-intervention (Fig. 19.3). Two unit transfusions decreased from 68% of all transfusions ordered to 23%, and the trend to decrease overall number and amount of transfusions has continued its downward slope to the present (Fig. 19.4). The percentage of patients transfused with a hematocrit ≥23% decreased from 60% to 34% over the same time period. The amount of cost avoidance was $2.5

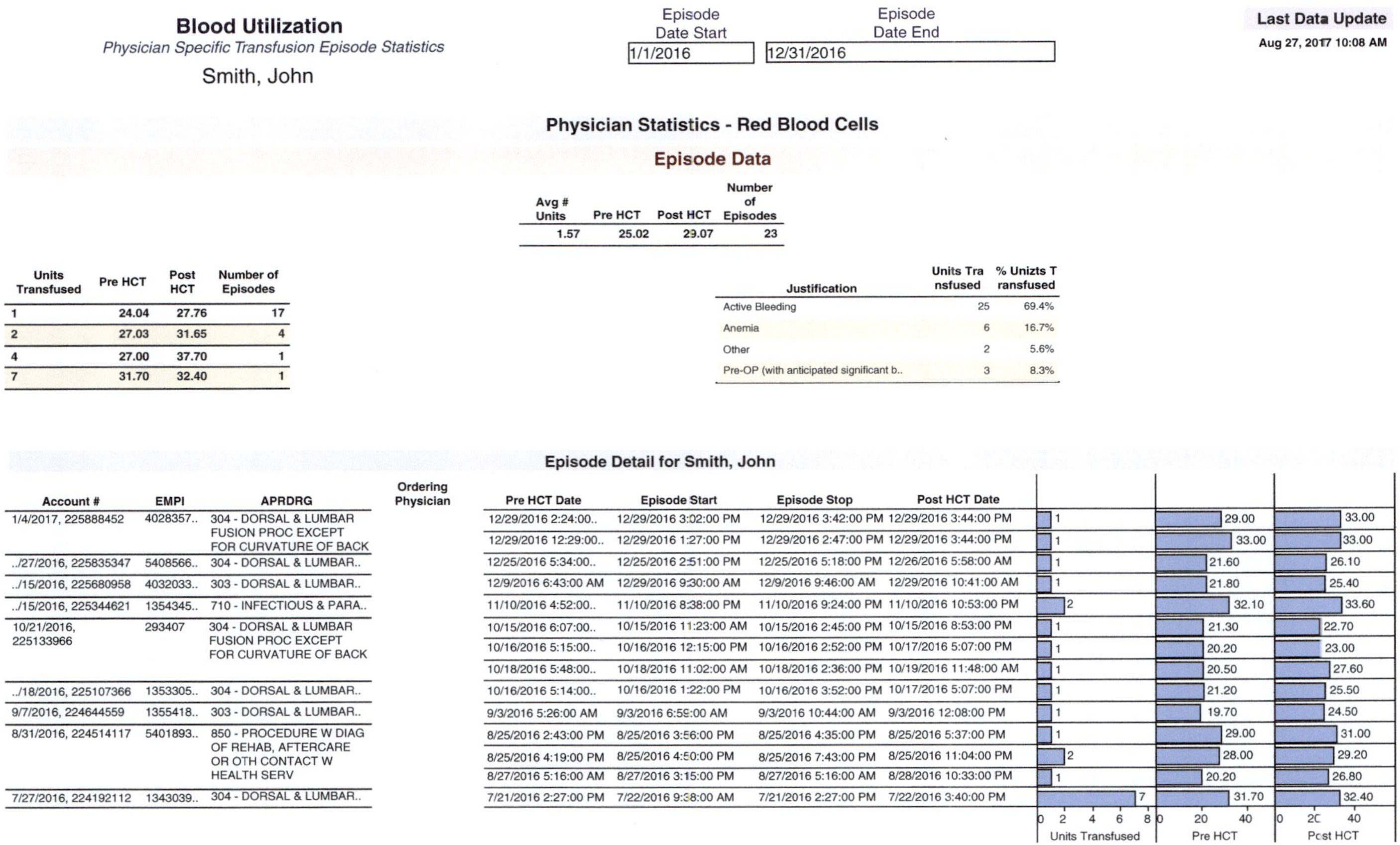

Blood Utilization
Physician Specific Transfusion Episode Statistics
Smith, John

Episode Date Start: 1/1/2016 Episode Date End: 12/31/2016

Last Data Update Aug 27, 2017 10:08 AM

Physician Statistics - Red Blood Cells

Episode Data

Avg # Units	Pre HCT	Post HCT	Number of Episodes
1.57	25.02	29.07	23

Units Transfused	Pre HCT	Post HCT	Number of Episodes
1	24.04	27.76	17
2	27.03	31.65	4
4	27.00	37.70	1
7	31.70	32.40	1

Justification	Units Tra nsfused	% Unizts T ransfused
Active Bleeding	25	69.4%
Anemia	6	16.7%
Other	2	5.6%
Pre-OP (with anticipated significant b..	3	8.3%

Episode Detail for Smith, John

Account #	EMPI	APRDRG	Ordering Physician
1/4/2017, 225888452	4028357..	304 - DORSAL & LUMBAR FUSION PROC EXCEPT FOR CURVATURE OF BACK	
../27/2016, 225835347	5408566..	304 - DORSAL & LUMBAR..	
../15/2016, 225680958	4032033..	303 - DORSAL & LUMBAR..	
../15/2016, 225344621	1354345..	710 - INFECTIOUS & PARA..	
10/21/2016, 225133966	293407	304 - DORSAL & LUMBAR FUSION PROC EXCEPT FOR CURVATURE OF BACK	
../18/2016, 225107366	1353305..	304 - DORSAL & LUMBAR..	
9/7/2016, 224644559	1355418..	303 - DORSAL & LUMBAR..	
8/31/2016, 224514117	5401893..	850 - PROCEDURE W DIAG OF REHAB, AFTERCARE OR OTH CONTACT W HEALTH SERV	
7/27/2016, 224192112	1343039..	304 - DORSAL & LUMBAR..	

Pre HCT Date	Episode Start	Episode Stop	Post HCT Date	Units Transfused	Pre HCT	Post HCT
12/29/2016 2:24:00..	12/29/2016 3:02:00 PM	12/29/2016 3:42:00 PM	12/29/2016 3:44:00 PM	1	29.00	33.00
12/29/2016 12:29:00..	12/29/2016 1:27:00 PM	12/29/2016 2:47:00 PM	12/29/2016 3:44:00 PM	1	33.00	33.00
12/25/2016 5:34:00..	12/25/2016 2:51:00 PM	12/25/2016 5:18:00 PM	12/26/2016 5:58:00 AM	1	21.60	26.10
12/9/2016 6:43:00 AM	12/29/2016 9:30:00 AM	12/9/2016 9:46:00 AM	12/29/2016 10:41:00 AM	1	21.80	25.40
11/10/2016 4:52:00..	11/10/2016 8:38:00 PM	11/10/2016 9:24:00 PM	11/10/2016 10:53:00 PM	2	32.10	33.60
10/15/2016 6:07:00..	10/15/2016 11:23:00 AM	10/15/2016 2:45:00 PM	10/15/2016 8:53:00 PM	1	21.30	22.70
10/16/2016 5:15:00..	10/16/2016 12:15:00 PM	10/16/2016 2:52:00 PM	10/17/2016 5:07:00 PM	1	20.20	23.00
10/18/2016 5:48:00..	10/18/2016 11:02:00 AM	10/18/2016 2:36:00 PM	10/19/2016 11:48:00 AM	1	20.50	27.60
10/16/2016 5:14:00..	10/16/2016 1:22:00 PM	10/16/2016 3:52:00 PM	10/17/2016 5:07:00 PM	1	21.20	25.50
9/3/2016 5:26:00 AM	9/3/2016 6:59:00 AM	9/3/2016 10:44:00 AM	9/3/2016 12:08:00 PM	1	19.70	24.50
8/25/2016 2:43:00 PM	8/25/2016 3:56:00 PM	8/25/2016 4:35:00 PM	8/25/2016 5:37:00 PM	1	29.00	31.00
8/25/2016 4:19:00 PM	8/25/2016 4:50:00 PM	8/25/2016 7:43:00 PM	8/25/2016 11:04:00 PM	2	28.00	29.20
8/27/2016 5:16:00 AM	8/27/2016 3:15:00 PM	8/27/2016 5:16:00 AM	8/28/2016 10:33:00 PM	1	20.20	26.80
7/21/2016 2:27:00 PM	7/22/2016 9:38:00 AM	7/21/2016 2:27:00 PM	7/22/2016 3:40:00 PM	7	31.70	32.40

Fig. 19.2 Individual physician blood utilization dashboard

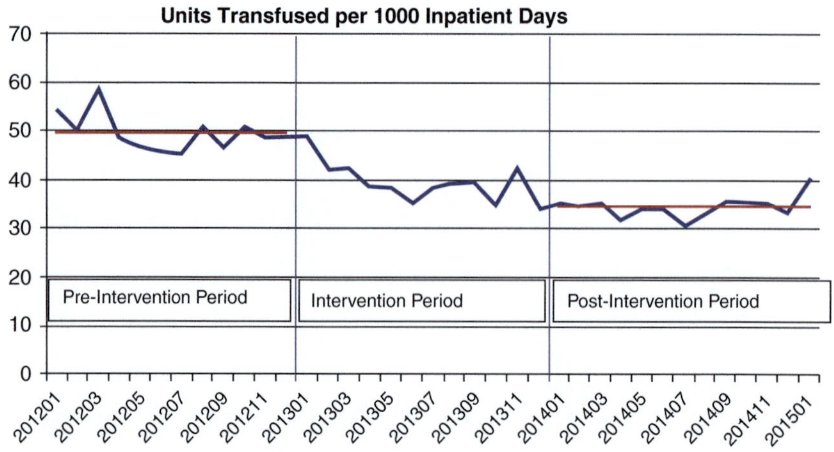

Fig. 19.3 Units transfused per 1000 patient days showing run rates for the pre-intervention, intervention, and post-intervention periods

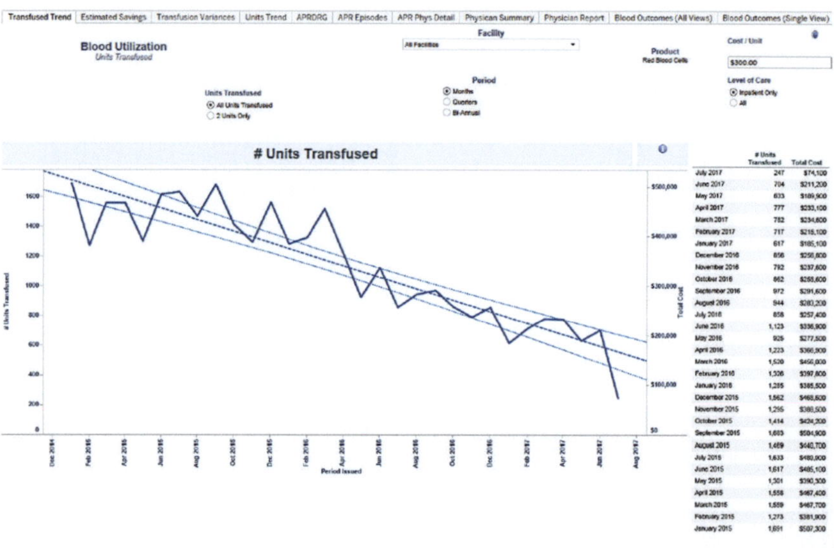

Fig. 19.4 Transfusion trends for total amount of RBC transfusion for inpatients in the Intermountain Healthcare system

million over the initial 2-year period, assuming each unit of RBC cost $300 and that cost avoidance continues (Fig. 19.5). Thirty-day mortality (Fig. 19.6) decreased in the same time period. For those patients that received RBC transfusions, their hospital acquired infection rate dropped from 10.85 to 8.73 per 1000 patient days, likely because they received fewer units of blood when a decision to transfuse was made. These results were achieved and sustained through

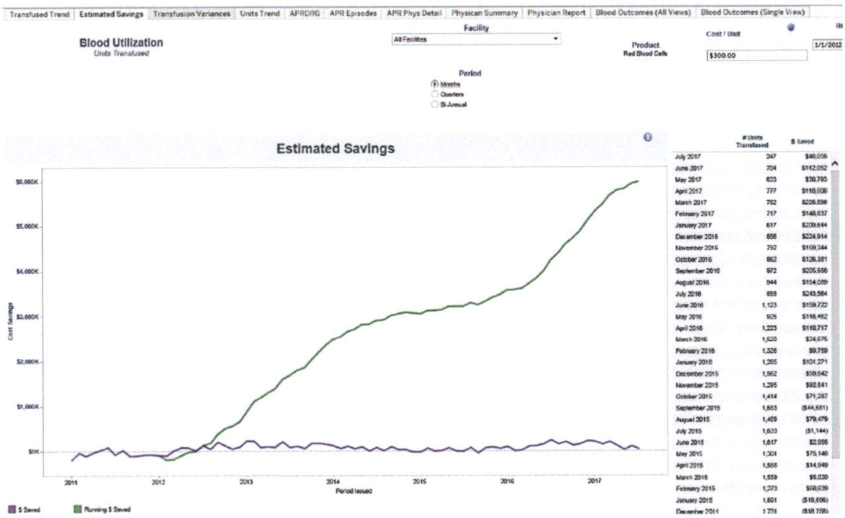

Fig. 19.5 Estimated cost saving for the Intermountain Healthcare system. This is calculated monthly based on the difference between the amount of RBC transfusion given at baseline prior to institution of the electronic blood ordering and tracking program and the current month. The purple line represents the savings per month, and the green line represents the cumulative savings since the program was instituted. The cost of a unit of blood to Intermountain Healthcare was set at $300 for the estimates

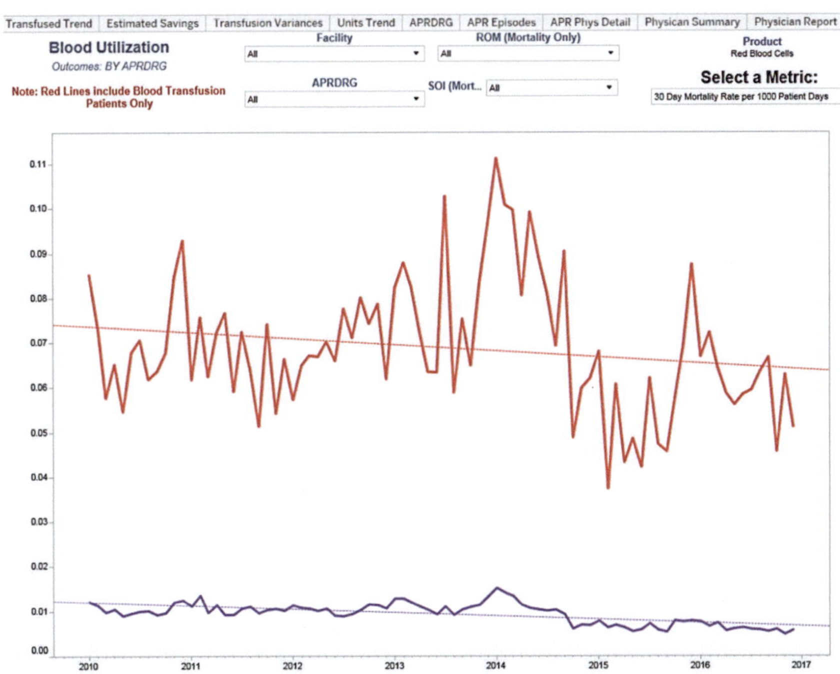

Fig. 19.6 30-day mortality rate per 1000 patient days for the Intermountain Healthcare system. The red line represents patient receiving RBC transfusions, and purple line represents all other patients not receiving RBC transfusions during inpatient admissions

physician and APC education, timely and repetitive feedback of each physician's personal transfusion practices, and the implementation of an automated data tracking and ordering system. The results of this were positive for patients, providers, payers, and for reducing the overall cost of healthcare delivery across the entire Intermountain Healthcare system.

Empiric Health

An area of intense focus in healthcare delivery is the rising cost of care. US healthcare spending increased 4.3 percent to reach $3.3 trillion or $10,348 per person in 2016. Healthcare spending growth decelerated in 2016 after the initial impacts of ACA coverage expansions and strong retail prescription drug spending growth in 2014 and 2015. The overall share of gross domestic product (GDP) related to healthcare spending was 17.9 percent in 2016, up from 17.7 percent in 2015 [5]. Addressing this "cost problem" is certainly one of the major issues of our society and frequently a topic of social and political dialogue. Many healthcare systems have reduced the number of vendors or required vendors to meet a price point to reduce the cost of implants, and these strategies have been effective in cost reduction [6]. Intermountain Healthcare has also employed these strategies by using surgeon committees who participate in the pricing and negotiation of these contracts. However, most of the items used in the daily care of patients and especially in the operating room are not amenable to this type of strategy and are truly "physician preference items." These daily decisions made by physicians and other care providers significantly drive the cost of healthcare. Yet, most clinicians are unaware of the cost of what they order or use every day in patient care.

The Surgical Services Clinical Program of Intermountain Healthcare sought to empower surgeons to make decisions on behalf of their patients by creating an automated system to allow surgeons and their care teams to know the cost of every item they chose to use at the point of care delivery. This system originally known as ProComp internally and now organized as a separate external company, Empiric Health, gives physicians and the care teams the ability to factor in cost as they make choices about quality and how to perform surgical procedures and all associated care. For example, a surgeon can decide which suture product A, B, or C, all of which perform similarly but have differing costs, is most appropriate for the care of the specific patient. If a surgeon decides that to use a 4.0 Vicryl on a FS2 needle instead of a PS2 needle (the needles are almost identical), the cost savings might be $2. That is not much, but if the surgeon uses this suture 300 times each year, that is a cost savings of $600/year. Sometimes a surgeon needs to decide to spend money on a supply item to save operating room time, which also has a cost. The surgeon might decide to use a particular disposable energy device to cut and seal tissue that cost $300 because it will save 20 min of operating room time at $40/min for a net savings of $500. One topical hemostatic agent costs $30 and other $150. If the surgeon believes they are equivalent, she/he will likely choose the $30 agent once they know the cost differential.

We believe the surgeon is the ideal person to determine the value of every item they want to have on their doctor's procedure card (DPC) for every procedure they perform. If the surgeon knows the cost of supplies, pharmaceuticals, radiology studies, operating room time, etc., they can factor in cost of those items along with the quality achieved by using these items and make better value decisions. There are thousands of decision points that a surgeon makes each year that result in significant cost differentials in the care of individual patients and in the cost to the healthcare system as a whole. When we began to use the ProComp/Empiric Health system in 2011, we purposefully never told the surgeons or surgical teams they need to use one item versus another. It was always a voluntary decision by each surgeon. The surgeons were quite interested in the information and began to change their DPCs to select less expensive items when appropriate. They wanted to decrease the cost of care for their patients. From 2012 through 2015 as we sequentially rolled out the system through all 22 hospitals in the Intermountain Healthcare system, we documented ~$100 million in cost savings over that 4-year period, including $2 million (2012), $16.8 million (2013), $42.9 million (2014), and $39 million (2015). To reassure the surgeons, who were also very concerned that the savings be passed on to the patients, we shared with them that in 2014 the total cost reduction was $42,965,516 and the reduction in charges to patients and payers was $37,977,462. Participation of the surgeons in cost saving and quality decisions did not require that any part of the savings be shared with the surgeons. They did this because they believed it was best for their patients.

The ProComp/Empiric Health system includes access to information in the operating room but also outside of the operating room and in departmental/divisional meetings. The computer in every operating room has a DPC icon on the desktop that contains the up-to-date cost of every supply item. The cost of an item is displayed along with comparable items and their cost. During the operation, the surgeon is able to ask the circulating nurse what a particular item costs and, in seconds, have that cost while the surgeon is operating. If the surgeon decides to use a different item and wants the DPC permanently changed, the circulating nurse can make the change on the DPC for that procedure and on all other similar procedure cards for that surgeon. The change is then active for all future cases with those DPCs.

Outside the operating room, the surgeon can use another component of the system, called Opportunity Explorer, to see the cumulative effect of a specific change over a years' worth of cases based on the surgeons known annual usage of the product in a specific case type or across multiple procedures (Fig. 19.7). The system also allows physicians in a department/division meeting to see how they compare to their colleagues for the exact same procedure. The information is presented in an unblinded fashion, so that each physician can see where they are in outcomes and cost. They can also see each specific component that affects their total cost (Fig. 19.8). Groups of physicians can use the system to optimally design a surgical procedure to give the best

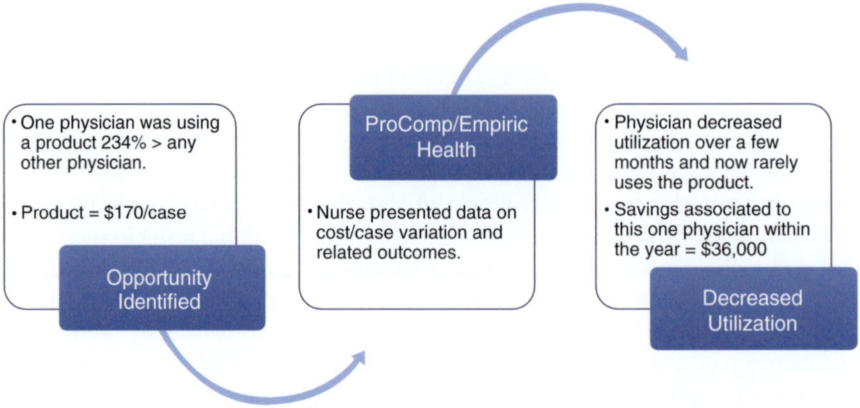

Fig. 19.7 Opportunity Explorer Methodology of the ProComp/Empiric Health system

Lap Chole														
Facility	Cases	Total Cost	Surg Time	OR Minutes	Trocars	Trocars Per Case	Clip Appliers	Cautery	Irrigator	Endoloop	Endocatch	Closure Dev.	Cholang. Set	Hemostatics
Colum	Colu	Colum	Colu	Colu	Colum	Colum	Colum	Colum	Colum	Colum	Colum	Colum	Colum	Colum
Physician	30	$998.29	60	91	$ 98.58	3.70	$410.47	$209.79	0.03	0.60	0.73	0.90	0.37	0.17
Physician	2	$885.53	28	55	$111.83	5.50	$282.37	$ 73.16	1.00	#N/A	1.00	1.50	#N/A	#N/A
Physician	1	$848.88	58	84	$109.99	5.00	$487.54	$ 16.73	1.00	#N/A	1.00	#N/A	#N/A	#N/A
Physician	61	$744.55	55	86	$ 64.55	4.08	$139.51	$165.20	#N/A	1.05	0.87	1.00	0.25	0.21
Physician	2	$549.98	54	87	$ 86.32	4.00	$115.71	$ 41.77	#N/A	1.00	1.00	1.00	#N/A	#N/A
Physician	85	$543.89	48	75	$101.80	4.07	$178.11	$ 0.09	0.48	0.34	0.49	0.94	0.54	#N/A
Physician	1	$525.33	45	78	$ 73.02	4.00	$243.77	$ 33.46	1.00	#N/A	#N/A	#N/A	1.00	#N/A
Physician	1	$514.35	27	51	$ 81.18	4.00	$243.77	$ 16.73	#N/A	#N/A	#N/A	#N/A	2.00	#N/A
Physician	6	$513.98	81	108	$ 78.79	3.67	$190.13	$ 20.28	#N/A	0.50	0.67	0.83	0.50	0.33
Physician	45	$499.01	69	102	$192.64	4.91	$ 85.41	$ 1.73	0.80	0.49	0.27	1.02	#N/A	0.02
Physician	23	$492.42	58	84	$ 72.55	4.04	$157.73	$ 2.65	0.35	0.57	0.74	1.00	0.09	0.13
IM	930	$478.30	48	74	$ 83.24	3.64	$159.53	$ 31.68	0.17	0.19	0.58	0.75	0.25	0.11
Physician	131	$473.96	51	78	$ 95.89	4.09	$159.47	$ 15.81	0.30	0.07	0.73	0.95	0.50	0.23
Physician	113	$447.09	42	67	$ 87.88	4.00	$162.53	$ 16.88	0.08	0.02	0.91	0.01	#N/A	0.30
Physician	157	$444.35	38	65	$ 89.98	4.02	$165.15	$ 16.76	0.01	0.03	0.53	0.88	0.08	0.03
Physician	2	$400.07	51	82	$ 66.75	4.00	$142.39	$ 48.22	#N/A	#N/A	0.50	#N/A	#N/A	#N/A
Physician	8	$397.75	64	111	$ 54.32	3.38	$ 78.14	#N/A	0.75	#N/A	0.75	#N/A	#N/A	0.63
Physician	7	$392.37	42	70	$ 83.25	4.00	$ 88.44	$ 95.81	0.29	#N/A	0.43	#N/A	#N/A	#N/A
Physician	17	$388.47	74	101	$ 88.79	4.18	$125.63	$ 2.05	0.06	0.06	0.82	0.82	0.06	0.06
Physician	184	$366.51	44	64	$ 41.45	1.92	$157.96	$ 0.17	0.05	0.05	0.30	0.92	0.42	0.04

Fig. 19.8 Facility procedure-specific presentation chart for laparoscopic cholecystectomy for department meeting presentation. The name of each surgeon is displayed unblinded in the left column. The row in yellow is the facility average cost for the procedure. Each surgeon can see their case volume, cost, and all resources used relative to each other to determine what accounts for their variation

outcome at the lowest cost. An example of this occurred at Primary Children's Hospital in our system. The pediatric general surgeons together developed a care process model for appendicitis that they felt would give the best outcomes at the lowest cost (Fig. 19.9). It also allows for comparison for the same procedure between hospitals using the system to see cost differentials and why they exist (Fig. 19.10). The graph shows that in 2013 the cost of a standard laparoscopic cholecystectomy varied among our own facilities from less than $1,000 to more than $3,700. Our goal as a system is to assure that patients in our system receive the same excellent care at the same low cost regardless of which of our facilities they use. That was not the case before we began sharing these data with our physicians and teams.

The system also includes quality outcome variables to help the surgeons identify and correct individual and hospital-wide deficiencies (Fig. 19.11). Across the top of

Year	n	Supply Costs	Direct Costs	Total Costs	Total Charges	Contractual Adjustments	Insurance Payments
2012	329	$840	$3,767	$6,720	$11,289	($2,779)	($6,870)
2013	319	$373	$2,744	$5,743	$9,909	($2,530)	($5,967)
2014	263	$275	$2,465	$5,481	$9,470	($2,736)	($5,306)

2014 costs and charges include encounters through November

2014 payments and adjustments include encounters through August

Comparing 2012 to 2014 shows

67.2% decrease in supply costs

34.6% decrease in direct costs

18.4% decrease in total costs

16.1% decrease in total charges

22.8% decrease in insurance payments

17.9% decrease in other payments

Fig. 19.9 Cost savings achieve by a redesign of the laparoscopic appendectomy operative care process model at Primary Children's Hospital in the Intermountain Healthcare system. The pediatric surgeons all agreed on standardization of the surgical procedure and supplies and care process and then instituted these with further refinements from 2012 to 2014

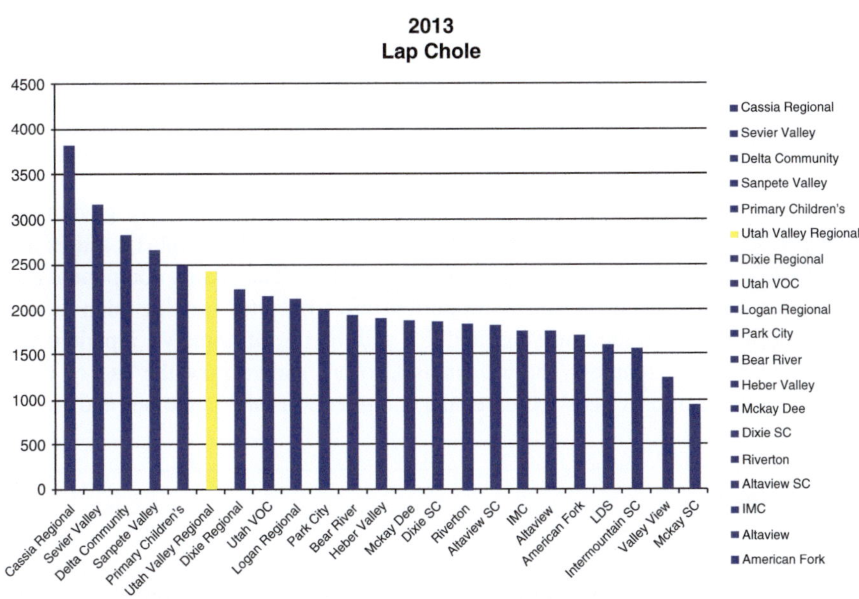

Fig. 19.10 Variation in cost (dollars) between Intermountain Healthcare facilities at the beginning of ProComp/Empiric Health implementation process. These data are share across the system with physicians so that they see how their facility compares to others in the region and system

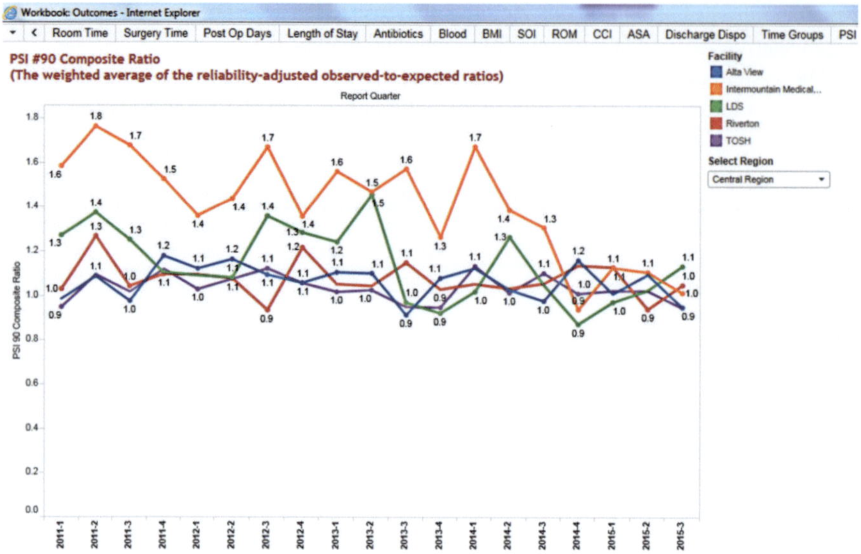

Fig. 19.11 Patient Safety Index #90 (PSI 90) tracking of several Intermountain Healthcare facilities displayed in quality section of the ProComp/Empiric Health system. Sharing of these data with clinicians at those facilities leads to improvement in quality metric performance over time. The bar across the top allows the selection from 19 different outcome variables

the quality dashboard are tabs for various quality metrics important to surgeons and their patients. By being able to easily see these outcomes, individual surgeons and groups of surgeons can become aware of their performance and make changes and design processes to continually improve them. In this particular example, the tab for Patient Safety Indicator 90 (PSI 90) is displayed. PSI 90 is a composite of multiple publicly reported quality outcome variables. One can see that the hospital depicted by the orange line was having a PSI 90 value 1.3 to 1.8 times expected, meaning that they were having complications 1.3 to 1.8 times more frequent than expected in that time period. When they became aware of this, they instituted multiple measures that lead to their PSI 90 value returning to 1.0 (as expected). The quality component also tracks for facilities and physicians important after hospital variable such as discharge to home vs. skilled nursing facilities and the use of home vs. inpatient and outpatient rehab resources. The clinicians also are shown how the use of these resources either improves or decreases the complications and outcomes and costs.

Conclusion

Within Intermountain Healthcare we have used these methods of data collection, analysis, sharing back with clinicians, and education to allow our clinicians to make choices about the care of their patients. The blood utilization and ProComp/Empiric Health systems are just two of many similar systems that have been developed by our teams of physicians, data analysists, and administrators to deliver high-value healthcare. We believe our success in improving quality and reducing costs for multiple care process models is attributable to the transparency of these data and the intrinsic desire of clinicians to provide excellent cost-effective care to their patients. The process has been voluntary and it has been effective. The process would be replicable within other healthcare systems and works for both physicians employed by that healthcare system and those in private practice. It did not require any sharing of the saving with the clinicians, as long as it was clear that the cost savings were leading to a similar decrease in billed charges and that the decision about quality and cost were made by the clinicians. This has been a success for patients, physicians, healthcare systems, payers, and our community.

References

1. Pfunter A, Wier LM, Stocks CA. Most frequent procedures performed in U.S. hospitals, 2010: Statistical Brief #149. Healthcare Costs and Utilization Project (HCUP) statistical brief. Rockville; 2013. Sponsored by the Agency for Health Care Policy and Research (US).
2. Rohde JM, Dimcheff DE, Blumberg N, Saints S, Langa KM, Kuhn L, et al. Healthcare-associated infections after red blood cell transfusions: a systematic review and meta-analysis. JAMA. 2014;311:1317–26.
3. Murphy GJ, Reeves BC, Rogers CA, Rizvi SI, Culliford L, Angelini GD. Increased mortality, postoperative morbidity, and cost after red cell transfusion in patients having cardiac surgery. Circulation. 2007;116:2544–52.
4. Hopewell S, Omar O, Hyde C, Yu LM, Doree C, Murphy MF. A systematic review of the effect of red blood cell transfusion on mortality; evidence from large-scale observational studies published between 2006 and 2010. BMJ Open. 2013;3(5). pii:e002154. https://doi.org/10.1136/bmjopen-2012-002154
5. National Healthcare Expenditures 2016 Highlights – CMS.gov. https://www.cms.gov/Research-Statistics-Data-and-Systems/...and.../highlights.pdf
6. Oren J, Hutzler LH, Hunter T, Errico T, Zuckerman J, Bosco J. Decreasing spine implant costs and inter-physician cost variation: the impact of programme of cost containment on implant expenditure in spine surgery. Bone Joint J. 2015;97-B(8):1102–5.

Impact of Quality Assessment on Clinical Practice, Kaiser Permanente

20

Kern H. Guppy, Jessica Harris, Johannes A. Bernbeck, and Harsimran S. Brara

Overview of Kaiser Permanente

The history of Kaiser Permanente began in the 1930s when Sidney R. Garfield, MD, acquired a small hospital in the Southern California and began providing care for employees of a Los Angeles Aqueduct building project [1]. Dr. Garfield had two concepts in mind: (1) prepaid medical care and (2) establish a multispecialty group practice rather than solo or small group practices. During the 1940s and 1950s, he collaborated with Henry J. Kaiser, a wealthy industrialist, to build the major components of the healthcare system now known as Kaiser Permanente (KP). Over the years KP grew and currently is made up of the Kaiser Foundation Health Plan (KFHP), the Kaiser Permanente Hospitals (KFH), and contracted medical groups collectively called the Permanente Medical Groups. Currently KP is the largest managed care organization in the United States insuring over 11.8 million members throughout eight states (California, Hawaii, Oregon, Washington, Georgia, Colorado, Maryland, Virginia) and the District of Columbia (Fig. 20.1).

K. H. Guppy (✉)
Neurosurgery, The Kaiser Permanente Medical Group, Sacramento, CA, USA
e-mail: Kern.H.Guppy@kp.org

J. Harris
Surgical Outcomes and Analysis, Southern California Permanente Medical Group, San Diego, CA, USA

J. A. Bernbeck
Orthopedics-Spine, Southern California Permanente Medical Group, Downey, CA, USA

H. S. Brara
Neurosurgery, Southern California Permanente Medical Group, Los Angeles, CA, USA

J. Ratliff et al. (eds.), *Quality Spine Care*,
https://doi.org/10.1007/978-3-319-97990-8_20

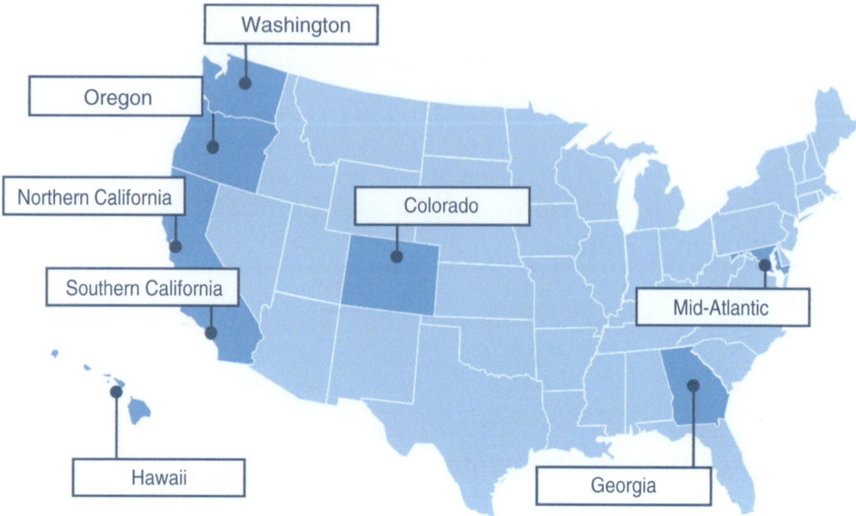

Fig. 20.1 The Kaiser Permanente healthcare system 2017

Electronic Health Record System

One of the hallmarks of an integrated healthcare system is the ability to share information across geographical regions instantaneously. In 2006 Kaiser Permanente implemented an electronic health record (EHR) system called HealthConnect™. This system is a customized EHR product, primarily managed by Epic Systems Corp (Verona,WI) but includes software applications from several other vendors. Software applications include clinical (such as ambulatory, inpatient, emergency room, operating room, etc.), access (admission, discharge, registration, scheduling), revenue, billing and claims optimization, financials, data integration (reporting, data repository, healthcare data management), and other applications (bar code scanning, mobile computing, etc.). The information collected from HealthConnect™ is stored permanently into a Clarity™ database (GridApp Systems, Inc., New York, NY). This national database is updated nightly and is organized into multiple tables, broken down by modules of the applications mentioned above. Specific encounter identifiers, transaction identifiers, and patient identifiers link all the information. This database allows, through secure connections, the extraction of the aggregate data using various database extraction tools, such as SQL (Structured Query Language; IBM Corp, Armonk, NY), SAS1 (SAS Institute Inc., Cary, NC), or Crystal Report (SAP America, Inc., Newtown Square, PA) [2].

Kaiser Permanente Registries

A registry is an organized system that collects uniform data (clinical and other data) to evaluate specified outcomes for a population defined by a particular disease, condition, or exposure and uses observational study methods to make conclusions [3].

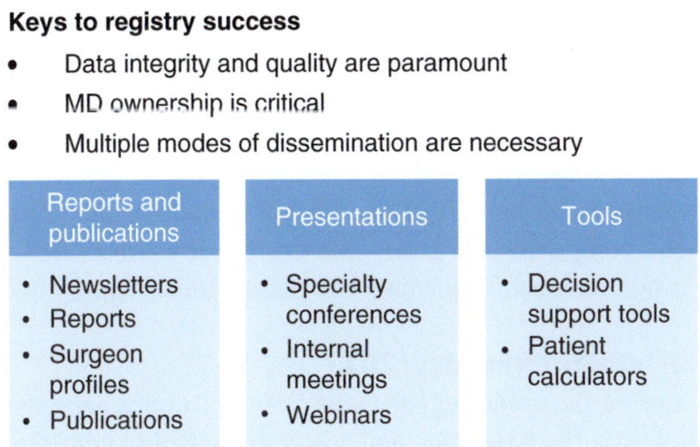

Fig. 20.2 Keys to Kaiser Permanente implant registries success

The EHR system is instrumental in providing a method to collect such data. Kaiser Permanente has created eight registries collectively known as the Kaiser Permanente implant registries [4]. The first, established in 2001, was the KP Total Joint Replacement Registry. It was designed as a post-market surveillance system for elective total hip and knee replacement and is now the largest total joint replacement registry in the United States. This model was replicated to create other registries, including the KP Anterior Cruciate Ligament (ACL) Reconstruction Registry, KP Hip Fracture Registry, KP Shoulder Arthroplasty Registry, KP Endovascular Stent Graft Registry, KP Cardiac Device Registry, and the KP spine registry [4, 5]. The keys to the success in our registries are multifactorial, but undoubtedly physician ownership and participation is vital to its success. It is also important that this information is disseminated to physicians via multiple modes (Fig. 20.2).

Kaiser Permanente Spine Registry

The KP spine registry has been one of Kaiser Permanente more successful registries. It is supported by both Neurosurgeons and Orthopedic spine surgeons who contribute their time and effort in collecting data to make it successful. Its present form has evolved over several years with several iterations from its initial development.

Historical Prospective

The KP spine registry was started in 2006 with the main purpose of collecting data on all KP patients undergoing spine surgery. Data collected included patients' demographics, clinical information, surgical procedures, spinal implant information, and patient outcome measures. Clinical data was extracted from HealthConnect™. Surgical information was obtained from surgeons using handwritten forms at the end of each spine procedures. Patient outcome questionnaires were distributed and collected during the patient's clinic visits. Patient outcome measures used were visual analog scale (VAS) scores, Oswestry disability questionnaires, modified Orthopedic Association Myelopathy (mJOA) questionnaires, neck disability questionnaires, and 36-Item Short-Form Survey (SF-36). This was done by standardized paper-based forms at preoperative and postoperative encounters. Between 2006 and 2009, the registry collected a large amount of data, but unfortunately the data acquisition fell short of our goals with compliances of <60%. From this initial endeavor, lessons learned included (1) any data collection for surgeons should be nonintrusive and be part of the normal workflow, and (2) more time was needed for patients completing the forms, and that hectic environment, such as during clinic visits, was not the ideal for patients completing these lengthy questionnaires.

Current Spinal Implant Registry: 2017

In 2009, the scope of the spine registry was limited to only patients who received spinal implants. Using the EHR data and a search algorithm combining spinal procedural codes from the *International Classification of Diseases, Ninth Revision, Clinical Modification (ICD-9-CM, now ICD-10 CM))* codes and manufacturers' implant catalogs reference numbers, all the instrumented spinal fusion cases were identified (Fig. 20.3).

Anomalies or miss-matches were reviewed by chart review and determinations made to their appropriateness for inclusion in the spine registry database. Patient's age, sex, body mass index, American Society of Anesthesiologists (ASA) score, operative time, diagnosis, region of the spine fused, number of spine levels fused, implant characteristics, and procedural information were all captured in the registry. Procedures were categorized based on spine region (cervical only, thoracic only, lumbar only (includes L5–S1), cervical-thoracic, and thoracic-lumbar) and fused column (anterior, posterior, combined). Automated computer algorithms flag data anomalies continuously and carry out rigorous quality control of the data. Data quality personnel using manual chart review then review these anomalies. These routines are supplemented by quarterly logical and cross-validation checks.

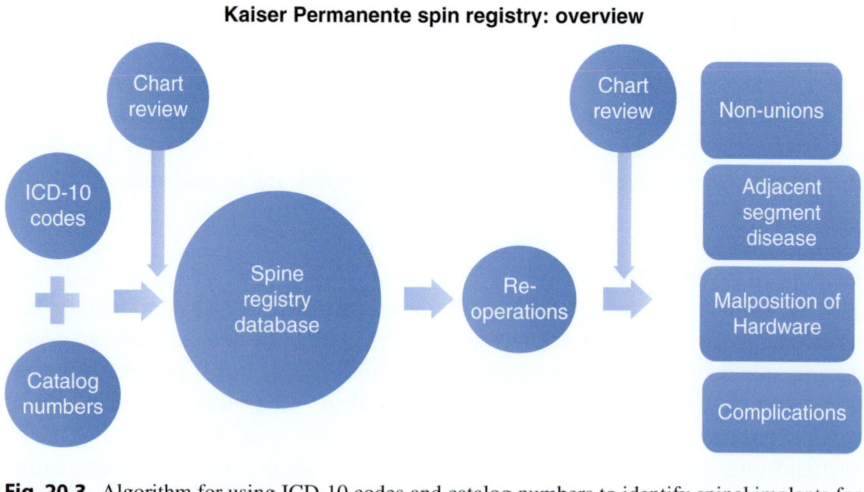

Fig. 20.3 Algorithm for using ICD-10 codes and catalog numbers to identify spinal implants for the Kaiser Permanente spine registry

Currently the spine registry has over 21,650 patients with over 80,000 spinal implants. Some characteristics of these patients include mean age of 58 years, 64% with BMI <30, 19% with diabetes, 10% currently smoking, and 61% with the admitting diagnosis of degenerative disc disease. Average length of stay of 1–3 days was 43%, with a 30-day readmission rate of 6% and a lifetime mortality of 5% [6].

Future Kaiser Permanente Spine Registry

Beyond 2017, the spine registry expanded to include all spine surgery cases. As Fig. 20.4 shows physician forms and patient outcome measures are obtained from four modules: preoperative module, intraoperative module, hospital stay module, and postoperative follow-up module.

Preoperative data is obtained by standardization of physician notes. Intraoperative data is obtained with the use of electronic forms (smart forms) that are completed by surgeons at the end of each surgical case which is somewhat integrated with the operative report. Currently compliance for the latter has reached 80%. Patient outcome measures are obtained electronically or by standardized paper-based forms. At some medical centers, we have introduced the electronic mailing of patient outcome questionnaires. These answered questionnaires are electronically scored and stored in the patient charts, which can be retrieved at a later date. Approximately 65% of our patients have accesses to electronic mailing systems. The remaining patients have the questionnaires filled out using electronic tablets or standardized paper-based forms at their clinic visit. The plan is for all outcome questionnaires to be electronically collected and scored in real time.

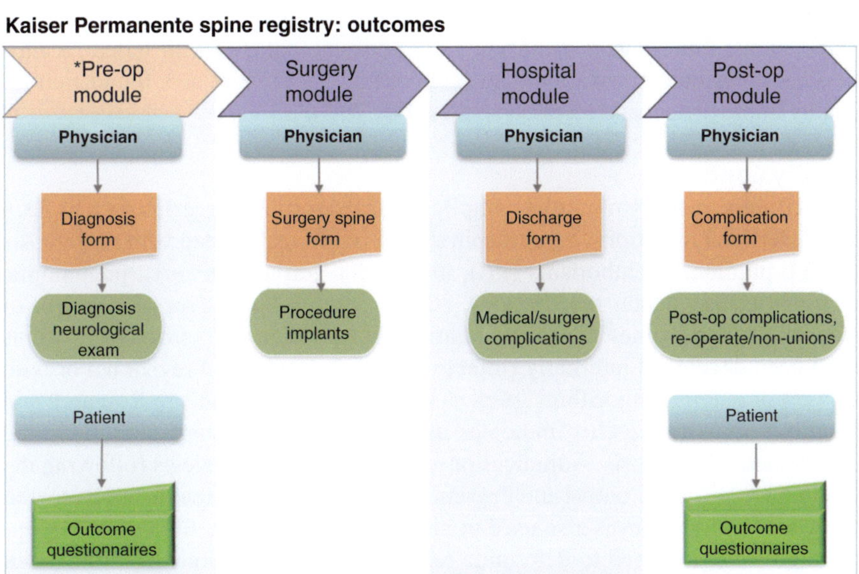

Fig. 20.4 Summary of Kaiser Permanente spine registry with different patient/physician points of contact and outcome questionnaires systems

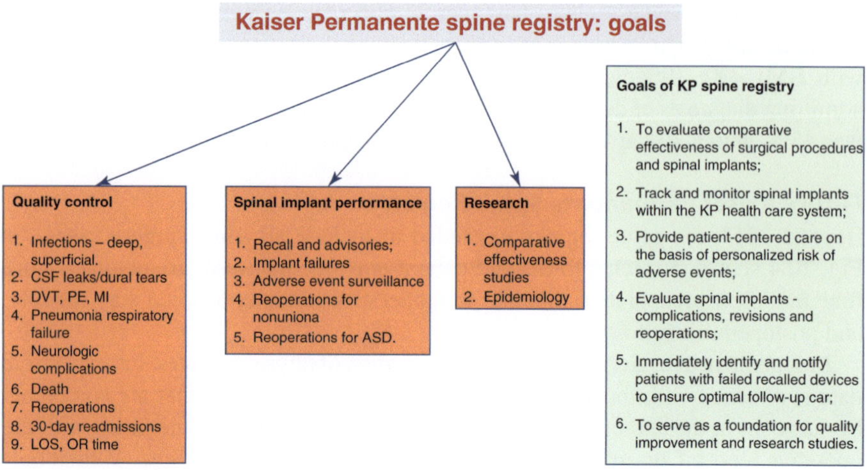

Fig. 20.5 Summary of goals and functions of Kaiser Permanente spine registry

Goals of Kaiser Permanente Spine Registry

The main objective of the KP spine registry is to monitor and assess the quality of spine care offered to our patients. This is done specifically by evaluating the comparative effectiveness of surgical procedures and the spinal implants used; tracking and monitoring these spinal implants used within the KP healthcare system during the patients' lifetime; providing patient-centered care on the basis of personalized risk of adverse events; evaluating spinal implants – complications, revisions, and reoperations; immediately identifying and notifying patients with failed recalled devices to ensure optimal follow-up care; and finally to serve as a foundation for quality improvement and research studies (Fig. 20.5).

Quality Control

The KP spine registry monitors complications from spine surgeries such as deep and superficial infections, cerebrospinal fluid (CSF) leaks, deep vein thrombosis (DVT), pulmonary embolisms (PE), myocardial infractions (MI), pneumonia, neurologic loss, death, reoperations, 30-day readmissions, excessive length of stay, or operating times. For postoperative complications, electronic algorithms have been developed internally (infections, reoperations, and revisions) or with support of external algorithms, such as the Agency for Healthcare Research and Quality's inpatient quality indicator algorithm for pulmonary embolism and deep venous thrombosis. Adjudication via medical record reviews following the Centers for Disease Control and Prevention and Agency for Healthcare Research and Quality guidelines is also used to identify complications. Electronic screening algorithms are used to determine reoperations and revisions from the index spinal procedure. Reoperations are defined as all spine surgical procedures subsequent to the index spinal fusion either at same level or adjacent levels.

Spinal Implant Performance

The spine registry monitors implant recalls/advisories, identifies risk factors for implants, and surveils implants to identify "outliers." An "outlier" is defined as an implant that is performing at a lower-than-expected rate compared with other similar spinal implants. Factors used to identify outliers include high complication rates from implant placement and high revision and reoperation rates. KP also monitors the US Food and Drug Administration (FDA) websites for public recalls/advisories of implant products, which they deem, are defective or contaminated, or otherwise have potential negative health implications.

Long-term reoperations are also monitored specifically for determining cases in which surgery is indicated for non-unions – at the same spinal level(s) as the index procedure or at an adjacent level(s) for "adjacent level disease (ASD)." Since these reoperations will occur in the 5 years that follow the index procedure, it is important that these patients be followed until death or no longer with KP.

Research

Registry data provides the basis for a myriad of research studies, including comparative effectiveness studies. Although randomized controlled trials (RCTs) are the gold standard for assessment of clinical effectiveness, strict inclusion and exclusion criteria limit their generalizability. Clinical trials are often not practical when long-term follow-up is necessary, complication rates are low, and random assignment to treatment conditions is unethical. Patient and spinal implant registries provide an alternative to RCTs in these situations for research [4, 5].

KP spine registry research focused initially on evaluating spinal implants and specifically looking at reoperations for non-unions (operative non-unions). One example of this research was on the use of bone morphogenetic protein (BMP). In 2002, the US Food and Drug Administration approved the use of recombinant human bone morphogenetic protein (BMP, rhBMP-2, INFUSE; Medtronic, Memphis, TN) for anterior lumbar interbody fusion surgery as an alternative to iliac crest bone graft [7, 8]. The purpose of this first study [6] was to determine the difference in the operative non-union rates with and without BMP at all spinal levels with anterior only, posterior only, or combined spinal fusions. Follow-up studies included operative non-union rates using BMP in C1–C2 fusions, O–C fusions, subaxial posterior cervical spine fusions, and posterior cervicothoracic fusions [9, 10]. Risk analysis for the relationship between BMP and cancer was also investigated and has been published [11]. KP spine registry has also studied reoperation rates for non-unions for single- and multiple-level anterior cervical discectomies [12], 30-day readmission rates after spinal fusions [13], and the risk factors for complications in spinal fusion patients such as obesity [14] and renal disease [15]. There are currently several large studies underway including comparing fusion rates for posterolateral lumbar spine fusions versus anterior lumbar spine fusion in the lumbar spine. We have also leveraged the other KP registries by combining several databases with outcome research topics such as effect of lumbar fusions on total hip replacements

Finally, the KP spine registry is unique in that it does not depend on outside funding for its research and therefore removes any perceived bias that have been associated with many recent publications on spinal instrumentation. It also has large cohort of patients with varying demographics and surgical indications and presents a more realistic assessment of routine spine fusion care.

Quality Assessment

As we have seen so far, KP spine registry provides objective data and analysis for assessing the quality of spine surgery. This data is used in several integrated steps to achieve clinical changes (Fig. 20.6). These steps include input for *quality improvement*, *outcome studies*, *cost-effectiveness*, and *physician feedback*. The continuous feedback system allows clinical changes to be re-evaluated and measures the effectiveness of these changes (Fig. 20.6).

Quality Improvement

As we have seen, KP spine registry monitors *quality control* and *spinal implant performance* as part of its goal for improving spine care. This data results in multiple reports/notifications that are issued to physicians to bring about clinical changes. These include quarterly quality scorecards, identifying risk factors, infection/revision, calculators, spinal implant surveillance reports, reports on outlier spinal implants and centers, risk-adjusted medical center reports, statistical process control charts, and interactive web-based reports (Fig. 20.6). Examples of these are presented.

Quality Reports

Using data from the KP spine registry, *quality control* information (Fig. 20.6) is used as a source for our quarterly quality monitoring reports displaying complication rates from various medical centers (regions) and nationally (Fig. 20.7). Reported complications include dural tears, pneumonia, epidural hematomas, infections (superficial and deep), deep vein thrombosis, pulmonary embolism, death, and reoperations. These types of reports are used to allow physicians to look closer at their complication rates and make corrective steps in their clinical practices.

Risk Factors

Specific research projects by KP spine registry have investigated risk factors for poor outcomes in spine surgery. For example, our data has shown higher mortality rates in patients with chronic kidney disease compared to patients with normal kidney function [15]. Another study concluded that there was no correlation between BMP usage in spine fusions and subsequent increased risk of cancer [11]. For 30-day readmission after spine surgery, we found the risks of readmission were increased when there were surgical complications (dural tear, deep infections,

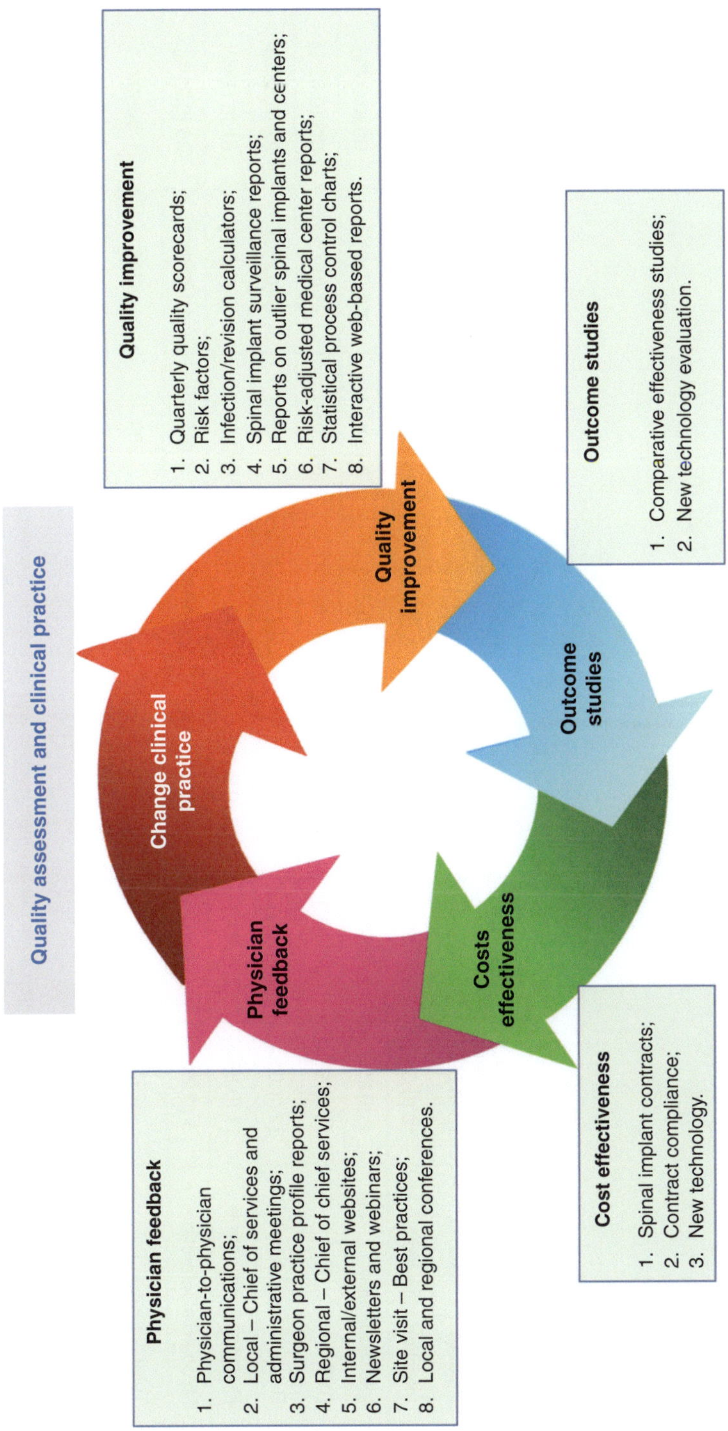

Fig. 20.6 Quality assessment and clinical practice algorithm at Kaiser Permanente

Region Complication[1]	Region #1 Cervical only N (%)	Thoracic only N (%)	Lumbar only N (%)	Region #2 Cervical only N (%)	Thoracic only N (%)	Lumbar only N (%)	All regions N (%)
Dural tear	16 (0.5%)	10 (2.6%)	238 (4.8%)	17 (0.6%)	1 (0.3%)	129 (4.0%)	462 (2.78%)
Pneumonia	36 (1.1%)	16 (4.1%)	64 (1.3%)	26 (0.9%)	8 (2.6%)	31 (1.0%)	185 (1.11%)
Epidural hematoma	16 (0.5%)	3 (0.8%)	76 (1.5%)	11 (0.4%)	2 (0.7%)	16 (0.5%)	135 (0.81%)
Infection-superficial	10 (0.3%)	1 (0.3%)	36 (0.7%)	6 (0.2%)	12 (3.9%)	34 (1.0%)	109 (0.66%)
Infection-deep	8 (0.2%)	2 (0.5%)	41 (0.8%)	9 (0.3%)	8 (2.6%)	20 (0.6%)	99 (0.60%)
DVT	15 (0.5%)	11 (2.8%)	24 (0.5%)	17 (0.6%)	6 (2.0%)	23 (0.7%)	103 (0.62%)
Respiratory failure	32 (1.0%)	7 (1.8%)	9 (0.2%)	34 (1.2%)	1 (0.3%)	6 (0.2%)	97 (0.58%)
Pulmonary embolism	11 (0.3%)	7 (1.8%)	28 (0.6%)	12 (0.4%)	6 (2.0%)	15 (0.5%)	87 (0.52%)
Myocardial infarction	5 (0.2%)	0%	14 (0.3%)	2 (<0.1%)	0%	10 (0.3%)	35 (0.21%)
Total N cases	3295	392	5001	2780	304	3248	16599

1. Percent are based on the column totals.

Fig. 20.7 Example of quality reports with complication rates comparing two regional medical centers to all regions

superficial infections, epidural hematoma), malignancy, lengthy operative and hospitalizations times, hypothyroidism, depression, rheumatoid arthritis, and malignancy [13]. Identification of variables that are associated with increased risk of non-unions in spinal fusions and adverse events are also reported. All these findings are shared with surgeons and are considered during preoperative assessment and surgical planning.

Infection and Revision Calculators

Internal web-based risk calculators are developed to identify patient-specific risk of complications and reoperations and can be used to advice patients and make clinical decisions for spine surgery. These risk factors are based on data obtained from the KP spine registry. These risks calculators have been published for several of our KP registries [15–18]. Currently, specific calculators are being developed for the KP spine registry. Example of this type of calculator currently being developed is shown in Fig. 20.8.

Spinal Implant Surveillance Reports

KP spine registry tracks any recall activities or advisories on its implants. When spinal implants are recalled and advisories occur, the spine registry will immediately identify patients with patient-specific adverse events and risks of implant failures and report these to the surgeons. The surgeons will advise or notify their patients. The KP spine registry works closely with the KP National Product Recall Department to provide accurate data on postoperative outcomes of those patients

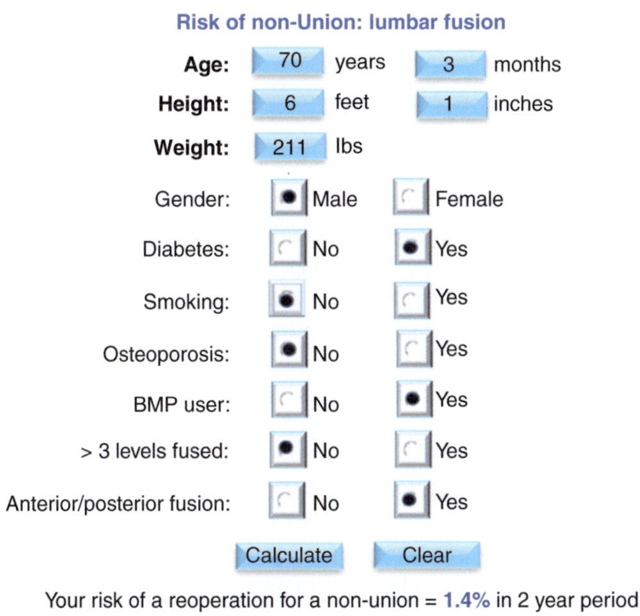

Fig. 20.8 A sample patient-specific risk calculator for reoperations for non-unions

with recall implants and develop case management tools for patient follow-up. An example of this was in 2008 when the KP spine registry was informed of the FDA warnings of the life-threatening complications associated with BMP in the cervical spine. We also stressed to our surgeons that of the FDA concern that the safety and effectiveness of BMP in the cervical spine had not been demonstrated and not been approved by FDA for this use [19].

As discussed previously, the KP registry also monitors implant "outliers" which have lower-than-expected outcomes or higher complications compared with other similar spinal implants. Once an outlier is identified, an expert panel of physicians reviews all information on the spinal implant for confirmation and interpretation of the clinical information. The panel of physicians then distributes their findings to other physicians within the KP system. To date we have not had any other FDA recalls for spinal implants nor spinal implant "outliers," although we are currently investigating several implants that we believe to be suboptimal.

Outcome Studies

One of the functions of the KP spine registry is to answer clinical questions that allow our surgeons to provide evidence that support or change their clinical practices to reflect the best spine care (Fig. 20.6). Comparative effectiveness studies are routinely carried out on topics suggested by physicians or on topics the registry has identified that result in less than expected outcomes. Similarly, studies are done on new technologies on a limited basis. These results are then shared with physicians and the procurement departments.

Comparative Effectiveness Studies

An example of this, as previously discussed, was our studies on the use of BMP. KP had noted increased in the use of BMP over the years following several articles published showing the beneficial effects of using BMP and expanding its use outside the Food and Drug Administration initial guidelines. Our surgeons were concerned about the increased use of BMP and KP began using the spine registry to investigate its complication rates and reoperation rates. The first study [6], using data from 9425 spinal fusion cases, found that reoperation rates for BMP versus non-BMP non-unions for all fusion cases with follow-up of 1 year or more (1.9% vs 2.2%) and follow-up of 2 years or more (2.3% vs 2.6%) were not statistically significantly different. The conclusion was that BMP did not change the operative non-union rate in spinal fusions at all spine regions (cervical, thoracic, lumbar) involving all fused columns (anterior only, posterior only, and combined). Using this information, KP surgeons changed their practices with the use of BMP. It should be noted that some of these studies are accepted for publication, but the goal of the registry is to support our patients and physicians and not necessarily to publish all our findings. As is shown later, many of these studies are shared in KP via multiple platforms.

New Technology Evaluation

It is imperative that for advancing spine care at KP, new technologies are introduced as they become available in the marketplace. However, not every new technology is as advertised. With this in mind at KP, the spine registry will evaluate new spinal implants and products in a limited manner with a review and outcome process so that recommendations can be made. An example of this was the coflex® product. This was evaluated among several surgeons across regional centers, and patients were followed for 1–2 years. Based on these outcomes, recommendations were made to the procurement departments.

Cost-Effectiveness

In attaining high quality, there must be a consideration of the value of the product – cost-effectiveness (Fig. 20.6). This can be done by standardizing device selections (formulary) and ensuring surgeon compliance. A spine formulary is formed to provide high-quality implants using cost efficiencies through inventory management and advantageous contracts.

Spinal Implant Contracts

In order to establish a spine formulary, it was important that we standardized device selection that come from few suppliers at reduced prices. The ability of KP to negotiate favorable spinal implant contracts with suppliers, benefits from its economies of scale. About 5–10 vendors supply the majority of spinal implants in the United States. So, with the help of KP spine surgeons (usually 8–10 spine surgeons, of which 1–2 also serve with the KP spine registry) and the procurement staff, a Sourcing and Standards Teams (SST) committee is formed. The committee function is to identify two or three vendors, in which 90% of their spinal implants will be used by KP spine surgeons at negotiated reduced price.

The process for selection of these 2–3 vendors is quite exhaustive and last over 1 year. It is first started with "Request for Information (RFI)" from 10 to 15 vendors. This is a method of collating information from different suppliers prior to formally sourcing products or services. It is normally used where there are many potential suppliers, and not enough information is known about them. With review of these RFIs, some of these vendors are eliminated to a manageable number – usually 4–6. Vendors are eliminated based on several factors including breadth of products, perception of quality, supporting staff, and KP previous experience with the vendors.

The second phase of the evaluation process requires a formal method of receiving detailed and comparable proposals for defined spinal implants with their associated services. Examples of spinal constructs (e.g., single-level anterior cervical discectomy construct or two-level posterior interbody fusion with pedicle screws construct) are used to compare pricing from the suppliers. Over a 3–4-month period, the third phase includes "champions" surgeons, identified from the SST committee, who use these implants in selected patients and report on the surgical techniques in placing these implants as well as other surgical information that is useful for its evaluation. Usually over 100 responses are collected from between 15 and 20 different spine surgeons that help the committee select the best vendors.

The SST committee reviews all the evaluations from surgeons, pricing, as well as input from the KP spine registry on current spinal implants especially identifying any "outliers" from its data base before a final decision is made. In the past, Dual Source National Standard agreement have been offered to vendors with a 5-year fixed pricing contract with a guaranteed 90% compliance with the right to terminate agreement in years 3 and 4.

Contract Compliance

It is important for the negotiated contracts to have 90% compliance. The SST committee produces timely device utilization reports that verify adherence to formulary guidelines and purchasing agreements and support monitoring of any unique contract features such as warranties, rebates, or volume discounts. The SST committee also reviews requests from surgeons for spinal implants outside of the formulary. By regulating the formulary compliance by physicians, this results in cost-effectiveness for the organization. The SST committee and administrative staff members notify surgeons not in compliance.

New Technology

Since the contracts can last for over 5 years, there may be advancements in new implant technology that should be made available to our surgeons. New technology spinal implants outside the spinal contracts may be added to our spine formulary if there is strong evidence that supports its use. For these implants exceptions are made and the implants placed temporarily on the formulary for a selected number of surgeons. With the assistance of the KP spine registry, these implants are evaluated. In some cases, if the contracted vendors develop similar products with comparable outcomes, the excepted implants will be removed from the formulary and replaced with the contracted vendors' implants.

Physician Feedback

The fourth and most critical part of the *quality assessment* process is the involvement of physicians to initiate clinical changes. This is accomplished by a *physician feedback* processes (Fig. 20.6) in which findings from our *quality improvement, outcome studies, and cost-effectiveness* endeavors are communicated to physicians. This is accomplished via a widespread audience of surgeons, administrators, and clinical staff through several methods: physician-to-physician communications; local, chief of services and administrative meetings; surgeon practice profile reports; regional, chief of chief services; internal/external websites; newsletters and webinars; site visits, best practices; and local and regional conferences. A few of these examples are presented.

Physician-to-Physician Communications

Quality reports are distributed quarterly at regional chiefs (neurosurgery and orthopedic spine surgery) meetings and then disseminated to the surgeons at each medical center. At local levels, direct communications by departmental/administrative meetings with chief of service discuss quality issues from these reports. Regionally, chief-of-chief services meet monthly and communicate on quality variations among medical centers regionally, and corrective steps may be taken including site visits to remedy these differences. Another mechanism of communication is from the KP spine registry directly to the physicians via physician leaders (that is, physicians responsible for communicating registry findings locally, championing registry participation, and monitoring registry strategic plans). The physician leaders notify the local physicians at each medical center. Physicians are encouraged to participate in the process to analyze and improve any quality issues. The KP spine registry physician leaders recommend that medical center physicians pursue the following activities in evaluating the quality issues: (1) review quality issues within the affected department, (2) designate a small group of surgeons within that specialty to evaluate the quality issues, and (3) enlist the assistance of a review team from other KP medical centers if needed.

Surgeon Profile Reports

KP spine registry provides surgeon-specific reports (Fig. 20.9) that outlines several benchmarks including the number of surgical cases completed during a certain period of time, the reoperation rates, the demographics of the surgical patients, their diagnosis, and quality measures such as 90-day pulmonary embolisms, 90-day deep vein thrombosis, 90-day deep surgical site infections, 30-day readmission rates, 30-day emergency department visit rates, and 90-day mortality rates.

These reports also include similar results from the physician's medical center, the region and nationally. The medical center-specific reports are also available via an internal KP website. Surgeon-specific reports can be obtained by secure communication if requested by the surgeon. These targeted reports are intended to compare information among regions, and nationally, creating an opportunity for benchmarking and learning and adjusting clinical practice to improve quality of care.

Internal/External Websites

Internal/external websites are used to distribute to all its surgeons information such as new publications, accessing quality reports and risk calculators and viewing recent recalls. A web-based report containing details on recalls and number of cases

Spine annual surgeon report

KP national implant registry

Surgeon name: Sample

Surgeon report covers data from 2005 through 2016				
Spine registry	Surgeon	Facility	Region	National
# of primary (revised) cases	34 (1)	428 (17)	1903 (53)	6027 (151)
Primary patient characteristics				
Age (year), Median (IQR)	70.0 (66.0–75.0)	69.0 (63.5–75.0)	69.0 (63.0–75.0)	69.0 (63.0–75.0)
Female	50.0%	47.9%	49.6%	49.7%
Diagnosis: Degenerative	100.0%	97.4%	95.3%	94.3%
Diagnosis: Spondylolisthesis	0.0%	0.5%	1.7%	2.0%
Diagnosis: Trauma	0.0%	0.5%	1.4%	1.5%
Reason(s) for revision	n (%)	n (%)	n (%)	n (%)
Adjacent segment disease	0 (0.0)	6 (35.3)	13 (24.5)	34 (22.5)
Nonunion	0 (0.0)	4 (23.5)	14 (26.4)	51 (33.8)
Staged procedure	0 (0.0)	5 (29.4)	20 (37.7)	48 (31.8)
Second spine procedure (unrelated)	1 (100.0)	4 (23.5)	12 (22.6)	36 (23.8)
Cumulative revision probability †	% (95% CI)	% (95% CI)	% (95% CI)	% (95% CI)
1 year	0.0 (0.0–0.0)	29.4 (13.4–56.9)	45.3 (33.1–59.6)	38.4 (31.2–46.7)
3 years	0.0 (0.0–0.0)	58.8 (37.4–81.4)	75.5 (63.4–86.0)	74.8 (67.7–81.4)
5 years	0.0 (0.0–0.00)	76.5 (55.1–92.7)	90.6 (81.0–96.5)	88.7 (83.1–93.2)
Primary 90-day outcomes	n (%)	n (%)	n (%)	n (%)
Pulmonary embolism	0 (0.0)	1 (0.2)	8 (0.4)	23 (0.4)
Readmission	0 (0.0)	3 (0.7)	10 (0.5)	26 (0.4)
Deep surgical site infection (lifetime)	0 (0.0)	8 (1.9)	18 (0.9)	42 (0.7)
Mortality	0 (0.0)	1 (0.2)	4 (0.2)	13 (0.2)

Fig. 20.9 Example of annual surgeon-specific report

Research Newsletter from Kaiser Permanente's Implant Registries
Surgical Outcomes & Analysis (SOA) SOA home contact us archive
As part of SOA's efforts to share findings from KP's registries, please find highlights from a recent study below.

Does Bone Morphogenetic Protein Change the Operative Nonunion Rates in Spine Fusions?

Reoperation Rates for Nonunion Cases

Reoperation time period	Total n (%)	No BMP n (%)	BMP n (%)	P Value
6 months (n=7285)	29 (0.4%)	13 (0.4%)	16 (0.4%)	0.69
1 year (n= 5681)	58 (1.0%)	21 (0.9%)	37 (1.1%)	0.57
2 years (n= 2559)	52 (2.0%)	22 (2.4%)	30 (1.8%)	0.37

Nonunion Rate by Spine Level

Spine region	Total cases		Nonunion cases		
	No BMP	BMP	No BMP n (%)	BMP n (%)	P value
Cervical only	2806	422	44 (1.6%)	4 (0.9%)	0.33
Thoracic only	182	97	1 (0.5%)	2 (2.1%)	0.24
Lumbar only	595	4418	12 (2.0%)	74 (1.7%)	0.55
Cervical/thoracic	224	135	5 (2.2%)	1 (0.7%)	0.41

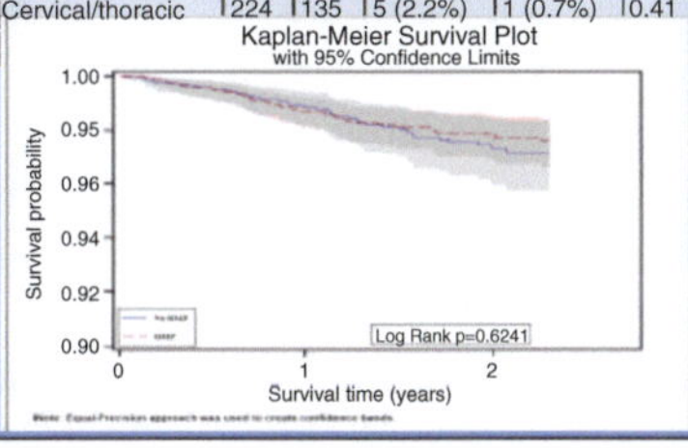

Why did you conduct this study?
Bone morphogenetic protein (BMP) has been used in spinal fusions to prevent nonunions and reduce re-operation rates. Several studies have examined nonunion rates based on radiographic findings which may or may not be symptomatic or require re-operations. Our study reported the operative nonunion rates in spinal fusion for the first time in a large and diverse community-based sample without any of the restrictive inclusion/exclusion criteria encountered in a clinical trial.

What were your findings?
In the study cohort, 5454 cases used BMP and 3967 did not. The mean age was 60.4 years (SD=12.9), with the majority being females (53 percent) and with median follow-up time of 1.2 years (IQR: 0.6–2.0). BMP and Non-BMP groups differed statistically in age, sex, ASA, operative time and length of stay. Differences in re-operation rates for non-BMP and BMP nonunions at 1 year (0.9% vs. 1.1%) and at 2 years follow-up (2.4% vs. 1.8%) were not statistically significant.
After controlling for differences in patient characteristics, operative time, diagnosis group, region of spine fused (cervical only, lumbar only, other) versus the non-BMP group was 0.64 (95% CI: 0.39–1.03).
Differences in BMP vs. non-BMP rates did not reach statistical significance within the lumbar only or cervical only sub-regions.

How can this affect practice?
This study raises important questions about the usefulness of BMP in spinal fusions. Nonunion is one outcome measure we can use, but operative time and cost are other factors we need to examine. Some surgeons may choose to change their practice by reducing the use of BMP We plan to continue to monitor the performance of BMP closely as we accumulate more cases and increase the follow-up time.

Guppy K, Bernbeck J, Harris J, Ake C, Paxton L, Phan K. Does Bone Morphogenetic Protein Change the Operative Nonunion Rates in Spine Fusion? Proceedings of the American Association of Neurological Surgeons; 2013 April 27-30; New Orleans.

Fig. 20.10 Example of newsletter used to communicate with KP surgeons on research done at KP spine registry on bone morphogenetic protein

affected is available for surgeons' reference on the internal KP website. The report lists the date of recall, name of the implant, manufacturer, alert type (recall, withdrawal, or advisory), and FDA classification (class I, high risk; class II, moderate risk; class III, low risk) [19].

Newsletters and Webinars

Newsletters and webinars are used to dessiminate key clinical findings. There are quarterly webinars and routine e-news promoting discussion of current presentations and publications (Fig. 20.10). Some of these are submitted to journals for publication, but many of these topics are for KP internal use.

Changes in Clinical Practice

The final result of the four input components of *quality assessment* should lead to change in clinical practice (Fig. 20.6). It is, however, also important that a dynamic feedback mechanism be implement so that the results of these clinical changes can be measured and evaluated. We present two examples of quality assessment that resulted in modification of clinical practice. As we described previously, KP spine registry in 2009 began looking into the operative non-union rates in all our spinal fusion patients with and without the use of BMP. The early findings of no difference in operative non-union rates between these groups of patients were shared with our surgeons via the several methods described. Guidelines for the use of BMP were initiated regionally and nationally in KP.

As Fig. 20.11 shows, after modifications in clinical practices, there was a downward trend in the use of BMP in the years following our preliminary results. In Q1 2009, 63% of all fusion procedures used BMP, and by the last quarter of 2015, the rate dropped to 30%. The northwest region demonstrated the most significant change in practice (41% vs. 0%). This is an example how the use of registry data presented clinical findings that led to feedback to our surgeons, which caused changes in their clinical practice that also resulted in cost savings.

Another example of changes in clinical practice was our study on 30-day readmissions among our spinal fusion cases. Between 2009 and 2013, we identified 14,939 patients that had spinal fusions, and using descriptive statistics, univariate, and multivariate logistic regression analysis (Fig. 20.12), we found that the 30-day readmission rate was 5.5%.

We also found a compact set of risk factors associated with an elevated risk for 30-day readmissions (hospital length of stay (LOS) > 5 days; operating (OR) time > 199 min, hypothyroidism, depression, rheumatoid arthritis, malignancy, and surgical complications). Our findings were shown to our surgeons (Fig. 20.12), initiating certain medical centers to institute guidelines for reducing 30-day readmissions (Fig. 20.13). Such guidelines included early postoperative follow-up (2-weeks) for high-risk patients.

Future Quality Assessment on Clinical Practice

Over the past 15 years, the healthcare industry has modeled techniques used in the manufacturing industry to maximize their efficiencies [20, 21]. One such industry has been the automobile industry and in particular one automobile manufacturer – Toyota. Toyota developed an integrated sociotechnical system called the Toyota Production System that comprises its management philosophy and practices resulting in enhanced productivity, decreased personnel costs, reduced waste, and increased financial performance [20]. From the Toyota Production System, "Lean" analysis (also known as Lean Production, Lean Enterprise, and Lean Thinking) was derived. Lean assessment requires a value stream mapping in which key people, resources, activities, and information flows required to deliver a product or service are made explicit and depicted graphically. The value stream map is a key tool for identifying opportunities to improve efficiency. Another technique used for process analysis is Six Sigma [21]. This technique, through the application of statistical methods, is similar to Lean and is used to improve the quality and efficiency of operational processes by making processes more uniform and precise. The

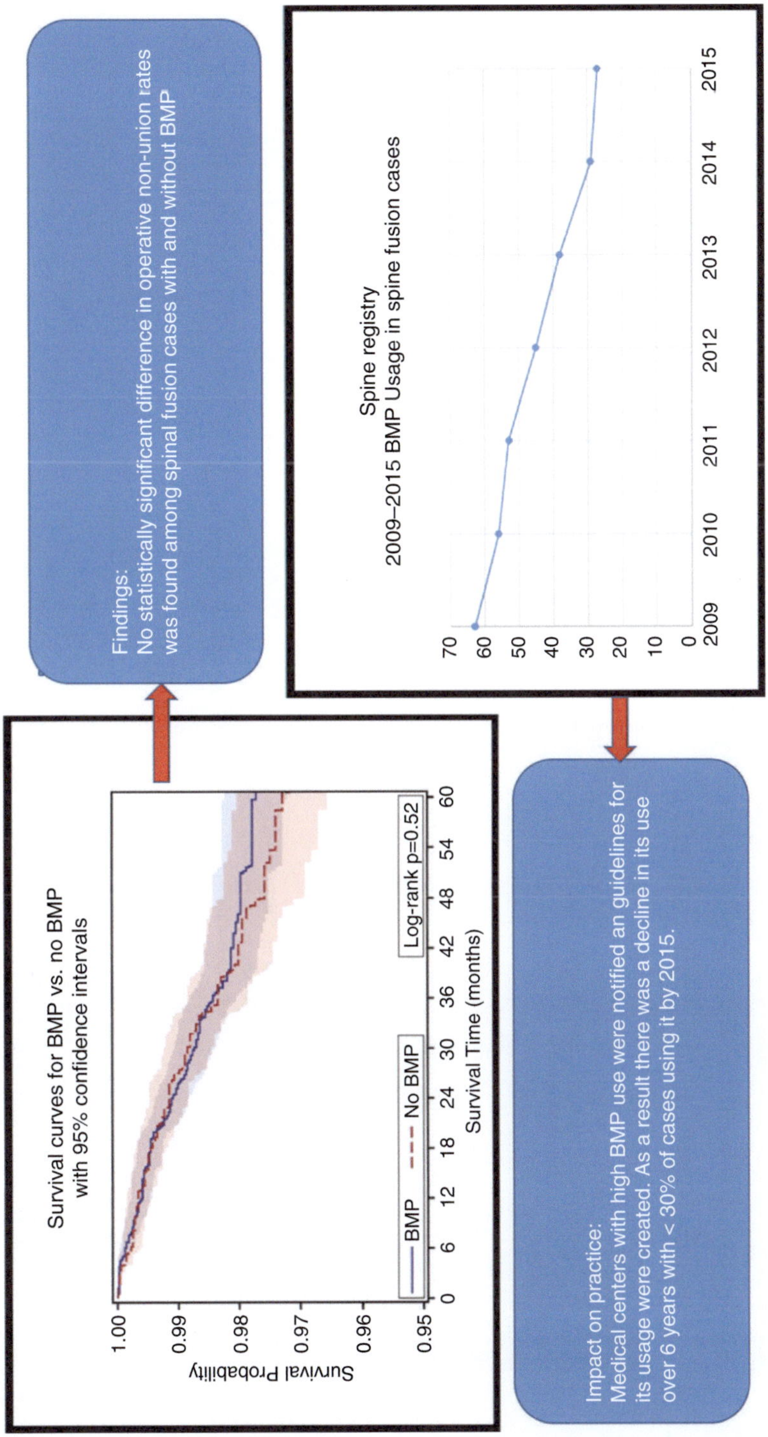

Fig. 20.11 Example of KP surgeons using research done at KP spine registry on bone morphogenetic protein to change their clinical practice

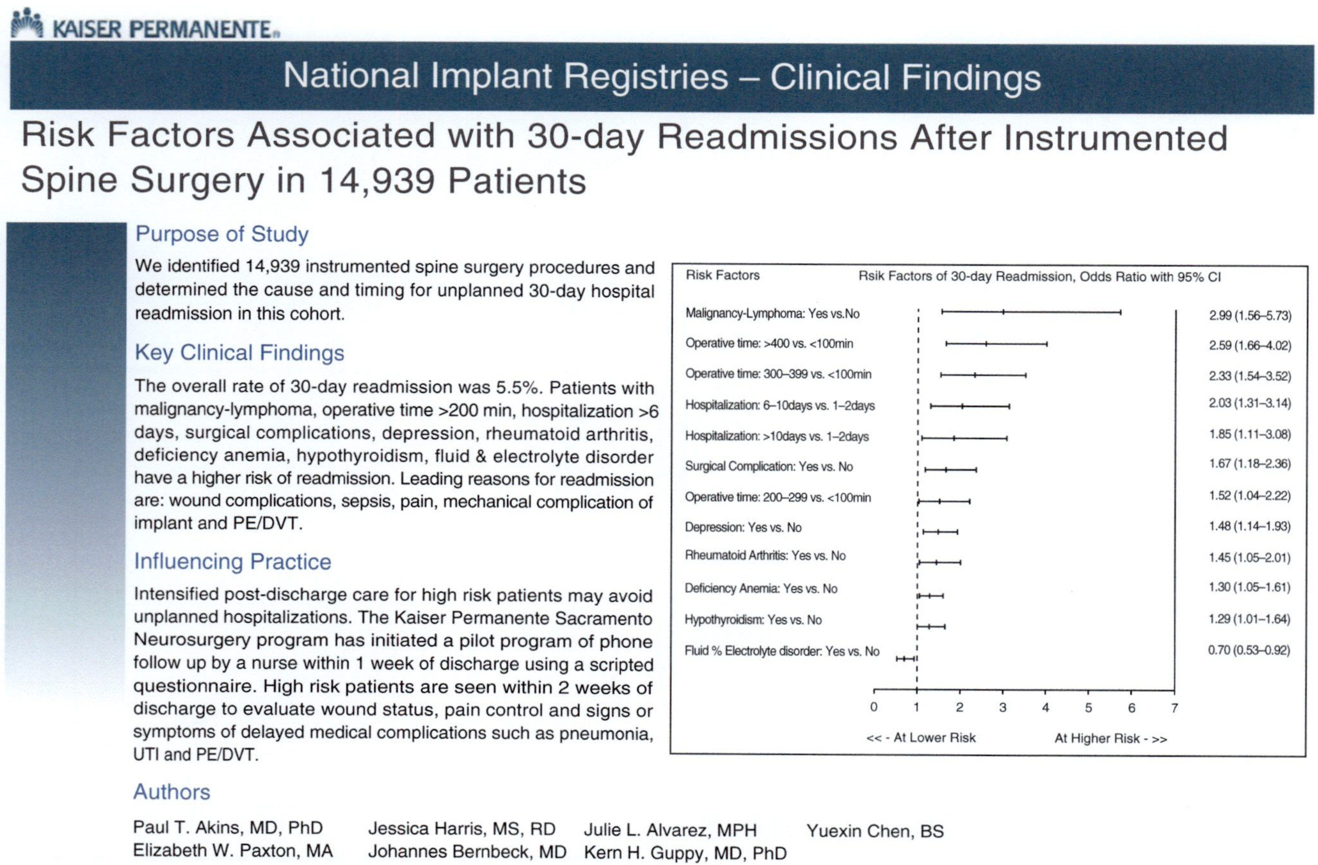

KAISER PERMANENTE

National Implant Registries – Clinical Findings

Risk Factors Associated with 30-day Readmissions After Instrumented Spine Surgery in 14,939 Patients

Purpose of Study

We identified 14,939 instrumented spine surgery procedures and determined the cause and timing for unplanned 30-day hospital readmission in this cohort.

Key Clinical Findings

The overall rate of 30-day readmission was 5.5%. Patients with malignancy-lymphoma, operative time >200 min, hospitalization >6 days, surgical complications, depression, rheumatoid arthritis, deficiency anemia, hypothyroidism, fluid & electrolyte disorder have a higher risk of readmission. Leading reasons for readmission are: wound complications, sepsis, pain, mechanical complication of implant and PE/DVT.

Influencing Practice

Intensified post-discharge care for high risk patients may avoid unplanned hospitalizations. The Kaiser Permanente Sacramento Neurosurgery program has initiated a pilot program of phone follow up by a nurse within 1 week of discharge using a scripted questionnaire. High risk patients are seen within 2 weeks of discharge to evaluate wound status, pain control and signs or symptoms of delayed medical complications such as pneumonia, UTI and PE/DVT.

Risk Factors	Rsik Factors of 30-day Readmission, Odds Ratio with 95% CI
Malignancy-Lymphoma: Yes vs.No	2.99 (1.56–5.73)
Operative time: >400 vs. <100min	2.59 (1.66–4.02)
Operative time: 300–399 vs. <100min	2.33 (1.54–3.52)
Hospitalization: 6–10days vs. 1–2days	2.03 (1.31–3.14)
Hospitalization: >10days vs. 1–2days	1.85 (1.11–3.08)
Surgical Complication: Yes vs. No	1.67 (1.18–2.36)
Operative time: 200–299 vs. <100min	1.52 (1.04–2.22)
Depression: Yes vs. No	1.48 (1.14–1.93)
Rheumatoid Arthritis: Yes vs. No	1.45 (1.05–2.01)
Deficiency Anemia: Yes vs. No	1.30 (1.05–1.61)
Hypothyroidism: Yes vs. No	1.29 (1.01–1.64)
Fluid % Electrolyte disorder: Yes vs. No	0.70 (0.53–0.92)

Authors

Paul T. Akins, MD, PhD · Jessica Harris, MS, RD · Julie L. Alvarez, MPH · Yuexin Chen, BS
Elizabeth W. Paxton, MA · Johannes Bernbeck, MD · Kern H. Guppy, MD, PhD

Fig. 20.12 Example of internal KP publication on our 30-day readmissions to KP surgeons

KP spine registry guidelines for reducing 30-day readmission rates (5.5%)

Risk factors for 30-day readmissions	Details
Hospital length of stay	> 6 days
Operative time	> 200 minutes
Surgical complications	Dural tear, superficial or deep infections, Epidural hematoma/seroma
Medical history	Recent malignancy, depression, rheumatoid arthritis, deficiency anemia

Practice change:

1. Pre-op clinic: PA/NPs will identify all patients with medical history risk factors(see above).
2. Hospital discharge: PA/NPs will identify patients with surgical complications, long operative time and long hospitalization (see above) as well as medical history risk factors (2nd check from pre-op).
3. Arrange clinic visit for all these high risks patients 2 weeks post-surgery.

Akins PT, Harris J, Alvarez JL, Chen Y, Paxton EW, Bernbeck J, Guppy KHO Risk Factors Associated with 30-day Readmissions After Instrumented Spine Surgery in 14,939 Patients. Spine 2015;40:1022-1032

Fig. 20.13 Guidelines for reducing 30-readmission study to our surgeons to initiate changes in their clinical practice

following are examples in which these techniques have been used to make system changes at KP and may impact spine care in the future.

High-Efficiency Operating Rooms

Developing high-efficiency operating rooms (OR) are both challenging and rewarding goal for any healthcare system. The OR is traditionally a high-cost/high-revenue environment, and therefore making it highly efficient is imperative. Using the analytical techniques described previously, we were able to identify several system problems that affected OR scheduling, OR turnover times, anesthesia procedures, time waiting for X-rays, OR prep time, and length of hospital stay for our spine patients. Making simple changes such as using historical performance data of surgeons to schedule cases in allocated block times with preference to scheduling similar cases on the same day resulted in more cases completed in an 8-h period. Completing spinal anesthesia, regional nerve blocks, or intravenous (IV) lines prior to transfer to the OR resulted in less OR time per case. Again, using historical performance data for our surgeons we were able to identify surgeons capable of performing specific procedures with high efficiency. In orthopedic surgery, for the past several years, we have implemented high-efficiency operating rooms in which 4–5 knee replacements can be done during an 8-h period. In spine surgery, we are in the process of implementing similar high-efficient rooms. At present, we have identified best practices among our surgeons who can complete four microdiscectomies with 30-min turnover times in an 8-h period.

In summary, an efficient and cost-effective OR that maximizes utilization is essential for reducing costs in spine surgery. This however must be tied to good outcomes with safe, reproducible, and high-quality care.

Step Cycle Analysis of Surgical Procedures

There is no doubt that the costly component in the operating room is the actual time spent during the surgical procedure. There is variation among surgeons for completing the same procedure. The ability to study this variation has been elusive until the application of techniques such *step cycle analysis.*

This technique breaks down a task (surgery) into procedural steps from the beginning of the surgery to the end. The analysis gives important information on steps in the process that are highly variable and in which corrective steps can be taken to achieve high efficiencies. This analysis has traditionally applied for identifying systemic problems; however as Fig. 20.14 shows, we have the opportunity to look closer at the surgical procedure itself.

This is an example of data collected on several surgeons as they perform single-level anterior lumbar interbody fusions (ALIFs) followed by posterior placement of pedicle screws. Several important steps are identified and the timing of each step is recorded. Analysis of the data shows there is a large variation between surgeons with respect to "mobilization of great vessel." This is helpful, since we can identify which surgeons are more efficient at this particular step and allow that surgeon to share his/her experience and technique with their colleagues. This approach may, however, have a negative impact in that it also appears to identify less efficient surgeons. We should again note, this method analyzes "time" and not necessarily surgical outcome. It definitely poses important questions on its future use. Will this be used to determine a surgeon's performance and if so who will determine this accountability?

In summary, time is the OR's most valuable resource. We believe that a consistent, almost automated attitude to procedures decreases variability and improves efficiency.

Conclusions

Kaiser Permanente has been in the forefront of innovation and efficiency in heath delivery over the past 70 years. One of the reasons for KP success in improving quality care with cost-effectiveness has been the involvement of our KP physicians at all levels in planning patient care. The development and implementation of our spine registry was a vital component in evaluating our quality of spine care. Several key factors were identified for its success. The most important was surgeon leadership and engagement with close involvement of state-wide, regional, and interregional chiefs' groups. Registry participation was found to increase significantly when local medical center chiefs made it their goal that their facility would

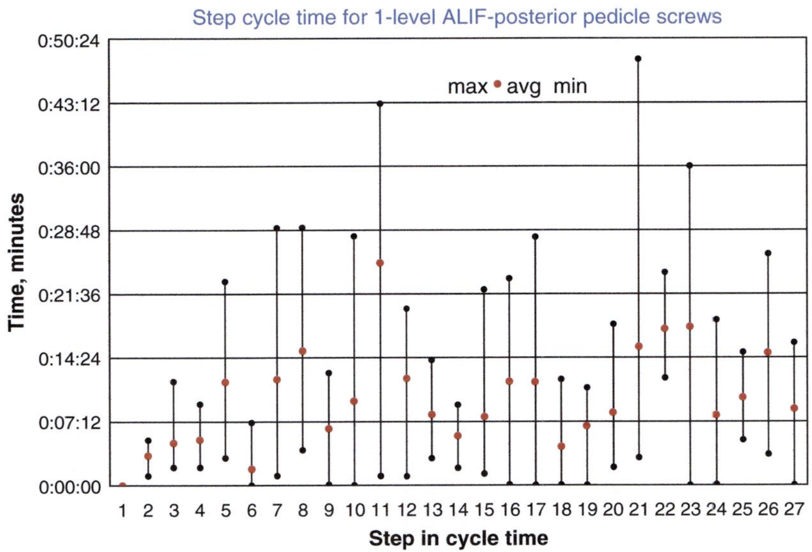

Step	Begin of step-----End of step
1	Patient in room
2	Patient in room ----- Time out
3	Time out ----- Intubation
4	Intubation ----- Neuro-monitoring set up
5	Neuro-monitoring ----- Foley placement
6	Foley placement ----- Position patient
7	Position patient ----- Skin prep/drape
8	Skin prep/drape ----- Skin incision
9	Skin incision ----- Incision of post rectus sheath
10	Incision of post rectus sheath -- Mobilize great vessels
11	Mobilize great vessels ----- Time of annulotomy
12	Time of annulotomy ----- First implant trial in disc space
13	First implant trial in disc space ----- End of cage placement
14	End of cage placement ----- Inspect of retroperitoneal
15	Inspection of retroperitoneal ----- End of fascia closure
16	End of fascia closure ----- End of skin closure
17	End of skin closure ----- Start of transfer to Jackson table
18	Start of transfer to Jackson table ----- End of positioning
19	End of positioning ----- Beginning of imaging for pedicles
20	Beginning of imaging for pedicles ----- Start of prep
21	Start of prep ----- Skin incision
22	Skin incision ----- Last K-wire placed
23	Last K-wire placed ----- End of bilateral rod placement
24	End of bilateral rod placement ----- End of fascia closure
25	End of fascia closure ----- End of skin closure
26	End of skin closure ----- Extubation
27	Extubation ----- Out of room

Fig. 20.14 Step cycle time for 1-level ALIF with posterior pedicle screws. (Courtesy of Dr. Ravi Bains, Kaiser Permanente, Oakland, California)

participate in the registry. Each geographical region also had surgeon champions who were critical for providing feedback on registry participation and disseminating registry findings.

Physician knowledge on the cost of health delivery is also very important. They must participate in the selection of the spinal implants and evaluating the quality of these implants. Ultimately physicians have to be at the forefront in driving quality assessments and change in their clinical practices to accommodate positive changes with patient safety and well-being as the ultimate goal.

References

1. Debly T, Stewart J. The story of Dr. Sidney R. Garfield: the visionary who turned sick care into health care. Oakland: The Permanente Press; 2009.
2. Paxton EW, Inacio CS, Khatod M, Yue EJ, Namba RS. Kaiser Permanente national total joint replacement registry: aligning operations with information technology. Clin Orthop Relat Res. 2010;468:2646–63.
3. Gliklich RE, Dreyer NA, editors. Registries for evaluating patient outcomes: a user's guide [monograph on the Internet]. (Prepared by Outcome DEcIDE Center [Outcome Sciences, Inc dba Outcome] under Contract No. HHSA29020050035ITO1.) AHRQ Publication No. 07-EHC001-1. Rockville: Agency for Healthcare Research and Quality; 2007 Apr [cited 2012 May 8]. Available from: www.effectivehealthcare.ahrq.gov/repFiles/PatOutcomes.pdf
4. Paxton EW, Inacio MC, Kiley ML. The Kaiser Permanente implant registries: effect on patient safety, quality improvement, cost effectiveness, and research opportunities. Perm J. 2012;16(2):36–44.
5. Paxton EW, Kiley ML, Love R, Barber TC, Funahashi TT, Inacio MC. Kaiser Permanente implant registries benefit patient safety, quality improvement, cost-effectiveness. Jt Comm J Qual Patient Saf. 2013;39(6):246–52.
6. Guppy K, Paxton L, Harris J, Alvarez J, Bernbeck J. Does bone morphogenetic protein change the operative nonunion rates in spine fusions? Spine (Phila Pa 1976). 2014;15:1831–9.
7. Boden SD, Zdeblick TA, Sandhu HS, et al. The use of rhBMP-2 in interbody fusion cages. Definitive evidence of osteoinduction in humans: a preliminary report. Spine. 2000;25:376–81.
8. Burkus JK, Gornet MF, Dickman CA, et al. Anterior lumbar interbody fusion using rhBMP-2 with tapered interbody cages. J Spinal Disord Tech. 2002;15:337–49.
9. Guppy KH, Harris J, Chen J, Paxton EW, Alvarez J, Bernbeck J. Reoperation rates for symptomatic nonunions in posterior cervical (subaxial) fusions with and without bone morphogenetic protein in a cohort of 1158 patients. J Neurosurg Spine. 2016;24:556–64.
10. Guppy KH, Harris J, Chen J, Paxton EW, Bernbeck JA. Reoperation rates for symptomatic nonunions in posterior cervicothoracic fusions with and without bone morphogenetic protein in a cohort of 450 patients. J Neurosurg Spine. 2016;25:309–17.
11. Bains R, Mitsunaga L, Kardile M, Chen Y, Guppy K, Harris J, Paxton E. Bone morphogenetic protein (BMP-2) usage and cancer correlation: an analysis of 10,416 spine fusion patients from a multi-center spine registry. J Clin Neurosci. 2017 Sep;43:214–9.
12. Guppy KH, Harris J, Paxton LW, Alvarez JL, Bernbeck JA. Reoperation rates for symptomatic nonunions in anterior cervical fusions from a national spine registry. Spine (Phila Pa 1976). 2015;40:1632–7.
13. Akins PT, Harris J, Alvarez JL, Chen Y, Paxton EW, Bernbeck J, Guppy KH. Risk factors associated with 30-day readmissions after instrumented spine surgery in 14,939 patients: 30-day readmissions after instrumented spine surgery. Spine (Phila Pa 1976). 2015;40(13):1022–32.

14. Flippin M, Harris J, Paxton EW, Prentice HA, Fithian DC, Ward SR, Gombatto SP. Effect of body mass index on patient outcomes of surgical intervention for the lumbar spine. J Spine Surg. 2017;3(3):349–57.
15. Bains RS, Kardile M, Mitsunaga L, Chen Y, Harris J, Paxton E, Majid K. Does chronic kidney disease affect the mortality rate in patients undergoing spine surgery? J Clin Neurosci. 2017;43:208–13.
16. Khatod M, et al. Pulmonary embolism prophylaxis in more than 30,000 total knee arthroplasty patients: is there a best choice? J Arthroplast. 2012;27(2):167–72.
17. Namba RS, Inacio MC, Paxton EW. Risk factors associated with surgical site infection in 30,491 primary total hip replacements. J Bone Joint Surg Br. 2012;94(10):1330–8.
18. Khatod M, et al. Prophylaxis against pulmonary embolism in patients undergoing total hip arthroplasty. J Bone Joint Surg Am. 2011;93(19):1767–72.
19. United States. U.S. Food and Drug Administration. Home Medical Device Safety Communications, Public Health Notifications (Medical Devices) – FDA public health notification: life-threatening complications associated with recombinant human bone morphogenetic protein in cervical spine fusion. Silver Spring: 2008. https://www.fda.gov/MedicalDevices/Safety/
20. Ohno T. Toyota production system: beyond large-scale production. New York: Productivity Press; 1988.
21. Bendell T. A review and comparison of Six Sigma and the Lean organizations. TQM Mag. 2006;18(3):255Y262.

How Quality Is Assessed in Insurance Markets

21

Catherine H. MacLean and Chad M. Craig

Introduction

While a standardized approach to quality assessment in healthcare can be traced to Codman in the early 1900s [1], contemporary interest in quality assessment arose from insurance markets. Frustrated by continually rising healthcare costs and no clear indication that they were getting value from their large expenditures on health insurance, employers led the current quality movement by demanding quality reporting [2]. The result of these demands was the establishment of the not-for-profit National Committee for Quality Assessment (NCQA) in 1990 which was tasked with measuring and reporting the quality of care delivered to beneficiaries enrolled in different health plans. NCQA's first product, the Health Plan Employer Data and Information Set (HEDIS), which measured and reported health plan performance on a small set of quality measures, demonstrated that quality could be assessed at large scale in a valid, reproducible way [2]. The explosion of quality assessment that has ensued is largely the result of this pioneering work by NCQA.

C. H. MacLean (✉)
Center for the Advancement of Value in Musculoskeletal Care, Hospital for Special Surgery, New York, NY, USA
e-mail: macleanc@HSS.EDU

C. M. Craig
Spine Service, Department of Orthopaedic Surgery and Department of Medicine, Hospital for Special Surgery, New York, NY, USA

J. Ratliff et al. (eds.), *Quality Spine Care*,
https://doi.org/10.1007/978-3-319-97990-8_21

The Rationale Behind Quality Assessment

The principle stakeholders within insurance markets include health benefits companies, employers, providers, and patients. These stakeholders have different and sometimes multiple interests in healthcare quality, which can best be understood by considering their roles within the healthcare ecosystem.

Health benefits companies in the United States started out as insurance companies, which for a fee, assumed the risk of costs associated with future health events [3, 4]. Over time, the role of these companies has evolved to also include developing packages of health benefits, networks of providers to deliver the benefits, and a way to process the claims for the benefits (i.e., obtain and pay the bills for health services rendered) [3, 4]. These companies may additionally provide disease and care management services. Like any business, health benefits companies answer to their clients – the individuals and employers who purchase health benefits on behalf of employees. While these purchasers are interested in the quality associated with different insurance products, they are also very price sensitive [5–7] and look to health plans to keep healthcare costs down. One way that quality assessment helps health plans meet the needs of its customers is by facilitating quality transparency. Health plans also look to quality assessment as a tool to reduce healthcare costs. Adhering to recommended preventive services such as vaccines and cancer screening, achieving better control of chronic conditions such as diabetes and hypertension, and reducing adverse events – all topics of quality assessment – will reduce healthcare costs and, hence, from a plan's perspective fulfill two interests of its clients, improved quality and reduced cost. Health plans have additional interest in quality based on regulatory requirements. These requirements vary by state and insurance product.

Employers' interest in quality assessment relates to understanding the value of any insurance products they are purchasing, reducing their direct medical expenditures, maintaining a healthy workforce that is more productive, and providing benefits that will help in hiring and retaining talent. In 2016, 56% of insured Americans had employer-based health insurance [8]. Prior to World War II, little health insurance in the United States was employer-based. The rise in employer-sponsored health plans was a result of wage controls imposed by the Federal Government during World War II [4]. Since other benefits, such as health insurance, were considered "fringe" and not subject to the price control, health benefit offerings served as, and continue to serve as, a differentiator among employers competing for a limited workforce.

Provision of health benefits to workers is a substantial expenditure for American companies accounting, on average, for 7.6% of the budgets of small companies in the United States [9]. Warren Buffet, the CEO of Berkshire Hathaway, has characterized these expenditures as "the tapeworm of American competitiveness" [10]. Consequently, quality initiatives that can reduce healthcare cost are of particular interest to employers.

Some employers are "self-insured," meaning they do not purchase coverage of risk from health plans, i.e., they don't pay into an insurance pool that will cover the cost of covered health costs *if* these costs arise. Rather these employers simply plan to cover the medical costs for their populations for covered events. These employers are often much more involved in developing the benefits, networks, and quality components of the insurance offerings for their employees. Self-insured employers contract with health plans to perform, at a minimum, "administrative services," (i.e., processing insurance claims) but may also purchase other services from a health plan including disease and case management. They may also contract directly with providers and others for various health and administrative services, many of which have a quality component. For example, a number of large employers utilize the Employee Centers of Excellence Network (ECEN) developed by the Pacific Business Group on Health (PBGH) to promote quality and cost savings for spine and other care.

***Spotlight:* PBGH – Employee Centers of Excellence Network – Harnessing Employer Clout to Improve Healthcare Value**

The Pacific Business Group on Health (PBGH) is an innovative not-for-profit organization representing the interests of more than 50 private and public employer organizations purchasing healthcare in the United States. They advocate from the employer stakeholder perspective and utilize the combined clout of large employers' numerous covered members – approximately ten million employees, including those of Walmart, Lowe's, McKesson, and JetBlue Airways – to provide high-value care through the reorganization of healthcare delivery.

As a large organization they have a number of initiatives; however, some of their more innovative programs include (1) a center of excellence network focused on select surgical episodes of care; (2) an intensive outpatient care program for high utilizers of healthcare services; (3) an enormous joint replacement registry used to provide feedback to surgeons, hospitals, and patients about their treatment decisions; and (4) a healthcare transparency center focused on sharing of outcomes and cost data [11].

Their Employee Centers of Excellence Network (ECEN), launched in 2014, has effectively combined episode-based bundled care with select centers of excellence. In the ECEN for spine surgical care, there are currently four highly vetted [12] centers of excellence in the United States where patients can (optionally) receive surgical care. Presently these are in Pennsylvania, North Carolina, Washington, and Texas. Travel for patients is coordinated through a third-party administrator, and all medical and travel expenses are included in a defined episode of care. One group of authors described spine care in this program as follows:

> *...all spine program patients are reviewed by a participating center and then scheduled for an in-person comprehensive spine evaluation including orthopedics and/or neurosurgery, physiatry, internal medicine, and psychology specialists to determine*

the best treatment plan. Neurology and interventional pain management services are available at participating sites on an ad hoc, patient need-dependent basis. If surgery is not appropriate, patients and their caregivers are counseled on nonsurgical options and recommendations and shared with the patient, companion, and home provider. For patients who do undergo surgery, the participating center completes a handoff to a home provider who has agreed in advance to participate in the patient's care upon their return home. [13]

The bet here is that care provided at such centers will be more appropriate, in line with best practices and associated with better long-term outcomes. This cost-sharing structure places some financial risk on the individual centers of excellence (in the event of say an undesired outcome within an episode of care) yet also functions to reward quality and appropriate utilization over volume. Included patients meet strict criteria, including certain BMI cutoffs and non-smoking status. Bundled rates are negotiated between participating centers and PBGH for both medical and surgical visits. Centers of excellence and affiliated providers benefit from exposure to a geographically larger patient base. Each ECEN center shares surgeon-level data, care-pathways, and patient-reported outcomes to in turn help drive adoption of best practices at other centers and hold one other accountable to high-quality care. This is part of PBGH's broader effort to advocate transparency of healthcare outcomes and costs.

The ECEN has demonstrated some encouraging outcomes. Charges for all spine-related care (both medical and surgical) have averaged 10–15% less than traditional fee-for-service charges for existing employers. Additionally, of patients who are recommended for surgery by providers in their home market, one-third to one-half of all spine cases reviewed by a center of excellence are counseled against surgery and provided with alternative treatment recommendations [12, 13]. The ECEN program has demonstrated success in total joint replacements as well, with significantly lower revision surgery rates, lower readmissions, and a higher number of patients discharged directly home versus to a skilled rehabilitation center [13]. The average out-of-pocket patient savings for joint replacement surgery was estimated at $3300 per patient by one employer [12].

PBGH is not alone in their recognition of their bargaining power to pursue bundled care and drive delivery of care to centers of excellence, as a cost-sharing strategy through their ECEN. Boeing and General Electric have separately pursued similar individual bundled care programs with other centers. Health Transformation Alliance is an employer-led organization, similar to PBGH, pursuing similar efforts at a regional level. As an organization PBGH carries enormous influence with payers, both government and private, and has influence in the health policy arena as well. They are an employer-led organization that has effectively positioned them to advocate on behalf of large companies and through their ECEN program drive care toward high-quality cost-efficient centers.

Healthcare providers (including physicians, hospitals, skilled nursing facilities, nurses, physical therapists) have varying degrees of professional, reputational, and financial interests in quality assessment. While all healthcare providers have a professional imperative to provide high-quality care to their patients, most quality assessment efforts linked to transparency and/or reimbursement have focused largely on hospitals, physicians, and skilled nursing facilities. Related, performance scores may influence whether providers are included in networks.

Patients, the object of care delivery, have, perhaps, the greatest stake in healthcare quality as it impacts their own personal health and financial well-being. As consumers, patients are interested to understand the quality of the care available from different providers in order to rationalize cost. For example, some consumers may be willing to pay a higher premium for higher-quality care. At the same time, healthcare quality can impact wages through lost work due to poorly treated disease or inefficient care that requires more time away from work.

Quality Assessment Framework

The framework within which healthcare quality is assessed derives from the work of Donabedian [14], who conceptualized high-quality healthcare as that which is expected to achieve the best balance of health benefits and risks. This framework considers technical and interpersonal care.

Technical care can be measured in three domains: structure, process, and outcomes. Structure refers to the relatively stable characteristics of the providers, the tools and resources available to them, and the physical environment and organizational characteristics of the health system. Examples of structural quality measures include board certification of physicians and accreditation of health organizations such as hospitals and health plans, case volumes of physicians and hospitals, and participation in registries.

Process refers to what healthcare providers do for patients. Examples of process measures include the delivery of preoperative antibiotics for certain procedures and provision of venous thromboembolus prophylaxis for certain hospitalized patients. Process measures are largely under the direct control of healthcare providers.

Outcomes pertain to a patient's health state. Currently, the most commonly assessed outcome measures pertain to complications such as surgical site infection rates, venous thromboembolism rates, and mortality rates. Increasingly, measures that assess gains in patient-reported outcomes such as pain, function, and quality of life are being adopted. Indirect outcome measures include those of *clinical parameters* such as blood pressure, blood sugar, and lipid levels and *utilization* such as hospital admissions, readmissions, and emergency room visits. Unlike some care processes, outcomes are not mostly under the control of providers. While care delivered will impact outcomes, the degree to which outcomes are impacted may be influenced by a number of factors beyond the control of the provider such as underlying disease severity, comorbidities, and socioeconomic factors. As such, outcome measures require risk adjustment.

Interpersonal care describes the "goodness" of interactions between patients and the healthcare system and includes patient experience or patient satisfaction. Examples of patient experience measures include Consumer Assessment of Healthcare Providers and Systems (CAHPS®) [15] and Press-Ganey [16] surveys.

Data Sources for Measuring Quality

How quality is measured within insurance markets depends on how it will be used and the availability of data elements needed to construct quality scores. Data elements used to construct quality scores may come predominantly from administrative data, medical records, and surveys. Increasingly, registries may serve as data sources, although the elements in registries generally come from medical records.

Administrative Data

Administrative data, or billing data, are the predominant type of data used to assess quality within insurance markets because they are broadly available to insurers. In order to get paid for services rendered, healthcare providers must submit claims to insurers using standard codes that describe the diagnoses associated with the visit and the specific procedures provided. International Classification of Diseases (ICD) codes are used to describe the diagnoses. Procedures maybe coded with Common Procedural Terminology (CPT) or Diagnostic Related Group (DRG) codes. Depending on the type of care delivered, professional (from clinicians) and/or facility (from hospitals and others) claims may be submitted. Claims for drugs include the unique National Drug Code (NDC) associated with the medication, the number of units dispensed, and a prescriber identifier. Durable medical equipment may be billed using CPT or Healthcare Common Procedure Coding System (HCPCS) codes.

Although administrative data are generated for billing, they contain enough information to measure quality for a number of diseases or health states. Codes for age, gender, and diagnoses can be used to identify populations who should or should not receive certain drugs, tests, or procedures which are also coded. For example, the proportion of patients with new-onset back pain who receive a radiograph within 6 weeks of the diagnosis. Similarly, procedure codes can identify groups of beneficiaries who have undergone certain procedures, while ICD codes can be used to determine if complications occurred. For example, the proportion of patients who underwent spinal surgery who had a subsequent venous thrombotic event can be identified using procedures codes to idntify the surgery and ICD codes to identify the complication.

Two of the biggest advantages of administrative data for quality assessment include availability and completeness. There is no extra work and hence no additional collection costs for plans or providers when administrative data are used since they are collected as a routine part of the insurance business. Additionally, they generally include a complete longitudinal record of all health services across all different providers for all beneficiaries within a health plan. While these data have great breadth, their level of clinical detail is limited. For example, while administrative data may describe whether a beneficiary has a disease, they generally do not describe the severity of the disease (e.g., degree of claudication or neurological deficits) or characteristics of the patient that may be relevant to risk adjustment and quality assessment (e.g., frailty, BMI, or tobacco use). Likewise, many details of procedures, such as number of levels for a spinal fusion procedure, are not readily available in claims data. In one study that developed a comprehensive set of 182 quality measures for older adults spanning 22 conditions, only 20% of the measures could be applied to administrative data; the rest required a level of clinical detail not available in claims data [17]. Furthermore, while performance as measured by administrative data did not differ from that measured using medical records for the same measures, summary scores from these data sources vary substantially when the totality of care that can be measured by each data source is measured.

Medical Records

Although rich in details important to quality assessment, medical records are seldom used as the primary data source for quality assessment in insurance markets because obtaining and abstracting data from those records are extremely resource intensive for both health plans and healthcare providers. Medical records are, however, routinely used as a supplementary data source for some administrative data-based measures. These "hybrid" measures use administrative data to identify eligible populations and then seek medical records to obtain data elements not available or reliably available in the administrative data. To further reduce the burden of collecting data from medical records, a random sample large enough to produce a statistically valid point estimate is drawn from the eligible population. Examples of hybrid measures include NCQA's Diabetic Retinal Exam measure (DRE) for which the eligible population of people with diabetes is identified from administrative data [18]. A random sample is drawn from this population. Beneficiaries in this sample who have evidence of a diabetic retinal exam in the administrative data are considered to have "passed" this measure. For those with no claims for a DRE, the health plan will pursue all medical records that might document a DRE. Unless documentation of a DRE is found, the measure is considered a "fail."

As electronic health records become standard, there is an opportunity to greatly enhance quality assessment. This will, however, require thoughtful consideration of the quality measures, which should be enhanced or developed, and the creation of discrete structured data fields to support those measures that are collected on a routine basis. Ideally, the future state of quality assessment will incorporate real-time quality assessment and reporting to clinicians at the time of service.

Surveys

Consumer Assessment of Healthcare Providers and Systems (CAHPS®) surveys [15], which ask consumers and patients to report on and evaluate their experiences with healthcare, are routinely collected and used for a variety of quality programs within insurance markets. Among these there are surveys that assess consumer and patient experience with health plans (CAHPS Health Plan Survey), hospitals (HCAHPS Survey), and clinicians or clinician groups (CG-CAHPS Survey). These surveys assess whether consumers/patients are able to get timely appointments, care, and information; how well providers communicate with patients; providers' use of information to coordinate patient care (CG-CAHPS); customer service from the plan or the provider staff; and how patients rate their plans or providers.

Surveys of hospitals, medical groups, and individual clinicians may also be used by insurance companies or employers to assess quality. This is typically done in the context of a specific quality recognition or payment program that requires information about structures or outcomes of care not available in the administrative data. For example, the Blue Distinction Specialty Care Program for Spine Surgery [19] survey requests information on the number of spine surgeons at a center and whether the center "commits to examine spine surgeon procedure volume with consideration for reviewing evidence linking volume and outcomes and establishing a surgeon level case volume minimum requirement." Although the health plan has information on volume and complication rates for its own members, it cannot discern overall center volume or complication rates and hence also requests this type of information in its survey.

Registries

Accelerated by financial incentives for participation and/or reporting, there has been a boom in the development of, and participation in, clinical registries in the United States. For a number of health plan sponsored programs, participation in registries is a requirement or a means to garner quality points [20–23].

What Measures Are Used/How Are Measures Selected

Consider the journey a health plan or other assessor might go through to develop a quality program. Interest in some sort of quality program arises from an account or potential account (e.g., a large employer or union); from a trade group representing account segments (e.g., the National Business Group on Health or a regional business group); or from the leadership of the plan/assessor. This request is brought to a specific group of quality measurement experts within the organization that is tasked to develop the program within some finite period of time, generally in the range of months and possibly up to several years for a strategic initiative. Within these time constraints, this group needs to define the measures that will be used and put into place processes to perform the quality assessment, report the performance, and in some instances, determine how to score performance for programs linked to reimbursement.

In practical terms, quality measures that will be used will be ones that already exist and can be easily measured. As discussed above measures based on administrative data are the easiest to measure and hence form the basis for most quality assessment within insurance markets. While the scope of administrative data measures is limited, these measures can generally be applied across a broad population and hence form the basis for programs that compare quality across entities (e.g., health plans, hospitals, physicians). These sorts of assessments can be done without active participation of those being assessed and hence can be applied (involuntarily) to all entities in the dataset. In contrast, quality assessment programs based on more detailed clinical data obtained from medical records, surveys, or registries generally require participation from those being assessed. These sorts of quality programs are generally voluntary and hence are generally used as quality designation programs.

Measurement Programs

Quality assessment programs within insurance markets include those that assess health plans and those that assess providers.

Health Plan Quality Assessment

The two largest and most transparent health plan quality assessment programs are the Healthcare Effectiveness Data and Information Set (HEDIS) [23] and Medicare Advantage 5-star programs [24]. Various business collaboratives and quality assessment entities may also assist purchasers in assessing the quality of health plans.

The Healthcare Effectiveness Data and Information Set (previously the Health Plan Employer Data and Information Set) (HEDIS), a standardized set of population performance measures and methodologies for assessment, is used by more than 90% of America's health plans to measure and report performance on important dimensions of care and service. This tool currently includes 94 predominantly administrative data-based measures across 7 domains of care [23]. Although "voluntary," participation in this program is expected by essentially all large purchasers who consider HEDIS scores across health plans when making health plan purchasing decisions. Health plan performance may be accessed by licensing NCQA's Quality Compass [25], which provides benchmarking data and allows users to compare the performance of different health plans. Population performance on the HEDIS measures is available to the public through NCQA's "State of Health Care Quality" reports [26] and measures [27].

The Medicare Advantage (MA) 5-star program provides information to Medicare beneficiaries on the quality of the plan and incentives to health plans to deliver high-quality care. Medicare Advantage with prescription drug coverage (MA-PD) plan are rated on up to 44 unique quality and performance measures; MA-only plan (without prescription drug coverage) are rated on up to 32 measures; and standalone Part-D Prescription Drug Plans (PDPs) are rated on up to 15 measures [24]. Most of these measures are based on administrative data, and many are HEDIS measures. Performance is reported on the CMS Plan Finder [28] along with information on benefits provided and plan cost including premium and co-pays.

Incentives to health plans to achieve high quality include transparency of quality to potential beneficiaries and financial incentives from CMS for achieving high quality. Additionally, beneficiaries may enroll in 5-star plans or switch out of poorly performing plans at any time, i.e., they do not need to wait until the annual open enrollment period to make these switches.

Other trade groups such as the National Business Group on Health and private consulting firms provide a variety of tools and resources to purchasers to assess the quality of health plans. In some cases, plans are expected to complete detailed requests for information about quality-related structures and programs that they have in place. In addition to information on performance on HEDIS measures, purchasers may be interested to understand how many quality- or value-based contacts plans have with providers, whether plans provide information to network providers on their quality and efficiency, and how plans engage members with quality gaps to close them.

Hospital Quality Assessment

Within insurance markets, hospital quality is assessed in a variety of ways by health plans. Individual health plans may apply measures to their own administrative data experience to assess and report the quality of hospitals within their networks in provider directories. The publicly reported CMS Hospital Compare program reports hospital performance on a number of measures and utilizes up to 57 administrative data-based measures across seven care domains (mortality, safety, readmissions, patient experience, effectiveness of care, timeliness of care, and efficient use of medical imaging) to derive a summary score on a 5-star scale [29, 30]. A limitation of this measurement program is that while all hospitals are rated and compared on the same 5-star scale, the specific measures assessed vary across hospitals with individual hospitals being assessed on anywhere from 9 to 57 measures, producing an apple to oranges comparison. In addition to hospital measures to promote transparency, CMS provided monetary incentives for high quality through its Hospital Inpatient Quality Reporting (IQR) and Hospital Outpatient Quality Reporting (OQR) Programs.

Beyond administrative data-based quality programs that are used to compare hospital quality broadly on a similar set of measures, health plans have developed a number of other more detailed quality assessment programs that require additional data from hospitals to complete quality assessments. For example, the Anthem Quality-In-Sights® Hospital Incentive Program (Q-HIP®) supplements administrative data-based measures with ones reported in Society of Thoracic Surgeons (STS) and American College of Cardiology (ACC) registries, with the permission of participating hospitals [20]. This program provides financial incentives for quality improvement to participating hospitals. More specialized, "centers of excellence" programs sponsored by different health plans [19, 21, 22] typically focus on a specific disease or procedure. These programs typically invite network hospitals to complete a standard application that requests information on a variety of structure, process, and outcome measures. Hospitals that meet quality criteria may be designated as "centers of excellence" in the plan provider directories. In some instances, such designation may be required to participate in specific "high performing" network. In such instances coverage for a certain procedure may be limited to designated hospitals.

Physician Quality Assessment

Physician quality assessment may be performed at the level of the medical group or individual physician. As with health plan- and hospital-level quality assessment, physician-level quality assessment is based largely on administrative data supporting quality transparency and incentive programs. The CMS has announced that by the end of 2018, through the Medicare Access and CHIP Reauthorization Act (MACRA) Quality Payment Program, 90% of Medicare fee-for-service payments to clinicians will be based on "value," which will be determined by scores on a number of performance measures. The CMS 2017 Quality Payment Program (QPP) includes 271 measures from which physicians can select for reporting in the program [31–33]. Many of these and other physician-level quality measures have been criticized as not being clinically meaningful [34] or valid [35]. For example, in a comprehensive evaluation of the 87 QPP measures relevant to general internists, the American College of Physicians rated only 33 (38%) as valid [35]. This calls out the importance of making sure that measures used to measure physician-level quality are indeed valid. Unlike for clinical practice guidelines [36], there is no single set of standards currently available that can be used to evaluate the trustworthiness of performance measures. Not to be confused with the precision of a point estimate or whether comparisons of the measured metrics across physicians are statistically significant, the starting point for physician – and indeed all quality measurement – should be to ensure the measure is valid and clinically useful.

In contrast to plan- and hospital-level performance assessment for which sample sizes are generally large even within a single health plan, physician-level assessment may be constrained by small sample sizes which produce unreliable results. Although individual physicians or groups may have an adequate sample size across their patient population to produce a reliable estimate of performance, the data available to individual health plans are limited to only a segment of that physician's or group's patient panel, which may be too small to produce reliable estimates. To get around this problem, some organizations, such as the Integrated Healthcare Association (IHA) in California [37] and the Wisconsin Collaborative for Healthcare Quality (WCHQ) [38], pool the administrative data from multiple health plans to produce more robust group-level performance measurement, which may be used for public reporting as well as in health plan quality- or value-based incentive programs.

Another way to get around the small sample problem when measuring at the level of individual physicians within individual plans is to utilize many measures, the performance on which can be pooled to develop composite measures. The

United Premium Designation Program assesses the quality of network physicians based primarily on a large set of administrative data-based quality measures [39]. Network physicians may gain additional "quality points" in this program if they participate in a qualifying American Board of Internal Medicine (ABIM) Practice Improvement Module (PIM) [40]. The efficiency of physicians relative to others in the same geography is also assessed as part of this program. Quality and efficiency scores are reported for physician in the plan network, who have a large enough sample size to calculate reliable estimates. Efficiency is reported only for physicians who attain a quality designation. Hence, high-quality physicians can be designated as efficient or not. Efficiency is not reported for physicians with low or no (due to small sample) quality assessment. Quality and efficiency designations are reported in the United Healthcare provider directory.

References

1. Donabedian A. The end results of health care: Ernest Codman's contribution to quality assessment and beyond. Milbank Q. 1989;67:233–56.
2. Iglehart JK. The National Committee for Quality Assurance. N Engl J Med. 1996;335:995–9.
3. HIAA Insurance Education. Fundamentals of health insurance, part A. Washington, DC: Health Insurance Association of America; 1997. isbn:1-879143-36-4.
4. Buchmueller TC, Monheit, AC. Employer-sponsored health insurance and the promise of health insurance reform. NBER working paper number 14839. http://www.nber.org/papers/w14839.pdf?new_window=1. Accessed 1 Feb 2018.
5. Brook RH, Ware JE Jr, Rogers WH, Keeler EB, Davies AR, Donald CA, Goldberg GA, Lohr KN, Masthay PC, Newhouse JP. Does free care improve adults' health? Results from a randomized controlled trial. N Engl J Med. 1983;309:1426–34.
6. Marquis MS, Buntin MB, Escarce JJ, Kapur K, Yegian JM. Subsidies and the demand for individual health insurance in California. Health Serv Res. 2004;39(5):1547–70.
7. Abraham JM, Feldman R, Braven P. Employers' changing economic incentives to offer health insurance under the Affordable Care Act. Am J Health Econ. 2016;2:273–99.
8. Barnett JC, Berchick ER. Health insurance coverage in the United States: 2016. United States Census Bureau Report number P60-260, 2017.
9. 2016 Healthcare benchmarking report. Society for Human Resource Management, 2016. https://www.shrm.org/hr-today/trends-and-forecasting/research-and-surveys/Documents/2016-Health-Care-Report%2D%2DAll-Industries-All-FTEs.pdf. Accessed 1 Feb 2018.
10. Sahadi J. Warren Buffet is right. Health care costs are swallowing the economy. CNN Money. http://money.cnn.com/2018/01/30/news/economy/health-care-costs-eating-the-economy/index.html. Accessed 10 Feb 2018.
11. Pacific Business Group on Health. Website: http://www.pbgh.org/about. Accessed 10 Feb 2018.
12. Slotkin JR, Ross OA, Coleman R, et al. Why GE, Boeing, Lowe's and Walmart are directly buying health care for employees. Harvard Business Review. 2017:1–7.
13. Slotkin JR, Ross OA, Newman ED, et al. Episode-based payment and direct employer purchasing of healthcare services: recent bundled payment innovations and the Geisinger Health System experience. Neurosurgery. 2017;80(4):S50–8.
14. Donebedian A. Definition of quality and approaches to its assessment, Vol 1: explorations in quality assessment and monitoring. Ann Arbor: Health Administration Press; 1980.
15. About CAHPS. Agency for Healthcare Quality and Research. https://www.ahrq.gov/cahps/about-cahps/index.html. Accessed 1 Feb 2018.

16. Patient satisfaction surveys. Press Ganey. https://helpandtraining.pressganey.com/resources/patient-satisfaction-surveys. Accessed 10 Jan 2018.
17. MacLean CH, Louie R, Shekelle PG, Roth CP, Saliba D, Higashi T, Adams J, Chang JT, Kamberg CJ, Solomon DH, Young RT, Wenger NS. Comparison of administrative data and medical records to measure the quality of medical care provided to vulnerable older patients. Med Care. 2006;44:141–8.
18. HEDIS Volume 2: Technical Specifications for Health Plans. National Committee for Quality Assurance, 2017.
19. Blue Distinction Specialty Care. Selection criteria and program documentation: knee and hip replacement and spine surgery. Cross Blue Shield association. https://www.bcbs.com/sites/default/files/file-attachments/page/Spine.SelectionCriteria_0.pdf. Accessed 30 Dec 2017.
20. Anthem Quality-In-Sights® Hospital Incentive Program (Q-HIP®). https://www.anthem.com/wps/portal/ahpmedprovider?content_path=shared/noapplication/f2/s3/t0/pw_b140403.htm&rootLevel=1&label=Hospital%20Quality%20and%20Safety. Accessed 20 Dec 2018.
21. Blue Distinction Specialty Care. Selection criteria and program documentation: Cardiac Care. https://www.bcbs.com/sites/default/files/file-attachments/page/Cardiac.SelectionCriteria_0.pdf. Accessed 20 Dec 2017.
22. Aetna Institutes of Quality. Cardiac facility program requirements. http://www.aetna.com/healthcare-professionals/documents-forms/cardiac-care-facility-program-criteria.pdf. Accessed 20 Dec 2017.
23. HEDIS and Performance Measurement. National Committee for Quality Assurance. http://www.ncqa.org/hedis-quality-measurement. Accessed 1 Feb 2018.
24. 2017 Star Ratings. Centers for Medicare and Medicaid Services. https://www.cms.gov/Newsroom/MediaReleaseDatabase/Fact-sheets/2016-Fact-sheets-items/2016-10-12.html. Accessed 1 Feb 2018.
25. Quality Compass. National Committee for Quality Assurance. http://www.ncqa.org/HEDISQualityMeasurement/QualityMeasurementProducts/QualityCompass.aspx. Accessed 1 Feb 2018.
26. The State of Health Care Quality Reports. National Committee for Quality Assurance. http://www.ncqa.org/report-cards/health-plans/state-of-health-care-quality. Accessed 1 Feb 2018.
27. NCQA. Report Cards » Health Plans » State of Health Care Quality » Table of Contents [online]. http://www.ncqa.org/report-cards/health-plans/state-of-health-care-quality/2017-table-of-contents. Accessed 1 Feb 2018.
28. Medicare Plan Finder. Centers for Medicare and Medicaid Services. https://www.medicare.gov/find-a-plan/questions/home.aspx. Accessed 1 Feb 2018.
29. About Hospital Compare. Centers for Medicare and Medicaid Services. https://www.medicare.gov/hospitalcompare/Data/About.html. Accessed 20 Dec 2017.
30. How the Hospital Compare overall rating is calculated. Centers for Medicare and Medicaid Services. https://www.medicare.gov/hospitalcompare/Data/Hospital-overall-ratings-calculation.html. Accessed 20 Dec 2017.
31. Centers for Medicare and Medicaid Services. Quality payment program. https://qpp.cms.gov/. Accessed 8 Feb 2017.
32. Centers for Medicare and Medicaid Services. MIPS scoring 101 guide. November, 2017. https://www.cms.gov/Medicare/Quality-Payment-Program/Resource-Library/Resource-library.html. Accessed 1 Feb 2018.
33. Burwell SM. Setting value-based payment goals – HHS efforts to improve U.S. health care. N Engl J Med. 2015;372:897–9.
34. Berwick D. Era 3 for medicine and health care. JAMA. 2016;315(13):1329–30.
35. MacLean CH, Kerr EA, Qaseem A. Time out – charting a path for improving performance measurement. N Engl J Med. 2018;378:1757–61.
36. Institute of Medicine. Clinical Practice Guidelines We Can Trust. Washington, DC. National Academies Press, 2011.

37. Integrated Healthcare Association. Value Based P4P. http://www.iha.org/our-work/accountability/value-based-p4p. Accessed 15 Dec 2017.
38. Wisconsin Collaborative for Healthcare Quality. https://www.wchq.org/. Accessed 15 Dec 2017.
39. UnitedHealth Premium Program. United Healthcare. https://www.uhc.com/health-and-wellness/take-control-of-your-care/choose-a-doctor/united-health-premium-program. Accessed 15 Dec 2017.
40. UnitedHealthPremiumPhysician Designation Program. Detailed Methodology. https://www.unitedhealthcareonline.com/ccmcontent/ProviderII/UHC/en-US/Assets/ProviderStaticFiles/ProviderStaticFilesPdf/Unitedhealth%20Premium/UnitedHealth_Premium_Detailed_Methodology_2012.pdf. Accessed 15 Dec 2017.

Centers of Excellence and Payer-Defined Quality Assessment

22

Daniel Burkett, Clayton Haldeman, Paul Samuel Page, and Daniel K. Resnick

Background

Low back pain is extraordinarily common and is ranked as the leading cause of disability worldwide. According to some reports, approximately 80% of all adults experience low back pain at some time in their lives. Spine and musculoskeletal disorders account for about 70 million physician visits in the United States every year. These disorders also account for almost 130 million outpatient and emergency room visits a year. Back pain is now the second leading cause of hospital admissions in the United States. Martin et al. estimated the cost of treating low back and neck pain at $86 billion dollars in 2005, and that spending had increased 65% from just 8 years prior [1]. Due to the significant health and economic impacts of chronic back pain, there is a strong need to define the value and the efficacy of a wide variety of treatments available. This chapter explores how centers of excellence may be used to help facilitate efficient diagnosis, treatment, and recovery for patients in a cost-effective manner. With systematic evaluation of the outcomes of various treatment strategies, centers of excellence my help payers assess healthcare quality more effectively as well.

D. Burkett · C. Haldeman · P. S. Page · D. K. Resnick (✉)
Department of Neurosurgery, University of Wisconsin School of Medicine and Public Health, Madison, WI, USA
e-mail: resnick@neurosurgery.wisc.edu

J. Ratliff et al. (eds.), *Quality Spine Care*,
https://doi.org/10.1007/978-3-319-97990-8_22

What Is a Center of Excellence?

By definition, centers of excellence are specialized programs within healthcare institutions that supply exceptionally high concentrations of expertise and related resources focused on a specific medical area, such as the treatment of spine problems. The goal of these centers is to deliver evidence-based care in a comprehensive, interdisciplinary fashion to create the best patient health and satisfaction outcomes possible. Many specialties, including cardiology, orthopedic surgery, oncology, and ophthalmology, utilize this format to create a competitive presence in the healthcare marketplace [2].

The "center of excellence" designation typically comes from accrediting bodies or third-party payers. Each organization has different, sometimes evidence-based, criteria to apply the designation. Criteria may include training background of providers, volume of cases performed, performance on process quality measures, structural features of the institution, and nursing-patient ratios. The classic goal of such centers is the achievement of exceptional quality and lower cost. A center of excellence designation may be important for institutions because it not only signifies that the organization is meeting certain performance standards but also allows the institution to market this designation and stand out among other area institutions.

How to Become a Center of Excellence

Depending on the definition used by a payer or certifying body, the creation of a center of excellence may require a significant amount of vision, design, coordination, and integration in order to be established. The assembly framework used to design centers of excellence in individual institutions is often kept confidential due to competitive advantage, but a diligent organization can develop a center with the knowledge of some common key characteristics and a design framework. The basic key components to centers of excellence are a defined mission and vision, physician leadership, a standardized multidisciplinary approach, and the creation of a unique and pleasant patient experience.

Vision and Validation

The first step for establishing a center of excellence is conceptualizing the vision. In the setting of spine care, this vision involves a model that incorporates several subspecialties and medical disciplines and creates an organized, coordinated approach to diagnosis, treatment, and recovery. In order to be an effective center of excellence, this model must also increase patient satisfaction, decrease the utilization of medical services and medications, reduce the overall cost of care, decrease the length of treatment, and provide a quicker return to work or regular activity for patients. Seamless coordination between neurological and orthopedic surgery, physiatry, physical medicine and rehabilitation, physical therapy, occupational therapy, pain management, nursing, radiology, acupuncture, behavior medicine, and multiple other specialties is critical to this success. Local factors such as the patient mix, payer mix, and availability of appropriate specialists must also be considered. A committee of consultants, engineers, healthcare administrators, and other experts are appointed and tasked with the coordination and implementation of the center's vision.

Design and Development

Centers of excellence are often designed around a "servicescape" model. A servicescape is a collection of elements that create the service environment of a center. The servicescape of a spine center of excellence should be tailored specifically to the diagnosis, treatment, and recovery of the spine. An ideal design would incorporate every aspect of spine injury and treatment. The architecture and ambiance of the center, parking, signage, equipment and technology present, ergonomics, etc. should all lend to a patient's experience. The development of the center itself is typically focused on a few core principles. These include personnel, medical care, marketing, and finance.

Medical Care

At the heart of these principles is the primary purpose of a center of excellence, to provide superior medical care. Centers of excellence should be well equipped with top-of-the-line technology and equipment. The workforce should be experts in spine care and be capable of providing world-class care to every patient. Patient outcomes should meet every quality assessment standard that payers and third-party organizations set. With so many specialties involved in each patient's care, efficiency and close coordination between these various personnel is necessary to provide optimal patient experience and the results necessary to be called a center of excellence.

Personnel

Coordinating the variety of personnel at a center of excellence is key to creating a smooth and comfortable experience for the patient. Specialized personnel should be present at every level. Nurses, doctors, secretaries, administrators, and potentially every employee of a center of excellence should have specific training or extensive experience in the treatment of spinal injuries and disorders. This is one of the defining characteristics of specialized spine centers from hospitals and should be an attraction for patients.

Marketing

Even with superior medical care, centers of excellence are most effective when they are treating the maximum number of patients. Excellent medical care will not be the only attracting force for patients. The job of marketing is to develop a plan to draw patients away from other institutions and to their center. A marketing plan should focus on the fact that from the moment the patients step into a spine center, they will be interacting with spine expert professionals. It should also highlight that patients can receive every aspect of their care at one center by integrated staff with streamlined communication. This eliminates the problem of patients going to outside facilities for their rehabilitation or follow-up care and having personnel who are not familiar with their condition or treatment. Marketing the patient advantages of centers of excellence is important to attracting a consistent patient population.

Finance

Underlying the superior medical care and coordination provided by centers of excellence is the financial productivity and sustainability of the center. For institution administrators, having a spine center that has consolidated staff, resources, and equipment allows for cutting costs without compromising care. These centers can provide a higher efficiency of care because of their dedicated staff and streamlined model. If the marketing side is successful, this product differentiation can drastically increase patient volume and positively impact the bottom line.

Completion and Commercialization

This is the final step in establishing centers of excellence. Once a spine center is completed and every component is functioning properly, management must focus on the future of the center. It must become an established provider in the area that is known for sustainable, superior patient care.

Spine Centers of Excellence

As discussed previously, spine injuries create a large physical and economic burden on the United States. Spine surgeons and the hospitals that treat these conditions have specific challenges as well. Previously, hospitals and spine specialists could build and offer a wide variety of specialized spine programs and treatments for patients with the understanding that they would eventually achieve sustained patient utilization. Delivery of care systems are transitioning toward a managed care model, with a focus on primary care physicians. This may introduce difficulties for specialists to create center of excellence programs without a sustainable business model. To be successful in today's environment, spine surgeons must now work closely with their facility to ensure that they are delivering state of the art, cost-effective care that provides revenue for the institution. In addition to this focus, the competition in spine care treatment is intense, even within the same healthcare institution. Uniting the different spine entities in one institution under one facility is beneficial to the healthcare institution and the individual practitioners.

The business model of centers of excellence can be tailored specifically for a spine center [1]. Just like other centers of excellence, the goal of creating operative/nonoperative spine centers of excellence is to establish a regional presence and a robust patient population. The most important principle behind this goal is to bring together all of the different specialties involved in spine care in a seamless and organized fashion. In one spine center, the number of specialties involved may include neurosurgery, orthopedic surgery, rehabilitation, occupational therapy and physical therapy, pain management, specialized nursing, radiology, behavior medicine, and physiatry.

Every level of care should be standardized throughout the center. Specific guidelines and streamlined interdisciplinary workflows should exist with constant evaluation and modifications. Treatment decisions are supported by continuous outcome analysis and patient satisfaction surveys. Center administrators are committed to increasing efficiency, coordinating care delivery between the different specialties, and enhancing the overall patient experience.

Developing spine centers of excellence requires years of planning, resource gathering, building, and implementation of a care model in addition to a substantial financial risk from the home institution. If mistakes are made and steps are done poorly, a center can fail and become a financial drain on the overall institution. Having experts who have a full understanding of the business and clinical aspects of medicine is the foundation of a successful center. When implemented efficiently, these centers can be beneficial to everyone involved in spine care.

Benefits of Spine Centers of Excellence

A multidisciplinary spine center can offer a comprehensive, innovative, and economically efficient approach to the diagnosis and treatment of spine conditions. Some of the benefits offered include:

- Operative and nonoperative treatment options offered within one delivery system
- Outcome-driven care with well-defined inter-specialty workflows
- Reduced utilization of healthcare resources, reduced overall cost of care, and increased savings for the patient, payers, and institution
- Decreased length of treatment, quicker return to work, and decreased disability
- Benefits of this healthcare delivery model extend to patients, employers, payers, and the healthcare institution itself.

Do Spine Centers of Excellence Improve Care?

Centers of excellence are held to specific quality metrics, while they have the "center of excellence" designation. These standards have caused some commercial and public payers to require patients to obtain care at centers with the designation. The question still remains if centers of excellence actually provide better care and outcomes for patients. There is still limited data on the health outcomes provided by centers of excellence. A study evaluating spine surgery centers of excellence from 2007 to 2009 compared the outcomes and costs between 369 centers of excellence and 1449 hospitals without that designation. They studied patients between the ages of 18 and 64 who underwent cervical simple fusions with or without discectomy/decompression, lumbar simple fusions with or without discectomy/decompression, and lumbar discectomy/decompression without fusion. A total of almost 30,000 surgeries in each group were identified. They evaluated the hospitals based on hospital-level data on patient experience and surgical quality measures. These surgical measurements included postsurgery complication rates, readmission rates, discharge mortality rate, post-discharge complication rate, and repeat surgery rates. The costs measured included the total costs for spine surgery itself and the hospitalization. Their study found that centers of excellence performed about the same or worse on patient experience measures compared to non-designated hospitals. Centers of excellence generally performed better on surgical care measures, but their complication and 30-day readmission rates were statistically similar to other hospitals. They also found that patients suffered similar financial costs whether they were at the centers of excellence or non-designated hospitals. This same group did a similar study on knee and hip replacement centers of excellence and found that the designated hospitals had lower complication and readmission rates compared to the non-designated hospitals [3].

This study does not detract from the concept of centers of excellence. The designation criteria for centers of excellence may need to be reevaluated by each organization and potentially standardized. It is also important to consider the patient and procedure mix in both settings. In some freestanding surgical centers, patients with substantial comorbidities should not be treated due to the inability for these centers to manage postoperative adverse events. If freestanding centers essentially "cherry pick" the healthiest patients, this would lead to a more sick surgical patient population in the hospital population. In such a case, superior outcomes would be expected from the freestanding "center" if even equivocal care was offered. The importance of appropriate risk adjustment and the ability to track patient-reported outcome measures cannot be overstated when establishing the efficacy of these centers of excellence compared to traditional care settings. More studies comparing centers of excellence and non-designated hospitals are needed.

Establishing a regional spine center of excellence requires a significant amount of work, planning, and coordination. There is an inherit risk involved, but the end result may be rewarding for patients and the hospital. As healthcare continues to emphasize improvement in healthcare quality, spine centers of excellence can be at the forefront of cost-effective superior spine care.

Payer-Defined Quality Assessment

The healthcare environment has undergone a strong shift toward a focus on cost-effective healthcare [4]. This movement has helped fuel the interest in developing centers of excellence to achieve economy of scale. Much of the pressure on hospitals has come in the form of financial incentives and penalties from payers. Since payers are determining the reimbursement rates for institutions based on definitions of quality, it is useful to understand how the payers define and assess healthcare quality and how this factors into the structure of centers of excellence.

Healthcare quality is a very difficult concept to define broadly. It can be loosely defined as the degree to which healthcare services for individuals increase the likelihood of desired health outcomes and are consistent with professional knowledge. When defining healthcare quality, the difference between individual patient and patient population levels of analysis should be distinguished while also focusing on the importance of both.

The assessment of healthcare quality is the attempt to evaluate health outcomes and to link these outcomes to the specific healthcare services that influence them. The goal is to evaluate which evidence-based healthcare interventions can be implemented to improve the overall quality of healthcare. Several entities can perform healthcare assessment including medical practitioners, patients, payers, and the community. Medical practitioners tend to focus on the technical knowledge and the amenities of care provided, patients tend to focus on their interactions with practitioners and their overall experience in addition to their level of care, and the community focuses on the costs of the healthcare provided and the access to care. The focus of this section will be how payers assess the quality of healthcare.

Defining Quality in Healthcare

To assess healthcare, an entity must first be able to define what comprises quality in healthcare. While this is difficult, some characteristics are commonly found in measures used to define high-quality healthcare [5]:

- The measure contains a scale of quality.
- The measure encompasses a wide range of elements of care.
- The measure targets individual patients and patient populations.
- The measure is goal-oriented.
- The measures reflect that a risk versus benefit trade-off often exists.
- The measure attempts to link the healthcare processes involved to outcome benefits.

It is important to recognize the limitation of any single measure to accurately capture all elements of health quality. There may also be technological or social constraints limiting the utility of a given measure.

High-quality healthcare has a few other common process characteristics that support these goals. These characteristics include effective communication, shared decision-making, and the implementation of services in a technically competent and efficient manner. The care that patients receive and the outcomes they experience should be the result of integration of all of these concepts. The patient may only notice certain aspects of their care, such as their interactions with doctors, but their overall experience will be a result of the success of these qualities.

The Payer

In most cases, the payer is an entity other than the patient that processes a claim and finances or reimburses the cost of the healthcare. In the United States, this group includes both health insurance companies and Medicare (Centers for Medicare and Medicaid Services). The role of the payer is also distinct from that of a health plan even though the role can be filled by one entity. In the United States, claims are sent from the healthcare institution to the payers responsible and a payment is made on the patient's behalf depending on the patient's insurance plan.

As a health insurance payer gathers more and more patients within their payment plan, they gain leverage with the providers. Payers can negotiate prices and reimbursement plans for various services rendered and encourage their patients to use a given healthcare system. For hospitals, this helps establish a robust patient population and consistent utilization of services. Hospitals fear losing these large patient pools because it means decreased revenue for the system. The payers realize this leverage and include quality standards within their plans that institutions must meet in order to receive certain reimbursement payments. These standards are intended to decrease the cost of care for the patient, reducing overall cost for the patient and the payer.

There are a variety of payment plans that can be negotiated between providers and payers, with some incorporating quality standards directly in the plan. These payment plans include fee-for-service, pay-for-performance, bundled payments, comprehensive care payments, and accountable care organizations [6].

Fee-for-service is the most traditional healthcare payment model. With this model, payers provide payment for all services rendered by the provider. There are no quality requirements or standards that providers need to meet. Therefore, there are no incentives for providers to reduce hospitalizations, utilize preventive care measures, or incorporate any cost-saving measures into their practice.

Pay-for-performance is a payment system designed to incentivize providers to achieve certain metrics with care. Providers are rewarded for reaching certain quality standards and penalized for failing to do so. These plans may create quality improvement in some settings, such as the administration of aspirin in the emergency room for suspected cardiac ischemia. However, outside of relatively simple process measures, this strategy has had limited success due to problems with attribution, the existence of comorbidities, and the reliance on false endpoints.

With bundled payments, a payer gives a single payment for all of the services provided during one episode of patient care. The payment amount is the same regardless of the amount of treatment and the number of specialists that the patient sees. The goal of this payment plan is provide predictable costs for the payer. Theoretically, the health system is incentivized to cut down on duplicate treatments and costs and to reduce waste. CMS provides information about the type of care episodes they will cover and an outline for what services constitute a single episode of care. Bundled payments are also becoming common among commercial payers such as Walmart and Lowe's for certain services such as orthopedic procedures [7]. Their plans allow them to negotiate savings and full health coverage with designated treatment centers, including centers of excellence.

While bundled payments attempt to reduce the costs of each episode of care and hospitalization, it does not incentivize a reduction in the number of hospitalizations. Comprehensive care payments are designed to prevent hospitalizations through more preventive care services such as patient education. The structure of comprehensive care payments defines a single payment amount to cover all of the services needed to treat and manage all of the conditions a patient may experience over a set period of time. This payment is fixed regardless of the amount of episodes of care the patient needs for treatment. Ideally this plan gives providers greater resource flexibility to try innovative approaches for treatment but to also reduce inefficient and excess care. Some research has shown that comprehensive care payment plans can reduce the number of surgeries and diagnostic imaging performed when neutral advisors are involved with shared decision-making between the providers and patients [8, 9]. This system should not penalize providers for taking care of sicker patients. Under this system, payment would depend on the number and severity of a patient's health conditions [10]. Currently, comprehensive payment plans are not common in the United States.

Accountable care organizations are a shared savings arrangement between a payer and institution that is based on the total cost of care for a certain patient population. The payer agrees to pay the institution a certain amount for their patient population, and it is up to the institution to keep their costs within that amount. This type of payment plan is growing in popularity and is a complex arrangement that systematically forces the institution to provide effective primary care to treat minor health issues before they become serious and require expensive hospitalizations. While a continued focus on primary care may prevent some avoidable hospitalizations, lack of support for specialty care may create limited access when complicated problems occur.

The goal of value-based payment is to give providers enough resources to deliver effective, high-quality care with efficient and reasonable costs. The episode-of-care and complex care payments described above give providers incentives to be proactive in preventing healthcare problems, improving the quality of healthcare delivered. Value-based payments intend to produce better health outcomes during acute episodes, to reduce complications and their associated costs, and to reduce the overall cost of successful treatment. Care must be taken, however, to avoid creating perverse incentives which negatively influence patient care. For example, the best way to avoid a catheter-associated urinary tract infection is to avoid placing a catheter. This reduces costs through avoiding the catheter and avoiding the potential for infection. In many cases, this strategy is viable. Policies which make it cumbersome to place catheters in patients who need them, such as patients with spinal conditions resulting in bladder dysfunction, lead to increased complications and costs.

Payer Quality Assessment

Assessing and measuring the quality of healthcare can help eliminate inefficient and unsafe use of medical services, may identify the treatments and services that stimulate improvement, can hold healthcare providers accountable for delivering quality service, and will help consumers make an informed decision about healthcare institutions. With more payers moving from a fee-for-service payment plan to bundled payments and accountable care organizations, healthcare quality and patient outcomes become a greater focus of how payments are distributed. Setting quality measures and goals allows stakeholders to play a part in determining how much they will pay for given healthcare services rendered by a hospital. In the payers' perspective, holding hospitals accountable for their care should improve outcomes and reduce complications, decreasing costs. If healthcare institutions do not meet certain requirements, payers can refuse to pay for what they view as "substandard" care. A critical and worrisome issue, however, is what the payer defines as "quality" as opposed to what a patient or provider would define as "quality."

Quality measurement is, in general, the process of using data to evaluate the performance of healthcare providers against a quality standard of care. Measures of "quality" can be assessed at every level and setting of care, including hospitals, outpatient centers, imaging facilities, and the overall healthcare system. When assessing the quality of healthcare, it is important to understand the components of healthcare and how they factor into quality. The components of healthcare can be broken down into structure, process, outcome, and patient experience.

The structure of healthcare includes the material and human resources used. This includes doctors, hospitals, and their equipment. The capability of the staff employed, the functioning ability of the equipment, and the availability of medical resources are all assessed. Payers evaluate the structure of an institution to determine if they are capable of delivering high-quality care. This can include whether a system has an electronic medical record or an emergency room has a dedicated CT scanner [11]. Spine centers typically build their facility with the equipment necessary to meet all of the structural quality requirements for a spine center of excellence. A solid structure supports high-quality care, but does not equal good care [12].

Process measures are commonly used to provide a surrogate for "quality" in procedures. These measures are used to determine if providers are giving services that are consistent with the evidence-based standard of care. Providers should be delivering care and recommending treatments that are known to efficiently improve patient health and reduce complications [13]. Unfortunately, the evidence supporting the use of many process measures is weak and the exercise becomes more of a "gaming of the system" than a true quality improvement. From a payer perspective, assessing whether or not this is occurring may be done by evaluating the treatment that patients receive. Spine centers of excellence commonly use evidence-based and cost-effective processes, so meeting these measures should not be difficult. Documenting the performance of these processes is time consuming, expensive, and negatively impacts the patient experience independent of the provision of healthcare. For payers, completely setting their quality assessment and provider payments based on process measures alone is problematic. Providers are rewarded for checking off the process measure boxes, not for providing care.

Outcome measures evaluate patients' health as a result of the care they received [14]. The two components of measuring health outcomes are health perceptions and patient satisfaction. Health perception measures the impact of the care on patients' overall health. Typically, morbidity, mortality, and health-related quality of life issues are included in health perception outcome measures. For payers, using these outcomes to determine whether to reward or penalize providers through their payments may be helpful if appropriate measures are available and patients can be incentivized to complete them. Payers can set specified goals for providers, such as keeping surgical complication rates below a certain percentage or decreasing length of hospital stays. Problems exist with using only health outcomes for determining reimbursement rate. The illness severity of a patient population can fluctuate and vary greatly even between neighboring hospitals. It can be difficult to assess the illness severity of a certain patient population, attempting to factor in multiple chronic comorbidities and how they influence outcome measures. Social determinants of health such as economic support have a significant impact on health outcomes. These are also very difficult for payers and providers to numerically determine their overall influence on health outcomes [15]. Further complicating the issue is that these easily measured factors may have no bearing on the appropriateness of the care received or any benefit the patient derived from a procedure. A facility which only treats otherwise healthy patients without significant comorbidities will appear to provide high-quality low-cost care whether or not the patients required treatment at all.

The other component to patient health outcomes is patient satisfaction. Patient satisfaction closely evaluates the interpersonal aspects of healthcare but additionally includes a wide range of elements that factor into a patient's overall experience. This may include how quickly a patient was seen in an outpatient center, whether providers tell patients about test results, and the accessibility of the information that providers do tell patients. Research has shown that positive patient experiences can lead patients to become more engaged in their care and result in improved patient-perceived outcomes and clinical quality [16]. Payers such as CMS distribute patient satisfaction surveys to patients after an episode of care and will use those results to either reward or penalize payments to hospitals [17]. Unfortunately, when patient satisfaction surveys are compared to objective health outcomes, the results often have an inverse relationship. In emergency care, patients who consume the most resources and suffer the greatest morbidity and mortality are most satisfied with their care [18]. Similarly, in spine care, patients who are offered surgery or prescribed narcotics are more satisfied than those who are not [19].

How Payers Incorporate Quality Measures

Before quality measures are used for the assessment of healthcare quality by payers, their worth needs to be approved, usually by other accrediting organizations. To become a validated quality measure, practices are researched and their outcomes analyzed. Data is gathered from administrations, providers, and health records by organizations such CMS and the Joint Commission on Accreditation of Healthcare Organizations (JCAHO) or a for-profit organization such as *US News and World Report* [14]. Measurable quality standards using the results from these evidence-based practices are then developed. Other organizations such as the National Quality Forum (NQF) or the Agency for Healthcare Research (AHRQ) will then evaluate the quality measures and decide whether or not to endorse them. Once a quality measure is endorsed, payers will insert them into their reimbursement guidelines.

Once quality measures are established, payers such as health insurance companies and CMS will use these quality measures to arrange reimbursement rates. Payers that use fee-for-performance, bundled payments, comprehensive care payments, and accountable care organization plans may base reimbursement rates or incentive schedules based on provider performance compared to these quality measures. Payers will elect to reward or penalize providers for meeting or failing to meet these measures, with the end goal of decreasing the cost to the payer.

Payers' pressure on providers to meet quality metrics has led institutions to focus on developing health systems that meet these measures efficiently. Centers of excellence were created to accomplish the goal of providing care that consistently surpasses these quality standards in a cost-effective manner. The end achievement of both payer quality assessment and centers of excellence is high-quality, cost-effective healthcare.

References

1. Rogers MT. Developing the Spine Center Business Model [Internet]. SpineUniverse. [Cited 8 Jan 2018]. Available from: https://www.spineuniverse.com/professional/practice-management/developing-spine-center-business-model
2. Elrod JK, Fortenberry JL. Centers of excellence in healthcare institutions: what they are and how to assemble them. BMC Health Serv Res. 2017;17(S1):15.
3. Mehrotra A, Sloss EM, Hussey PS, Adams JL, Lovejoy S, Soohoo NF. Evaluation of a center of excellence program for spine surgery. Med Care. 2013;51(8):748–57.
4. Lohr KN. Concepts of assessing, assuring, and improving quality. In: Medicare: a strategy for quality assurance. Washington, DC: National Academies Press; 1990. p. 45–64.
5. Lohr KN. Defining quality of care. In: Medicare: a strategy for quality assurance: a report of a study by a committee of the Institute of Medicine, Division of Health Care Services. Washington, DC: National Academy Press; 1990. p. 116–39.
6. (U.S.) Iof M, (U.S.) NAP, Yong PL, Saunders RS, Olsen LA. Payment and payer-based strategies. In: The healthcare imperative: lowering costs and improving outcomes: workshop series summary, Learning health system series. Washington, DC: National Academies Press; 2010. p. 359–406.
7. Healthcare Payers and Providers: Best System for Process Improvement [Internet]. Health Catalyst, 2017. [Cited 8 Jan 2018]. Available from: https://www.healthcatalyst.com/healthcare-payers-providers-system-process-improvement
8. O Connor AM. Modifying unwarranted variations in health care: shared decision making using patient decision aids. Health Aff. 2004 Jul;23:63–72.
9. Bottles K. Decision-support alternative to prior authorization for ordering high-tech diagnostic imaging scans. Institute for Clinical Systems Improvement; 2009.

10. Miller HD. From volume to value: better ways to pay for health care. Health Aff. 2009;28(5):1418–28.
11. Selecting Structure Measures for Clinical Quality Measurement. National Quality Measures Clearinghouse. [Cited 8 Jan 2018]. Available from: https://www.qualitymeasures.ahrq.gov/help-and-about/quality-measure-tutorials/selecting-structure-measures
12. Cleary, P, O'Kane, M. Evaluating the quality of health care [Internet]. OBSSR e-Source – Evaluating the quality of health care. [Cited 8 Jan 2018]. Available from: http://www.esourceresearch.org/tabid/794/default.aspx
13. Cromwell J, Trisolini M, Pope G, Mitchell J, Greenwald L. Pay for performance in health care: methods and approaches. Research Triangle Park: Research Triangle International; 2011.
14. Measuring Health Care Quality: An Overview. Families USA [Internet]. Families USA. [Cited 8 Jan 2018].
15. Berenson RA, Pronovost PJ, Krumholz HM. The Potential of Health Care Performance Measures [Internet]. RWJF. Washington, DC: Urban Institute; 2017. [Cited 8 Jan 2018].
16. Case for Patient Experience [Internet]. Aligning Forces for Quality. [Cited 8 Jan 2018]. Available from: http://forces4quality.org/case-patient-experience
17. Annual Progress Report to Congress: National Strategy for Quality Improvement in Health Car. Annual Progress Report to Congress: National Strategy for Quality Improvement in Health Car. 2012.
18. Fenton JJ, Jerant AF, Bertakis KD, Franks P. The cost of satisfaction. Arch Intern Med. 2012;172(5):405–11.
19. Mazur MD, Mcevoy S, Schmidt MH, Bisson EF. High self-assessment of disability and the surgeons recommendation against surgical intervention may negatively impact satisfaction scores in patients with spinal disorders. J Neurosurg Spine. 2015;22(6):666–71.

Reporting Quality Results

23

Julian L. Gendreau, Allen L. Ho, Arjun Vivek Pendharkar, Eric S. Sussman, and Atman M. Desai

Introduction

Beginning in 1986, the US federal government began publicly reporting mortality rates of surgical outcomes for enrolled Medicare patients at the hospital level. This was the first public reporting of the quality of surgery outcomes [1]. In 1989, the New York Department of Health created the first state registry for reporting mortality rates of surgical outcomes when they began publishing data on coronary artery bypass grafting (CABG), which was also at the hospital level [2]. Following a Freedom of Information Act lawsuit by *Newsday*, the state of New York became the first entity to publish surgeon-specific data on surgery outcomes by publishing complications of CABG operations [2, 3]. Over a decade later in 2013, the United Kingdom became the first European country to mandate large-scale quality reporting of key procedures across nine surgical specialties [4]. Here in the United States, large-scale quality reporting across all specialties was introduced in July 2015, when the website ProPublica began publishing complication rates of over 17,000 surgeons in the United States [5]. This effort summarized publically available data maintained by CMS into a searchable web portal.

Concurrent with these changes in public reporting, several systems have been developed for the internal reporting of quality results to hospitals and physicians. Relevant to spine surgery, two prominent databases include the National Surgical Quality Improvement Program (NSQIP) and, the more recently introduced, National

J. L. Gendreau
Mercer University School of Medicine, Macon, GA, USA

Department of Neurosurgery, Stanford University School of Medicine, Stanford, CA, USA

A. L. Ho · A. V. Pendharkar · E. S. Sussman · A. M. Desai (✉)
Department of Neurosurgery, Stanford University School of Medicine, Stanford, CA, USA
e-mail: atman@stanford.edu

J. Ratliff et al. (eds.), *Quality Spine Care*,
https://doi.org/10.1007/978-3-319-97990-8_23

Neurosurgery Quality and Outcomes Database (N^2QOD). Another form of public quality reporting has also recently surfaced in the form of online consumer rating websites in which patients are able to rate physician and healthcare experiences. Such online rating services include Healthgrades, Yelp, Vitals, and RateMDs.

Further improving our healthcare system's ability to report data on surgical outcomes will allow us to better implement quality improvement initiatives, demonstrate transparency among physicians, facilitate patient choice, allow for identification of poor surgeon performance, and assist in academic research [6]. Most other major industries already use systemic data collection for quality improvement purposes. High-quality clinical data gathering systems should also be developed in the medical community. Improving these measures of quality in healthcare will greatly enhance our ability to maximize the value of medical intervention, including that of spine procedures.

Quality Reporting in Hospital Systems

Factors to consider when interpreting quality reporting data are sample size, risk adjustment, and accuracy of sources. Sample size is particularly important when looking at quality data of spine surgeons, as they generally perform fewer procedures and have lower mortality rates relative to other medical specialties. Consequently, the chance of finding a surgeon with an increased mortality rate is lower. Reporting solely on mortality data will be of little benefit to patients or hospitals for this reason; focusing on mortality as a reported surgical outcome significantly lowers the statistical power of any judgments made based off this data. However, if data is analyzed for mortality, hospital-wide data is preferable for analysis and more likely to be representative given the larger sample size [6]. Overall, examining records for mortality alone will not determine the extent of treatment effectiveness or the level of patient satisfaction in individual surgical procedures.

Therefore, in spine surgery, outcome reporting should ideally be directed toward more frequent outcomes such as surgical complications. Assessing rates of various complications is clearly more challenging than assessing mortality rates, but there have been no studies analyzing specific costs and resources required to study complication rates. Future studies should be focused on devising the most cost-effective strategies to collect complication data [6].

Efficient methods for data acquisition are crucial to quality reporting efforts. Some studies suggest that registries gathering information on spine treatments should provide questionnaires and take data at least 12 months after a given intervention, to accurately assess treatment benefit. With this longer follow-up period, patient responses regarding outcomes and complications are more representative; this approach will allow for a better description of which treatment options are most effective [7].

The Scoliosis Research Society has proposed a system for effectively acquiring complication data from spine surgery. In their model, they gather data solely on surgery for correcting scoliosis. To reduce the time required for surgeons to be compliant in data entry, they collect data from only a few major complications (death, neurological deficit, and blindness), and they collected information only from cases with complications. This led to significantly higher surgeon compliance rate in reporting complications of spine surgery [8]. From a statistical viewpoint, to best adjust for risk among patients, hierarchical multilevel models are preferable to logistic regression to best analyze the clustering of patients by surgeons, as well as surgeons within institutions [9].

Standard measures also need to be developed for measuring complications of spine surgery. The definition of complication and complication severity (minor versus major) in spine surgery has been found to be vague in past literature and needs to be better defined. When reviewing spine literature and quality reporting data from federal agencies, complication rates ranged from 5% to 19%, 7% to 18%, and 4% to 14% for cervical, thoracic, and lumbar spine surgery, respectively [10]. A 6-question Core Outcome Measures Index (COMI) was created to help document outcomes associated with spine surgery in order to better standardize the reporting to national registries. Using standardized documents for reporting spine surgery complications will improve our ability to collaborate in the scientific community, assess effectiveness of new treatments, and assess effectiveness of quality improvement initiatives [11, 12].

The rate of poor outcomes in spine surgery may depend on how the outcome was assessed by the surgeon performing the operation. Formal standardized methods are wanted [11]. It has been reported that surgeons are likely to downgrade the severity of an incident when reporting their own adverse events [13]. A recent study proposes that a Clinical Events Committee (CEC) should be developed in hospitals performing large numbers of spine operations to better independently classify and asses the complications. This report found establishing a third-party CEC, consisting of independent surgeons, is more likely to accurately assess a given incident [13]. In addition to a professional opinion from independent surgeons, many researchers suggest that patient-reported personal experiences of surgical outcomes may be of greater value than measuring the complication of surgery in isolation [11, 14, 15]. When reporting surgeon-specific surgical outcomes, it is also important to note that a single physician often does not control all aspects of patient care. Future quality reporting systems should recognize that outcomes are influenced by the multidisciplinary teams involved with patient treatment [16].

Centers for Medicare and Medicaid Services (CMS)

CMS is attempting to improve the nation's quality of healthcare by transforming their programs from a fee-for-service system to a value-based payment (VBP) system [17]. The value-based payment modifier results in differential payments for both individual physicians and group practices based on evaluations of quality cost and care measures. Currently, physicians can get bonuses or penalties of up to 4% of total Medicare billing, based upon quality and cost assessment [18]. These systems and percentages may be anticipated to change with ongoing legislative reform of CMS quality reporting and payment models.

In 2016, CMS launched a Physician Compare website to the public that publishes physician-specific quality data recorded by this program [19]. This website can be found at: https://www.medicare.gov/physiciancompare/. As a part of this transition to a VBP, the Physician Quality Reporting System (PQRS) was implemented in 2006, which enables eligible professionals (EPs) to report a variety of process measures and qualities of their patient interactions. EPs consist of physicians and other health professionals paid under the Medicare physician fee schedule, including nurse practitioners and physician assistants. PQRS is currently the primary data source in the quality reporting option of CMS's VBP payment system [20].

Many metrics in the PQRS system are endorsed by the National Quality Forum (NQF) after review and assessment from stakeholders. Assessing quality measures is a lengthy and expensive process, typically requiring approximately 3 years for a given measure [17]. NQF uses an 8-step Consensus Development Process that endorses consensus standards, uses evidence-based best practice recommendations, and includes quality frameworks and reporting guidelines. CMS is required to consider NQF-endorsed measures, but it can also adopt non-NQF-endorsed measures when gaps are present in high-priority quality reporting areas [19]. Participation in the PQRS is voluntary, but providers can earn incentives for reporting PQRS measures and penalties for not reporting. The exact amount of incentives and penalties has undergone various revisions, as legislation has been used to revise and replace portions of the program. Before 2015, to earn incentives, physicians had to report at least three quality measures on at least 50% of beneficiaries to obtain a bonus of up to 2% of their Part B allowed charges. In 2016, the system switched from giving bonus payments to only penalizing physicians up to 2% for non-participation [21]. With passage of the Medicare Access and CHIP Reauthorization Act (MACRA), the previous CMS model with penalties will again be replaced for an incentive payment-based value system, the Merit-Based Incentive Payment System (MIPS). This system consolidates the PQRS, electronic health records (EHR) meaningful use regulation, and value-based modifier programs for rating physician quality, and it allows for both penalties and incentives. Beginning in 2019, bonuses and penalties will be determined by a composite score of 0–100 based off 30% for quality reporting, 30% for resource use, 25% for meaningful use of EHR, and 15% for specialty-specific resource use [22]. These percentages may be anticipated to change with future regulatory modification of the system.

The PQRS, as well as modifier programs of the VBP and the EHR meaningful use regulation, is poorly applicable to surgical and other procedural subspecialists because it requires quality reporting on generic medical measures to avoid penalties. These qualities are often not measured in the offices of spine surgeons and may not be under the control of the surgeon at all

Another option for reporting through the MIPS system is through the Qualified Clinical Data Registry (QCDR) option enacted in 2014. In this option, the PQRS requirements can be fulfilled by CMS-approved QCDR entities that may include a distinct registry, certification board, or another collaborative effort that collects clinical data. A QCDR is not limited by only reporting measures in the traditional PQRS set, but it can only offer 20 measures that are non-PQRS. Recently in 2016, when MACRA was passed, it was a major step toward shifting to subspecialty-specific reporting requirements, and the new QCDRs play a large role in the new plan. The National Neurosurgery Quality and Outcomes Database (N^2QOD) provided data for the first neurosurgery-specific QCDR quality metrics. Neurosurgery is one of the first specialties to establish a QCDR, thus highlighting this specialty's leadership in improving the way medicine reports quality outcomes [19].

Physicians can report by individual providers or at the group level for group practices. Physicians can also report through a variety of systems such as using a PQRS-qualified registry, through their Part B claims, through web interfaces, through CMS-certified survey vendors, through participation in QCDR, or through an EHR [21]. In total, there are 284 quality measures available to report [17]. In its first years, participation was minimal. Since penalties are being assessed for non-participators, and with its incorporation into the VBP system, participation levels are expected to significantly increase in the future [20].

As part of these regulations passed in the previous years, physicians are required to meaningfully use EHR in a way that improves healthcare and better reports quality information. EHR systems have been used primarily to aid in effectively transmitting summaries of care documents and to protect against drug interactions [19].

Veterans Health Administration (VHA)

Public law 99–166 was enacted by Congress in 1985 mandating the Department of Veterans Affairs to begin reporting patient mortality and morbidity rates for every surgical operation performed. It also mandated the comparison of these numbers to the national averages and applied risk adjustment to account for patient illnesses. In 1994, the Veterans Affairs (VA) launched the first National Surgical Quality Improvement Program (NSQIP) in the nation to comply with this law [23]. This NSQIP reports annually on both risk-adjusted morbidity and mortality rates that occur within 30 days postoperatively for procedures in the eight surgical subspecialties to the Veterans Affairs Medical Centers (VAMCs) and the 23 Veterans Integrated Service Networks (VISNs), which distribute many resources to VAMCs. This database reports on every major non-cardiac procedure [23, 24]. The VA also has a separate Continuous Improvement in Cardiac Surgery Program (CICSP), which is equivalent to the NSQIP but only for cardiac surgery. In institutions where rates are high, evaluations can be initiated of the surgical care practices of that particular facility, and when a facility has low rates, they disseminate case studies to other facilities [24].

Chiefs of staff of VAMCs can analyze this data to find better ways to improve their medical center. Since the first NSQIP was created, many internal investigations have been performed sending nurse coordinators to the different VAMCs and re-abstracting raw data of cases to confirm accuracy of the reporting at that particular hospital. The program was found to be accurate and well performing [24].

Internal Quality Reporting Systems

Modern Internal Reporting: National Surgical Quality Improvement Program (NSQIP)

To drive quality improvement initiatives and for academic research, hospitals require strong systems for internal reporting [6]. In the United States, the National Surgical Quality Improvement Program assists with quality improvement of surgical cases (NSQIP) [24]. Developed by the VA, NSQIP has been widely used in private hospitals as well [24]. Eligible patients for inclusion in the NSQIP include all those that undergo general, spinal, or epidural anesthesia [24]. Studies have shown that the NSQIP can be adequately used in the private sector, with some reports noting reduction of both 30-day morbidity and mortality rates [25]. NSQIP is potentially a valuable tool for research, making the process of gaining access to large amounts of clinical data more efficient. NSQIP data has been shown to be reliable and accurate and have little interrater variability [24]. This system does not provide data on surgeons specifically, only hospitals. Hence NSQIP may be used to help identify issues outside of the operating room and issues outside of surgeon control [6].

The American College of Surgeons has adopted and widely implemented NSQIP, and it has been shown to lead to higher-quality care and lower costs at many private institutions [26]. In December 2017, CMS announced that data from the American College of Surgeons NSQIP will soon be made public to patients on the Hospital Compare website. Most surgeons do not support public release of the NSQIP data [27].

National Neurosurgery Quality and Outcomes Database (N^2QOD)

In 2012, NeuroPoint Alliance launched the National Neurosurgery Quality and Outcomes Database (N^2QOD, presently referred to as QOD), which is a collaborative registry of quality and outcome reporting for both cranial and spinal neurosurgical operations performed in the United States [28, 29]. Available to practicing neurosurgeons, the data is hosted at the Vanderbilt University Medical Center.

QOD is designed to establish risk-adjusted morbidity and complication rates that occur within 1 year postoperatively in spine procedures [28, 29]. The database looks primarily at five spinal diagnoses: disc herniation, stenosis, spondylolisthesis, revision for recurrent disc herniation, and adjacent segment disease. Data is gathered from patients at 30 days, 3 months, and 12 months. The main goals of this database include establishing risk-adjusted benchmarks for safety of neurosurgical procedures, allowing hospitals to analyze individual clinical outcomes, generating quality data to demonstrate value of medical care, developing risk models for patient procedures, and facilitating cooperative multicenter clinical studies [28, 29]. In its first years in operation, this system has served as a robust data collection platform [30].

Currently, NeuroPoint Alliance is in the process of developing the Spine Quality Outcomes Database (SQOD) in collaboration with the American Academy of Physical Medicine and Rehabilitation. This new database will collect quality data specific to spine patients and longitudinally track patient outcomes over their remaining lifespan. This database began enrolling new members in 2017 [31].

Quality Reporting Through Electronic Health Records (EHR) in Kaiser Permanente

Kaiser Permanente uses its EHR software, KPHealthConnect, for automatic quality reporting. KPHealthConnect manages over nine million members in a highly integrated and computerized way that has both quality and efficiency benefits. In 2010, Kaiser Permanente retooled its core measures for automatic quality reporting [32]. Using a "5-step process," this system uses discrete data values for reducing the chances of inaccuracies [32]. Kaiser also has a data interpretation staff consisting of groups of domain experts, abstractors, analysts, and legal and compliance employees. Once produced, the quality reports are thoroughly validated.

Quality Reporting Directly to Patients

Hospital Compare

Along with the recent additions to the federal healthcare systems, CMS has begun releasing yearly data of hospital quality measures obtained from Department of Defense hospitals, VA hospitals, and private hospitals. The Hospital Compare website is open to the public and can be found at: hospitalcompare.hhs.gov.

CMS assesses patient experiences of different hospitals by disseminating the Hospital Consumer Assessment of Healthcare Provider and Systems (HCAHPS) [33]. This is used in the value-based purchasing metric for CMS. HCAHPS is gathered from patients randomly through non-internet measures such as telephone or mail surveys [33]. US hospitals receive incentive Medicare payments based on different quality measures assessed [34]. Scores on the HCAHPS dictate up to 30% of financial incentives in the Medicare value-based purchasing program, and it can potentially penalize poor performance by up to 2% of payments [35, 36]. These results get published in risk-adjusted models and are also published on the Hospital Compare website [37].

Authors note that HCAHPS has significant potential for improvement. HCAHPS has been criticized for being expensive to use, having low response rates, having significant delay from patient hospitalization to survey response, and rarely actually identifying the source of the problems in the hospital system [38–41]. The Hospital Compare website has been criticized for its inaccuracies of the hospital data posted after its launch [42]. As CMS continues to publish more data publically, questions remain on accuracy of identification and attribution in these systems.

Open Payments

Open Payments is a federal program mandated by the Physician Payment Sunshine Act, Section 6002 in the Patient Protection and Affordable Care Act. Open Payments was officially launched in 2014, and it can be found at: openpaymentsdata.cms.gov. Publishing yearly, this program was designed to increase transparency of financial payments in the healthcare system. It gathers information on payments that physicians and teaching hospitals receive from drug and medical device companies. In addition, this report includes ownership interests that physicians or their immediate family have in drug and medical device companies. The program reports payments in three different categories: general payments, ownership interests, and research payments. Open Payments maintains an impartial role in payment reporting and does not identify beneficial relationships or conflicts of interest in their reports. Before its implementation, only eight states had laws requiring public disclosure of financial payments received by physicians and institutions. The effort sought to increase transparency for patients [43].

Open Payments has recently made available the first sets of data; studies have found inaccuracies in the first years after launch. In a study published in 2016, Babu et al. found that Open Payments only identified 2020 of 3240 neurosurgeons as having their specialty correctly listed in the database as neurosurgeon [44]. Another study found that at the 2014 American Academy of Orthopedic Surgeons Annual Meeting, 39% of surgeons made financial disclosures; however, only 28% of disclosures were in Open Payments. Eleven percent of presenters should have had disclosures in Open Payments but were not included. Surgeons with the most inconsistencies in their disclosures on Open Payments were those who had the most poster presentations and oral presentations among their colleagues [45].

Regarding spine surgery, this program indicates notable financial relationships between spine surgeons and industry. A significant 91.6% of spine surgeons reported at least one financial relationship with industry with a median payment of $994.07, and as many as 6.6% of surgeons received over $1,000,000 from industry. Payments from industry were most associated with orthopedic surgeon, academic practice, male gender, and west or south area of practicing [46]. When comparing payments across all specialties, orthopedic and neurological surgeons were the recipients of the most payments for travel and royalties than any other specialty [47, 48].

Consumers' Checkbook

The Consumers' Checkbook website recently released the option for its users to search and compare rates of surgical volume and surgical outcomes among surgeons. Rates were generated based on data released by CMS. The website compares both surgeon case volumes and complication rates among their colleagues to help patients make the most informed decisions. For spine surgery, patients can look up data for spinal cord exploration and spinal fusion operations. Consumers' Checkbook assesses overall surgeon quality and reports in the form of a star grading system with a scale of 1–5 stars. The website also claims that it provides rates of "complications," but this measure only included prolonged length of stay, readmissions and death, and not specific surgical complications. Linear regression is used to produce a probability rate of an adverse outcome for each surgeon; however the algorithm is not provided by Consumers' Checkbook [49]. Consumers' Checkbook created its algorithms based on methods that are proprietary and not peer reviewed, and they perform minimal or no risk adjustments of patients in the dataset [50].

ProPublica

Similar to Consumers' Checkbook, ProPublica has also released surgical complication rates from data released by CMS [5]. They also compare case volume and complication rates of surgeons among their colleagues to allow patients to make the most informed decisions. ProPublica's database is larger and more robust than Consumers' Checkbook, as surgeons are 2.8 times more likely to be found on ProPublica than on Consumers' Checkbook [50]. For spine surgery, they included both anterior and posterior column lumbar spinal fusion and cervical spinal fusion operations. ProPublica reports on death during hospital stay and 30-day readmission [51]. Similar to Consumers' Checkbook, this website also does not provide information on any specific surgical complications, but they provide information on events that result from complications [50].

The literature indicates that significant problems are found in the method of which ProPublica rates their surgeons. The "health score" coined by ProPublica is actually a modified Elixhauser comorbidity score [51, 52]. They also use a Charlson comorbidity score, which has been suggested by previous work to not be a reliable predictor of complication risk in spine surgery [53]. Like Consumers' Checkbook, ProPublica created these algorithms based on proprietary methods that are not peer reviewed [50]. When looking at the actual data reported, ProPublica reports only a 5% rate of readmission for lumbar fusion, while conservative estimates from literature reviews report rates closer to 20% [50, 54]. This illustrates discrepancies in the data used to compile the ProPublica rates. They also do not incorporate hospital-to-hospital reporting variation in their analysis, which has been found to significantly affect rates of adverse surgery outcomes [55].

Evaluating Consumers' Checkbook and ProPublica

A recent study by Xu et al. suggests that both websites have significant issues in their sources of high-quality input data, definitions of measured complications, definitions of patient preoperative risks, and sample sizes [50]. Both websites use ICD-9 procedural codes in defining patient cohorts, and these codes often combine a number of different procedures that are either high risk, such as reconstructive surgery, or low risk procedures such as lumbar fusion. Therefore, surgeons performing higher-risk procedures would have poorer results on these two websites. ProPublica and Consumers' Checkbook also do not adjust for patient comorbidities or other medical conditions that could predict or confound complications after surgery. These have been shown that they should be adjusted when measuring quality outcomes, especially when measuring spine surgery outcomes [56]. The sample size is small in the datasets used for each of the websites; therefore any deaths and readmissions can have a large effect in surgeon ratings. The authors note these websites cannot adequately predict which surgeons are below or above average, as it would require a larger sample size [50].

These shortcomings may explain the inconsistent representation of both neurosurgeons and orthopedic surgeons from top-ranked institutions on ProPublica and Consumers' Checkbook. Most surgeons from top institutions are not on either website, and many of them are ranked poorly. Only 4 out of 510 surgeons from top institutions had high volume rates with 5 stars on Consumers' Checkbook as well as low complication rates on ProPublica, further evidence that the ability of these websites to recommend surgeons may be poor. Surgeons with higher ratings in Consumers' Checkbook had lower complication rates in ProPublica; however this was a finding that was not statistically significant in the study by Xu et al. The misuse of the data provided by these websites can potentially have adverse effects on both surgeons and patients [50].

Impact on Healthcare: Lessons from New York's Coronary Artery Bypass and Grafting (CABG) Public Data Release of Mortality Rates

With recent effort to improve quality reporting systems in the United States, there is still little in the literature about the effect of reporting of surgical outcomes on the overall healthcare system. One study reports observations made from past publications of cardiac surgery mortality data to the public by the state of New York [6].

In 1989, cardiothoracic surgery began releasing datasets of surgical mortality rates for coronary artery bypass and grafting (CABG). Some negative consequences were reported after this release [6]. Cardiac surgeons began turning down operations for the sickest patients for fear of getting lower ratings [6, 57, 58]. In comparison, very sick candidates receiving repair for aortic dissection, which was an operation not publically reported, continued to receive operations [6, 57]. Some authors report that cardiac surgeons began exaggerating preoperative comorbidities in order to manipulate patient risk assessments to get higher ratings [9]. Reporting surgeon outcomes was shown to reduce the ability for trainees to take an active role in operative cases, as the complications of the trainee would fall under the record of attending surgeons. These changes might impact the ability to successfully train junior surgeons [4, 6, 59, 60].

Monetary effects also resulted from the release of CABG surgical outcome data. Patients from high socioeconomic levels became more likely to be treated by a surgeon with lower mortality rates, and patients from low socioeconomic levels became more likely to be treated by surgeons with a high level of mortality rates [61]. Both surgeons and hospitals that had low rates of mortality were able to charge more for their services [6].

The impact of this reporting program for CABG on overall mortality is not clear. Some researchers claim they did not decline and that there was limited impact of the reporting effort [61]. Other authors noted mortality decreased, but not as a result of public reporting [62]. Other reports focused upon the impact of surgeon risk aversion and the development of new procedures [63]. Overall, recent studies measuring the effectiveness of reporting surgical outcomes publically are largely inconclusive in establishing if reporting of outcomes improves patient care and lowers complications [61, 64].

Consumer Rating Websites

An increasing number of patients are turning to the internet when making healthcare decisions, including the decision to undergo surgery. Consumer rating websites are quickly emerging as one of the most used internet resources. Patients can rate and review physician quality from the patient's perspective of the patient-physician interaction. When looking at spine surgeons, a large study published in 2017 of 208 providers found that 99.52% had at least one rating on Healthgrades, Vitals, RateMDs, WebMD, or Yelp [65]. Advocates for these websites claim they provide invaluable data from the consumers' perspective of the patient-physician interaction [66]. Critics argue that these websites will be utilized by few disgruntled patients and could have detrimental effects on physician reputation [67].

Previous literature indicates that surgeon reviews on these consumer ratings sites have minimal correlation with quality of surgical care. Interestingly, in a large study by Godil et al. of 420 patients undergoing surgery of the lumbar spine, there was no correlation found between patient satisfaction of the clinical experience and actual effectiveness of the surgical spine care [68]. A prospective study of 160,235 patients undergoing spine surgery by Missios and Bekelis found that patient satisfaction was not associated with decreased discharge to rehabilitation, lower hospitalization charges, or less mortality [69]. However, it was found to be associated with decreased length of stay [19].

It is important to note that these websites do not require authentication of raters; therefore manipulation of reviews is possible. Additionally, patients may lack the medical expertise necessary to judge the quality of the healthcare being delivered [70]. Several studies have shown that greater physician work experience seems to lead to lower patient satisfaction. Ratings of orthopedic surgeons on consumer rating websites are significantly increased in surgeons who have had less than 10 years of board certification compared to the more experienced orthopedic surgeons (>10 years of board certification) [65, 71]. As these websites emerge as popular information sources of physicians, more critical attention should be given to these consumer rating websites to improve their ability to deliver accurate information to patients [72].

Healthgrades

Founded in 1998, this website provides ratings of physicians by patients as well as yearly hospital rankings derived from risk-adjusted mortality and in-hospital complications. Patients have the option to rate physicians on a scale from 1.0 to 5.0 and also write a brief review of their experience. This website is one of the most widely used consumer rating sites for healthcare, and a recent study found that as many as 94.7% of medical school clinical faculty members were found to have a profile on Healthgrades [73].

Vitals

Founded in 2007, Vitals provides physician ratings by patients. This website provides the option to rate providers on a scale from 1.0 to 5.0, and it also allows for the option to write a brief review of patient experiences. A recent review of faculty ratings at large institutions found that as many as 87.9% had a profile on the Vitals website [73].

Yelp

Founded in 2004, Yelp is a robust website hosting a wide variety of online consumer reviews of medical professionals, restaurants, retail stores, and other local businesses. Consumers are able to rate their experiences on a scale of 1–5 stars and submit brief reviews of interaction experiences. It has been shown that high ratings on Yelp are associated with lower mortality in hospitals from complications such as MI or pneumonia, and future studies should be conducted comparing Yelp rankings to spine surgery [70]. Ratings on this website are also found to correlate well with HCAHPS patient reviews disseminated by the CMS [70].

RateMDs.com

Founded in 2004, users review doctors on four dimensions of care: helpful, knowledge, staff, and punctual on a scale of 1.0–5.0. It also allows for patients to write brief reviews. In 2010, it was found that one in six physicians had online ratings in RateMDs.com. Interestingly, from 2004 to 2010, there was a 100-fold increase in physician ratings, and 16% of surgeons received a rating during this time [74].

Doximity

Doximity is the largest social networking service for health professionals in the United States. The network includes physicians, nurse practitioners, physician assistants, and pharmacists, and its database was found to include 1,078,305 physicians in 2016 [77]. Doximity is not a significant source for reporting surgical outcomes or patient experiences, but it does report on the quality of residency programs. Doximity began releasing the "Residency Navigator" in September 2014. Since then, studies have shown Doximity to have a significant effect on MATCH residency program rankings by residency applicants. However, the information on this website seems to be based on reputational data rather than accurate reporting of objective outcome criteria [75–77].

Conclusions

As the federal government transitions from a fee-for-service to a value-based incentive program, quality and outcome reporting becomes increasingly important to physicians. The Centers for Medicare and Medicaid Services' Hospital Compare, Physician Compare, and Open Payments websites could potentially become tools for increasing transparency and reporting accurate data directly to patients in an online setting. However, significant improvements to each of these portals are necessary. Private reporting systems have also emerged, such as ProPublica and Consumers' Checkbook, but the accuracy and quality of reported data are questionable. These web resources therefore should be utilized with caution. Recently developed internal quality reporting systems such as the National Surgical Quality Improvement Program (NSQIP) and the National Neurosurgery Quality and Outcomes Database (QOD) are becoming more widely utilized for hospital improvement and research and have significant potential to help lower healthcare costs and increase quality of care.

References

1. Health Care Financing Administration. Medicare hospital mortality information. Washington, DC: Government Printing Office; 1986.
2. Hannan EL, Kilburn H Jr, Racz M, et al. Improving the outcomes of coronary artery bypass surgery in New York State. JAMA. 1994;271(10):761–6.
3. Society of Thoracic Surgeons. STS public reporting online. Chicago; 2015. Available from: http://publicreporting.sts.org. Accessed 2 Jan 2018.
4. Radford PD, Derbyshire LF, Shalhoub J, et al. Publication of surgeon specific outcome data: a review of implementation, controversies and the potential impact on surgical training. Int J Surg. 2015;13:211–6.
5. Allen M, Pierce O. Making the cut: why choosing the right surgeon matters even more than you know. ProPublica; 2015. Available from: https://www.propublica.org/article/surgeryrisks-patient-safety-surgeon-matter
6. Burns EM, Pettengell C, Athanasiou T, et al. Understanding the strengths and weaknesses of public reporting of surgeon specific outcome data. Health Aff. 2016;35:415–21.
7. Parker SL, Asher AL, Godil SS, et al. Patient-reported outcomes 3 months after spine surgery: is it an accurate predictor of 12-month outcome in real-world registry platforms? Neurosurg Focus. 2015;39(6):17.
8. Shaffrey E, Smith JS, Lenke LG, et al. Defining rates and causes of mortality associated with spine surgery: comparison of 2 data collection approaches through the Scoliosis Research Society. Spine. 2014;39(7):579–86.
9. Shahian DM, Normand SL, Torchiana DF, et al. Cardiac surgery report cards: comprehensive review and statistical critique. Ann Thorac Surg. 2001;72:2155–68.

10. Dekutoski MB, Norvell DC, Dettori JR, et al. Surgeon perceptions and reported complications in spine surgery. Spine. 2010;35(9):9–21.
11. Mannion AF, Porchet F, Kleinstück FS, et al. The quality of spine surgery from the patient's perspective. Part 1: the Core Outcome Measures Index in clinical practice. Eur Spine J. 2009;18(3):367–73.
12. Deyo RA, Battie M, Beurskens A, et al. Outcome measures for low back pain research. A proposal for standardized use. Spine. 1998;23(18):2003–13.
13. Auerbach JD, McGowan KB, Halevi M, et al. Mitigating adverse event reporting bias in spine surgery. J Bone Joint Surg Am. 2013;95(16):1450–6.
14. Bream E, Black N. What is the relationship between patients' and clinicians' reports of the outcomes of elective surgery? J Health Serv Res Policy. 2009;14(3):174–82.
15. Varagunam M, Hutchings A, Black N. Relationship between patient-reported outcomes of elective surgery and hospital and consultant volume. Med Care. 2015;53(4):310–6.
16. Vincent C, Moorthy K, Sarker SK, et al. Systems approaches to surgical quality and safety: from concept to measurement. Ann Surg. 2004;239(4):475–82.
17. Koltov MK, Damle NS. Health policy basics: physician quality reporting system. Ann Intern Med. 2014;161(5):365–7.
18. Centers for Medicare & Medicaid Services. Value-based payment modifier. 2016. Available from: https://www.cms.gov/medicare/medicare-fee-for-service-payment/physicianfeedback-program/valuebasedpaymentmodifier.html. Accessed 2 Jan 2018.
19. Bekelis K, McGirt MJ, Parker SL, et al. The present and future of quality measures and public reporting in neurosurgery. Neurosurg Focus. 2015;39(6):3.
20. Dowd B, Li C, Swenson T, et al. Medicare's Physician Quality Reporting System (PQRS): quality measurement and beneficiary attribution. Medicare Medicaid Res Rev. 2014;4(2):1–14.
21. Centers for Medicare & Medicaid Services. 2010 reporting experience including trends (2007–2011). 2012. Available from http://www.mdinteractive.com/files/uploaded/2010%20PQRS%20and%20eRx%20Experience%20Report_03162012.pdf. Accessed 2 Jan 2018.
22. Medicare Access and CHIP Reauthorization Act of 2015, Public Law 114–10.
23. Daley J, Khuri S, Henderson WG, et al. The Department of Veterans Affairs' NSQIP: the first national, validated, outcome- based, risk-adjusted, and peer-controlled program for the measurement and enhancement of the quality of surgical care. Ann Surg. 1998;228(4):491–507.
24. Davis CL, Pierce JR, Henderson W, et al. Assessment of the reliability of data collected for the Department of Veterans Affairs national surgical quality improvement program. J Am Coll Surg. 2007;204(4):550–60.
25. Khuri SF, Henderson WG, Daley J, et al. Successful implementation of the Department of Veterans Affairs' national surgical quality improvement program in the private sector: the patient safety in surgery study. Ann Surg. 2008;248(2):329–36.
26. Lawson EH, Zingmond DS, Stey AM, et al. Measuring risk-adjusted value using Medicare and ACS-NSQIP: is high-quality, low-cost surgical care achievable everywhere? Ann Surg. 2014;260(4):668–77.
27. Neuman HB, Michelassi F, Turner JW, et al. Surrounded by quality metrics: what do surgeons think of ACS-NSQIP? Surgery. 2009;145:27–33.
28. Asher AL, McCormick PC, Selden NR, et al. The national neurosurgery quality and outcomes database and neuropoint alliance: rationale, development, and implementation. Neurosurg Focus. 2013;34:2.
29. McGirt MJ, Speroff T, Dittus RS, et al. The National Neurosurgery Quality and outcomes database (N^2QOD): general overview and pilot-year project description. Neurosurg Focus. 2013;34:6.
30. Asher AL, Speroff T, Dittus RS, et al. The national neurosurgery quality and outcomes database (N^2QOD): a collaborative North American outcomes registry to advance value-based spine care. Spine. 2014;39(22):106–16.
31. NeuroPoint Alliance. Spine Quality Outcomes Database (SQOD) fact sheet. 2017. Available from http://www.neuropoint.org/-/media/Files/NPA/PDF/SQOD-Fact-Sheet-20170623.ashx?la=en&hash=0BB203B6821D75327988BF353D8B92481E2F936F. Accessed 29 Dec 2017.

32. Garrido T, Kumar S, Lekas J, et al. E-measures: insight into the challenges and opportunities of automating publicly reported quality measures. J Am Med Inform Assoc. 2014;21(1):181–4.
33. Center for Medicaid and Medicare Services. HCAHPS: patient's perspectives of care survey. 2017. Available from http://www.cms.gov/Medicare/Quality-Initiatives-Patient-Assessment-Instruments/HospitalQualityInits/HospitalHCAHPS.html. Accessed 27 Dec 2017.
34. Centers for Medicare & Medicaid Services. What is hospital compare? 2014. Available from http://www.medicare.gov/hospitalcompare/About/What-Is-HOS.html. Accessed 27 Dec 2017.
35. 78 FR 50700 (Aug. 19, 2013).
36. 78 FR 51023 (Aug. 19, 2013).
37. Hospital Consumer Assessment of Healthcare Providers and Systems. Mode and patient-mix adjustment page. 2017. Available from http://www.hcahpsonline.org/en/mode%2D%2Dpatient-mix-adj/. Accessed 27 Dec 2017.
38. Jordan H, White A, Joseph C, et al. Costs and benefits of HCAHPS: final report. Cambridge, MA: Abt Associates Inc;2005. Available from: https://www.cms.gov/Medicare/Quality-Initiatives-Patient-Assessment-Instruments/HospitalQualityInits/downloads/HCAHPSCostsBenefits200512.pdf
39. Centers for Medicare & Medicaid Services. Summary of HCAHPS survey results. 2014. Available from: http://www.hcahpsonline.org/globalassets/hcahps/summary-analyses/summary-results/july-2014-public-report-october-2012%2D%2D-september-2013-discharges.pdf
40. Centers for Medicare & Medicaid Services. HCAHPS public reporting. Baltimore. Available from: http://www.hcahpsonline.org/files/HCAHPS%20Public%20Reporting_April2015_Dec2016.pdf
41. Schlesinger M, Grob R, Shaller D, et al. Taking patients' narratives about clinicians from anecdote to science. N Engl J Med. 2015;373(7):675–9.
42. Austin JM, Jha AK, Romano PS, et al. National hospital ratings systems share few common scores and may generate confusion instead of clarity. Health Aff. 2015;34:423–30.
43. Chimonas S, Rozario NM, Rothman DJ. Show us the money: lessons in transparency from state pharmaceutical marketing disclosure laws. Health Serv Res. 2010;45(1):98–114.
44. Babu MA, Heary RF, Nahed BV, et al. Does the open payments database provide sunshine on neurosurgery? Neurosurgery. 2016;79(6):933–8.
45. Hannon CP, Chalmers PN, Carpiniello MF, et al. Inconsistencies between physician-reported disclosures at the AAOS annual meeting and industry-reported financial disclosures in the open payments database. J Bone Joint Surg Am. 2016;98(20):90.
46. Weiner JA, Cook RQ, Hashmi S, et al. Factors associated with financial relationships between spine surgeons and industry: an analysis of the open payments database. Spine. 2017;42(18):1412–8.
47. Iyer S, Derman P, Sandhu HS. Orthopaedics and the physician payments sunshine act: an examination of payments to U.S. orthopaedic surgeons in the open payments database. J Bone Joint Surg Am. 2016;98(5):18.
48. Marshall DC, Jackson ME, Hattangadi-Gluth JA, et al. Disclosure of industry payments to physicians: an epidemiologic analysis of early data from the open payments program. Mayo Clin Proc. 2016;91(1):84–96.
49. Consumers' Checkbook. Consumers' checkbook: more about our measures of outcomes. 2015. Washington, DC. Available from: http://www.checkbook.org/surgeonratings/?action=article&articleID=more-about-our-measures-of-outcomes
50. Xu LW, Li A, Swinney C, et al. An assessment of data and methodology of online surgeon scorecards. J Neurosurg Spine. 2017;26(2):235–42.
51. Pierce O, Allen M: How we measured surgical complications. ProPublica. 2015. Available from https://www.propublica.org/article/surgeon-level-risk-short-methodology. Accessed 2 Jan 2018.
52. Van Walraven C, Austin PC, Jennings A, et al. A modification of the Elixhauser comorbidity measures into a point system for hospital death using administrative data. Med Care. 2009;47:626–33.

53. Whitmore RG, Stephen JH, Vernick C, et al. ASA grade and Charlson Comorbidity Index of spinal surgery patients: correlation with complications and societal costs. Spine J. 2014;14:31–8.
54. Veeravagu A, Cole TS, Azad TD, et al. Improved capture of adverse events after spinal surgery procedures with a longitudinal administrative database. J Neurosurg Spine. 2015;23:374–82.
55. Friedberg MW, Pronovost PJ, Shahian DM, et al. A methodological critique of the ProPublica surgeon scorecard. Santa Monica: RAND Corporation; 2015.
56. Schoenfeld AJ, Ochoa LM, Bader JO, et al. Risk factors for immediate postoperative complications and mortality following spine surgery: a study of 3475 patients from the National Surgical Quality Improvement Program. J Bone Joint Surg Am. 2011;93:1577–82.
57. Burack JH, Impellizzeri P, Homel P, et al. Public reporting of surgical mortality: a survey of New York State cardiothoracic surgeons. Ann Thorac Surg. 1999;68(4):1195–200.
58. Epstein AJ. Effects of report cards on referral patterns to cardiac surgeons. J Health Econ. 2010;29(5):718–31.
59. Khan OA, Iyengar S, Pontefract DE, et al. Impact of surgeon specific data reporting on surgical training. Ann R Coll Surg Engl. 2007;89:796–8.
60. Sheldon GF, Ricketts TC, Charles A, et al. The global health workforce shortage: role of surgeons and other providers. Adv Surg. 2008;42:63–85.
61. Fung CH, Lim YW, Mattke S, et al. Systemic review: the evidence that publishing patient care performance improves quality of care. Ann Intern Med. 2008;148:111–23.
62. Ghali WA, Ash AS, Hall RE, et al. Statewide quality improvement initiatives and mortality after cardiac surgery. JAMA. 1997;277(5):379–82.
63. Jarral OA, Kidher E, Patel VM, et al. Quality of life after intervention on the thoracic aorta. Eur J Cardiothorac Surg. 2016;49(2):369–89.
64. Hibbard JH, Stockard J, Tusler M. Hospital performance reports: impact on quality, market share, and reputation. Health Aff. 2005;24(4):1150–60.
65. Zhang J, Omar A, Mesfin A. On-line ratings of spine surgeons: analysis of 208 surgeons. Spine. 2017; https://doi.org/10.1097/BRS.0000000000002488. [Epub ahead of print].
66. Lagu T, Lindenauer PK. Putting the public back in public reporting of health care quality. JAMA. 2010;304(15):1711–2.
67. McCartney M. Will doctor rating sites improve the quality of care? No. BMJ. 2009;338:1033.
68. Godil SS, Parker SL, Zuckerman SL, et al. Determining the quality and effectiveness of surgical spine care: patient satisfaction is not a valid proxy. Spine J. 2013;13(9):1006–12.
69. Missios S, Bekelis K. How well do subjective hospital compare metrics reflect objective outcomes in spine surgery? J Neurosurg Spine. 2016;25(2):264–70.
70. Bardach NS, Asteria-Penaloza R, Boscardin WJ, et al. The relationship between commercial website ratings and traditional hospital performance measures in the USA. BMJ Qual Saf. 2013;22(3):194–202.
71. Jack RA, Burn MB, McCulloch PC, et al. Does experience matter? A meta-analysis of physician rating websites of orthopaedic surgeons. Musculoskelet Surg. 2017; https://doi.org/10.1007/s12306-017-0500-1. [Epub ahead of print].
72. Emmert M, Sander U, Pisch F. Eight questions about physician-rating websites: a systematic review. J Med Internet Res. 2013;15(2):24.
73. Sobin L, Goyal P. Trends of online ratings of otolaryngologists: what do your patients really think of you? JAMA Otolaryngol Head Neck Surg. 2014;140(7):635–8.
74. Gao GG, McCullough JS, Agarwal R, et al. A changing landscape of physician quality reporting: analysis of patients' online ratings of their physicians over a 5-year period. J Med Internet Res. 2012;14(1):38.
75. Rolston AM, Hartley SE, Khandelwal S, et al. Effect of Doximity residency rankings on residency applicants' program choices. West J Emerg Med. 2015;16(6):889–93.
76. Peterson WJ, Hopson LR, Khandelwal S. Impact of Doximity residency rankings on emergency medicine applicant rank lists. West J Emerg Med. 2016;17(3):350–4.
77. Ashack KA, Burton KA, Dellavalle RP. Dermatology in doximity. Dermatol Online J. 2016;22(2).

Achieving Success in Quality Reporting

24

Brian L. Anderson, Pratik Rohatgi, and Robert E. Harbaugh

Introduction

The ability to gauge the success of any process requires a clear understanding of the goals and outcomes expected and achieved. All the previous chapters have provided the historical framework behind the foundation and implementation efforts to organize quality measures in spine care. As unsustainable cost has driven the healthcare industry to prioritize the value of care, the ability to assess meaningful outcomes data has become essential. To determine the value of the healthcare delivered, one must know the resources utilized and the benefits provided [1]. Hospitals can easily determine the cost of a patient encounter, but assessing the impact of care is far more difficult due to numerous influences unique to each clinical situation. As the medical community and regulatory agencies embrace a quality-driven system and payers require documentation of value, implementing a quality assessment and improvement system has become essential for the success of any practice.

The burden is placed on providers and increasingly enforced through reimbursement strategies. The benefits of value-directed care are significant but cannot be realized with providers functioning in isolation. We cannot determine value when we lack the objective data needed to optimize care.

A system-wide approach, directed by physicians who understand the complexities of their own field, is needed. Organized neurosurgery has made efforts to establish such a program. The NeuroKnowledge program was established to address the question of value in the field of neurosurgery. The evolution of this program and other value-directed efforts over the past decade have made significant strides in establishing a system capable of furthering understanding and improving the quality of patient care.

B. L. Anderson · P. Rohatgi · R. E. Harbaugh (✉)
Department of Neurosurgery, Penn State University, Milton S. Hershey Medical Center, Hershey, PA, USA
e-mail: reh21@psu.edu

J. Ratliff et al. (eds.), *Quality Spine Care*,
https://doi.org/10.1007/978-3-319-97990-8_24

In 2001, the Department of Health and Human Services (HHS) and the Centers for Medicare and Medicaid Services (CMS) instituted quality initiatives (QI) in an effort to improve patient safety and increase performance transparency for healthcare organizations. The metrics and assessment strategies employed in these initiatives created confusion and frustration and failed to foster participation [2]. The ability to evaluate quality outcomes data in the context of multiple covariates (i.e., risk stratification) was not possible with the existing database infrastructure [3, 4]. This resulted in efforts to assess quality focusing on the processes used to provide care, rather than the outcomes of care. Concerns were voiced over the ability of these initiatives to actually determine the quality of care, as opposed to merely tracking process measures. Causal relationships between processes of care and patient outcomes are often assumed without objective confirmation. While the belief that adhering to a process actually improves outcome may be widespread and process measures easy to capture, this correlation in many clinical settings remains unproven. As reimbursement strategies shift to quality-driven models, the ability to obtain accurate outcomes data has become essential.

Organized neurosurgery, initially through the efforts of the NeuroKnowledge program (which has now evolved into a separate corporation, the NeuroPoint Alliance) and the Quality Improvement Workgroup (presently known as the Neurosurgery Quality Council), has worked diligently over the last 20 years to develop the infrastructure and expertise needed for quality assessment in neurosurgery through registries with patient-reported outcomes. We realized that if we were to be held accountable for the quality of the care we deliver, we needed to ensure the reliability of our assessment methods by meticulous planning before launching our outcomes initiative. Some of the critical aspects of this planning follow.

NeuroPoint Alliance

In an effort to participate in the national focus on registry-driven patient care improvements, the American Association of Neurological Surgeons (AANS) became an organizational member of the Physician Clinical Registry Coalition (PCRC) [5]. The PCRC represents over 20 society and physical-led registry projects. They play a key role as sponsors and advocates for public policy that encourages registry growth. In an effort to obtain neurosurgery-specific data, the AANS formed the NeuroPoint Alliance (NPA) in 2008 to collect, analyze, and report on clinical data from neurosurgical practices nationwide [6]. One program of the NPA, originally created as the National Neurosurgery Quality and Outcomes Database (N^2QOD), now known as the Quality Outcomes Database (QOD) is a multifaceted tool that allows practices to participate in quality initiatives, satisfy Centers for Medicare and Medicaid Services (CMS) reporting requirements, and facilitate case collection for board certification and maintenance of certification. Subspecialty registries exist for spine surgery, and neurovascular surgery. A tumor surgery registry is set to launch in 2018 [7].

In a review of 25 spine registries performed by van Hooff et al. in 2015, the QOD-Spine registry was one of only three that included patient reportable outcomes measures (PROMs) [8]. In 2017, Karhade et al. reviewed the 18 national databases commonly used for neurosurgical outcomes research and found that only the QOD outcomes measures specifically related to neurosurgical care [9]. One key feature of the QOD-Spine is the ability to provide longitudinal outcomes data to provide a more complete evaluation of treatment options for patient with spine pathology.

Another key focus of the QOD efforts was addressing the regulatory factors put into place by governmental agencies. The reporting requirements established by the Centers for Medicare and Medicaid Services (CMS) highlight how a well-designed registry system can help mitigate increasing administrative demands on clinical practices. The CMS Physician Quality Reporting System (PQRS) was founded on several pieces of congressional legislation in the 2000s to reduce healthcare costs through quality improvement incentive programs [10, 11]. In 2014, the CMS Qualified Clinical Data Registry (QCDR) reporting option was created to allow medical specialty groups to develop registries that contain clinically relevant healthcare quality metrics that meet PQRS requirements [12]. To satisfy the PQRS requirements, the sponsoring organization must submit the proposed QCDR for review and must capture nine measures across two National Quality Strategy domains and two outcomes measures.

To remain in compliance, in November of 2014, the NPA brought together a multidisciplinary team of healthcare policy experts, clinicians, qualified scientists, medical administrators, and epidemiologists to survey how existing PQRS-approved measures captured care metrics related to neurosurgical care [12]. The working group proposed to collect 21 metrics unique from existing PQRS measures through the QOD, which was accepted as a QCDR in the spring of 2015. Thus, neurosurgery practices now could use a single tailored tool for both quality improvement projects and CMS reporting. Practices using the QOD could elect to authorize NPA to submit their data to CMS as a QCDR to satisfy PQRS requirements. The QOD was statistically designed for sampled data entry from the first six patients cared for by a submitting provider on rotating 6-day cycle. As such, electing to submit data to CMS may require a provider to collect and record more clinical data from patients to meet the CMS requirement of data capture from 50% of eligible serviced patients.

In 2015, the Medicare Access and CHIP Reauthorization Act (MACRA) further changed reporting requirements for providers participating in Medicare programs. The passage of MACRA suspended the sustainable growth rate (SGR) formula used to determine Medicare Part B reimbursement rates [11, 13]. The SGR was established by President Clinton through the Balanced Budget Act of 1997. In practice, the SGR routinely threatened substantial cuts in Medicare reimbursement each year and placed considerable and costly administrative burdens on providers. To replace cost-control pressures of SGR, CMS created the Merit-Based Incentive Payment System (MIPS) and the Alternative Payment Models (APM). Participating providers must comply with one of the two options which vary to address differences in practice type. The more common MIPS program is tailored for traditional care delivery systems while APM is generally used for innovative model strategies.

MIPS replaces existing incentive programs such as PQRS with a reimbursement adjustment based on a provider composite performance score (CPS). The CPS is a weighted score based on activity on four measured domains: quality improvement, resource use, clinical practice improvement activities, and advancing care information. For those participating in MIPS, reporting metric on these domains will become mandatory starting in 2019. The NPA QOD can fulfill all the reporting requirements of MIPS, thus greatly simplifying practice overhead and providing motivation for participation [6].

Registry Structure

The scope of the registry had to be clearly defined. If the validation of specific treatment strategies was needed, a more rigorous process was required than if a simple assessment of practice patterns was desired. Careful attention to the quality and measurability of desired data was essential. Large amounts of meaningless data would be of no value. Similarly, the patient population had to be appropriately focused, and patients enrolled needed to provide an appropriate representation of the target population. The registry structure had to address the integrity of the reported data including who, what, and for how long included patient data were to be collected and analyzed. This integrity was assured through careful consideration of how data would be obtained and reported. Regular evaluation for system error was also addressed.

Data Management

The strength of any registry-based system lies within the data itself. The system must be integrated and able to obtain, evaluate, archive, review, and monitor the data while maintaining the registries predetermined scope. As data integrity is at the core of any scientific process, particular attention was given to how this would occur for our registry efforts. The first step was to consider the source of data. Data can be primary (obtained initially for the registry) or secondary (obtained initially for another purpose but incorporated into the registry). Use of secondary data sources may reduce cost and improve enrollment but the integrity of the data would always be questioned. For this reason, we decided that a prospective registry needed to be developed and that regular evaluations of the registry scope and data integrity would be needed.

It was tempting to include as many possible data points as possible, but some data elements may be more harmful than helpful. Data elements with poor integrity will weaken the integrity of the registry. Several factors had to be considered, including how each data element correlated with the outcomes in question, the burden of obtaining the particular element, and how reliable the data element really was. Each data element should be determined from the outset and quality assurance efforts able to affirm the integrity of the process. A risk-based approach is required to evaluate the cost limitations of each aspect of quality assurance with a focus on the intended registry goals.

Recruitment and Retention

The ideally structured registry would have no value if providers and patients could not be recruited to participate. Several motivating factors were used to encourage participation. A committed group of surgeons who were driven to provide the best care possible were recruited to launch our initiative. This group was convinced that participation in the registry would help provide evidence of the present value of our care and help to make it even better. It was clear from the start that only the participation of committed surgeons would assure the success of the registry and every effort was made to make participation valuable to the practices. The key factors affecting active participation and retention in any registry include minimizing the data management burden, confidence in the registry's validity, and relevance of the registry to the practices involved. Considerable attention was paid to each of these factors as our registries were developed. We knew that the product produced must provide sufficient value for the cost and time required by the participants.

Analysis

The data produced by any registry is a direct result of the integrity of the process used initially to produce it. The rigorous standards discussed were followed, paying careful attention to several key questions: Who is the population? How was the data collected and verified? How were inconsistencies handled? What analysis was performed? The registry provided consideration of covariates, patient characteristics, outcomes, and patient exposures. Each of the relevant data elements were established in the study design.

Registry in Action

The stereotactic radiosurgery registry was created as a joint effort between the AANS and American Society for Radiation Oncology (ASTRO) [14]. Stereotactic radiosurgery treatment requires collaboration between different medical specialties and thus was ideally positioned to benefit from this partnership. Most clinical studies in stereotactic radiosurgery are published as single-center retrospective studies due to challenges in effective patient accrual in randomized multicenter clinical trials. In this regard, registry-based research possesses an inherent advantage over a randomized control trial. ASTRO determined that the National Radiation Oncology Registry did not sufficiently address stereotactic radiosurgery. To address this concern, the Stereotactic Radiosurgery (SRS) registry was created with the aims of defining patterns of care, identifying gaps in coverage, and creating benchmark data for quality improvement, providing evidence to support clinical decision-making, improving clinical outcomes and costs, and tracking longitudinal data for outcome-related research. The SRS registry board created a common data dictionary of 135 metrics to improve comparisons across treatment centers. The registry takes advantage of the computer sophistication of SRS to automate many of these perimeters, leaving 25 parameters to be entered manually. Unlike the subscription model adopted by the QOD, the SRS registry is funded through corporate educational grants to the AANS.

A true measure of a successful registry is the ability to provide useful clinical insights related to the intervention provided. The QOD-Spine registry has now accrued enough patient information for such analysis with an increasing rate of publication to address such questions (see Table 24.1). As a recent example, Chan et al. reviewed the QOD-Spine database for patients who underwent surgery for grade 1 degenerative lumbar spondylolisthesis from July 2014 to December 2015 [33]. Of 477 patients in the registry who met this criterion, 255 patients identified as most satisfied while 25 identified as least satisfied 12 months after surgery, based on the NASS satisfaction questionnaire measures. There were no differences in baseline PROMs, but the most satisfied patients had lower pain and disability PROMs 12 months after surgery. Patients who identified as most satisfied had lower mean body mass index (BMI) and lower rates of coronary artery disease. Contrasting prior studies, women were found to be more likely satisfied with the outcome of surgery than men as an independent variable based on multivariate analysis, though the effect was small. These studies may drive more refined indications and selection of surgical treatments for spine patients.

Another recently reported project using the NeuroPoint Alliance's Quality Outcomes Database (QOD) data highlights the strengths of a mature registry. This paper takes into account the role that patient-reported outcomes play in determining the effectiveness of intervention but also notes the difficulty of interpreting the various grading scales used for reporting. A certain numerical increase on one scale does not correlate with a similar change on another or even with a different part of the same scale. The value derived from these various reported scales comes from the clinical relevance that coincides with the change. The authors recognized that a change which results in a clinically significant difference for the patient should be set as the threshold for meaningful change. Traditional efforts used to determine the minimal clinically important difference (MCID) require significant cost and resource utilization with review of patient history, assessment, intervention, and follow-up. Patient characteristics and comorbidities must be considered, and the study population must be powered to show a meaningful result. When considering spinal surgery, this must be done for each pathology encountered and perhaps even separated by disease severity within the same condition. They are often single-center trials or require the retrospective review of incongruent data collected across various sources.

Using the QOD data, the authors were able to collect 12-month outcomes data for a selected patient population diagnosed with spondylolisthesis and confirmed by review of preoperative imaging. They chose to frame the scope of the study to evaluate degenerative Meyerding grade I spondylolisthesis patients who underwent a posterior surgical approach. The reported primary outcomes included the Oswestry

Table 24.1 Key publications 2015–2018

Title	Journal
Lumbar Surgery in the Elderly Provides Significant Health Benefit in the US Health Care System: Patient-Reported Outcomes in 4370 Patients From the N2QOD Registry [15]	*Neurosurgery*
Inception of a national multidisciplinary registry for stereotactic radiosurgery [14]	*Journal of Neurosurgery*
Predictive value of 3-month lumbar discectomy outcomes in the NeuroPoint-SD Registry [16]	*Journal of Neurosurgery: Spine*
Using Clinical Registries to Improve the Quality of Neurosurgical Care [17]	*Neurosurgery Clinics of North America*
Benefit of Transforaminal Lumbar Interbody Fusion vs Posterolateral Spinal Fusion in Lumbar Spine Disorders: a Propensity-Matched Analysis From the national neurosurgical quality and Outcomes Database Registry [18]	*Neurosurgery*
Defining, measuring, and predicting quality in neurosurgery. Can big data bridge the chasm? Issues, opportunities, and strategies for the evolving value-based healthcare environment [19]	*Neurosurgical Focus*
The present and future of quality measures and public reporting in neurosurgery [20]	*Neurosurgical Focus*
The National Neurosurgery Quality & Outcomes Database Qualified Clinical Data Registry: 2015 measure specifications and rationale [12]	*Neurosurgical Focus*
Neurosurgery value and quality in the context of the affordable care act: a policy perspective [21]	*Neurosurgical Focus*
Effect of complications within 90-days on the patient-reported outcomes 3-months and 12-months following elective surgery for lumbar degenerative disease [22]	*Neurosurgical Focus*
Quality analysis of anterior cervical discectomy and fusion in the outpatient vs. inpatient setting: analysis of 7288 patients from NSQIP database [23]	*Neurosurgical Focus*
Patient-Reported Outcomes 3-Months after Spine Surgery: is it an Accurate Predictor of 12-Month Outcome in Real World Registry Platforms [24]	*Neurosurgical Focus*
Prediction model for outcome after low-back surgery: individualized likelihood of complication, hospital re-admission, return to work, and 12-month improvement in functional disability [25]	*Neurosurgical Focus*
Anterior cervical discectomy and fusion in the outpatient ambulatory surgery setting: analysis of 1000 consecutive cases and comparison to hospital inpatient ACDF [26]	*Journal of Neurosurgery: Spine*
Modeled cost-effectiveness of transforaminal lumbar interbody fusion compared with posterolateral fusion for spondylolisthesis using N(2) QOD data [27]	*Journal of Neurosurgery: Spine*
Inadequacy of 3-month Oswestry Disability Index outcome for assessing individual longer-term patient experience after lumbar spine surgery [28]	*Journal of Neurosurgery: Spine*
Predictors of extended length of stay, discharge to inpatient rehab, and hospital readmission following elective lumbar spine surgery: introduction of the Carolina-Semmes Grading Scale [29]	*Journal of Neurosurgery: Spine*

(continued)

Table 24.1 (continued)

Title	Journal
An analysis from the Quality Outcomes Database, Part 1. Disability, quality of life, and pain outcomes following lumbar spine surgery: predicting likely individual patient outcomes for shared decision-making [30]	*Journal of Neurosurgery: Spine*
An analysis from the Quality Outcomes Database, Part 2. Predictive model for return to work after elective surgery for lumbar degenerative disease [31]	*Journal of Neurosurgery: Spine*
Defining the minimum clinically important difference for grade I degenerative lumbar spondylolisthesis: insights from the Quality Outcomes Database [32]	*Neurosurgical Focus*
Women fare best following surgery for degenerative lumbar spondylolisthesis: a comparison of the most and least satisfied patients utilizing data from the Quality Outcomes Database [33]	*Neurosurgical Focus*

Disability Index (ODI), EQ-5D (EuroQoL Group), and numeric rating scale for back and leg pain (NRS-BP, NRS-LP). The authors were able to review 441 patients from 11 institutions. The QOD provided patient demographics, intervention, and all the follow-up data used in the assessment. They were able to perform relevant statistical analysis to determine the MCID for the study population. Additional subgroup analysis was completed to compare those undergoing arthrodesis with those undergoing decompression alone [32]. Utilizing the QOD database, the authors were able to evaluate a group across multiple organizations with a study size ten times larger than the most comparable previously reported group. A similarly structured randomized control trial to address this question would simply be cost and time prohibitive.

Conclusion

The continued transition to outcome-focused care will undoubtedly require the US healthcare system to make significant changes over the next decade. Both ethical and legal considerations are required to address concerns regarding the escalating cost of healthcare delivery as well as the impact interventions are having on the care of the patient. Public skepticism has increased over recent years with reports highlighting medical errors and questioning physician motivations [34–36]. If the past is any indicator, we are likely to see continued changes to the regulations and practices that shape healthcare delivery in the USA. The ability to adapt and address currently unknown concerns represents one of the greatest strengths of a well-established and appropriately maintained patient registry. The rate at which clinical understanding can be improved is accelerated compared to traditional research strategies. Accurate and transparent data collection and assessment across varying practice patterns can provide collaborative insight to more appropriately manage patients.

References

1. McCauley JL. Guidelines and value-based decision making: an evolving role for payers. N C Med J [Internet]. 2015 [cited 2015 Dec 19];76:243–6. Available from: http://www.ncbi.nlm.nih.gov/pubmed/26509518.
2. Keswani A, Uhler LM, Bozic KJ. What quality metrics is my hospital being evaluated on and what are the consequences? J Arthroplasty [Internet]. 2016 [cited 2016 May 6]; Available from: http://www.ncbi.nlm.nih.gov/pubmed/27101770.
3. Mitchell PH, Lang NM. Framing the problem of measuring and improving healthcare quality. Med Care [Internet]. 2004 [cited 2018 Jan 3];42:II-4-II-11. Available from: http://content.wkhealth.com/linkback/openurl?sid=WKPTLP:landingpage&an=00005650-200402001-00002.
4. Dimick JB, Welch HG, Birkmeyer JD. Surgical mortality as an indicator of hospital quality. JAMA [Internet]. American Medical Association; 2004 [cited 2018 Jan 3];292:847. Available from: http://jama.jamanetwork.com/article.aspx?doi=10.1001/jama.292.7.847.
5. Physician Clinical Registry Coalition. About – Physician clinical registry coalition [Internet]. [cited 2018 Jan 14]. Available from: http://www.registrycoalition.net/about/.
6. Neuropoint Alliance. Spine Quality Outcomes Database (SQOD) [Internet]. [cited 2018 Jan 14]. Available from: http://www.neuropoint.org/en/NPA-SQOD/.
7. AANS. NeuroPoint alliance expands quality outcomes database [Internet]. AANS E-News. 2017 [cited 2018 Jan 14]. Available from: http://www.aans.org/AANS-E-News/November-2017/NeuroPoint-Alliance-Expands-Quality-Outcomes-Database.
8. Hooff ML van, Jacobs WCH, Willems PC, Wouters MWJM, Kleuver M de, Peul WC, et al. Evidence and practice in spine registries. Acta Orthop [Internet]. 2015 [cited 2018 Jan 14];86:534–44. Available from: http://www.ncbi.nlm.nih.gov/pubmed/25909475.
9. Karhade AV, Larsen AMG, Cote DJ, Dubois HM, Smith TR. National databases for neurosurgical outcomes research: options, strengths, and limitations. Neurosurgery [Internet]. 2017 [cited 2018 Jan 14]. Available from: http://www.ncbi.nlm.nih.gov/pubmed/28950367.
10. CMS. The Physician Quality Reporting System [Internet]. CMS.gov. 2017 [cited 2018 Jan 14]. Available from: https://www.cms.gov/Medicare/Quality-Initiatives-Patient-Assessment-Instruments/PQRS/index.html?redirect=/pqri.
11. Swartz KR, Cheng JS. Anticipated changes in spine practice with advancing center for medicare and medicaid services-required changes. Neurosurgery [Internet]. 2017 [cited 2018 Jan 14];80:S28–33. Available from: https://academic.oup.com/neurosurgery/article-lookup/doi/10.1093/neuros/nyw149.
12. Parker SL, McGirt MJ, Bekelis K, Holland CM, Davies J, Devin CJ, et al. The national neurosurgery quality and outcomes database qualified clinical data registry: 2015 measure specifications and rationale. Neurosurg Focus [Internet]. American Association of Neurological Surgeons; 2015 [cited 2017 Dec 28];39:E4. Available from: http://thejns.org/doi/10.3171/2015.9.FOCUS15355.
13. CMS. The quality payment program [Internet]. [cited 2018 Jan 14]. Available from: https://qpp.cms.gov/.
14. Sheehan JP, Kavanagh BD, Asher A, Harbaugh RE. Inception of a national multidisciplinary registry for stereotactic radiosurgery. J Neurosurg [Internet]. 2016 [cited 2018 Jan 14];124:155–62. Available from: http://thejns.org/doi/10.3171/2015.1.JNS142466.
15. McGirt MJ, Parker SL, Hilibrand A, Mummaneni P, Glassman SD, Devin CJ, et al. Lumbar surgery in the elderly provides significant health benefit in the US health care system: patient-reported outcomes in 4370 patients from the N2QOD registry. Neurosurgery [Internet]. 2015 [cited 2018 Jan 14];77 Suppl 4:S125–35. Available from: https://academic.oup.com/neurosurgery/article-lookup/doi/10.1227/NEU.0000000000000952.
16. Whitmore RG, Curran JN, Ali ZS, Mummaneni P V, Shaffrey CI, Heary RF, et al. Predictive value of 3-month lumbar discectomy outcomes in the NeuroPoint-SD registry. J Neurosurg. Spine [Internet]. 2015 [cited 2018 Jan 14];23:459–66. Available from: http://thejns.org/doi/10.3171/2015.1.SPINE14890.

17. Asher AL, Parker SL, Rolston JD, Selden NR, McGirt MJ. Using clinical registries to improve the quality of neurosurgical care. Neurosurg Clin N Am [Internet]. 2015 [cited 2018 Jan 14];26:253–63. Available from: http://linkinghub.elsevier.com/retrieve/pii/S1042368014001454.
18. Glassman SD, Carreon LY, Ghogawala Z, Foley KT, McGirt MJ, Asher AL. Benefit of transforaminal lumbar interbody fusion vs posterolateral spinal fusion in lumbar spine disorders. Neurosurgery [Internet]. 2016 [cited 2018 Jan 14];79:397–405. Available from: https://academic.oup.com/neurosurgery/article-lookup/doi/10.1227/NEU.0000000000001118.
19. Asher AL, McGirt MJ, Ghogawala Z. Introduction: defining, measuring, and predicting quality in neurosurgery. Neurosurg Focus [Internet]. 2015 [cited 2018 Jan 14];39:E1. Available from: http://thejns.org/doi/10.3171/2015.9.FOCUS15502.
20. Bekelis K, McGirt MJ, Parker SL, Holland CM, Davies J, Devin CJ, et al. The present and future of quality measures and public reporting in neurosurgery. Neurosurg Focus [Internet]. 2015 [cited 2018 Jan 14];39:E3. Available from: http://thejns.org/doi/10.3171/2015.8.FOCUS15354.
21. Menger RP, Guthikonda B, Storey CM, Nanda A, McGirt M, Asher A. Neurosurgery value and quality in the context of the Affordable Care Act: a policy perspective. Neurosurg Focus [Internet]. 2015 [cited 2018 Jan 14];39:E5. Available from: http://thejns.org/doi/10.3171/2015.9.FOCUS15376.
22. Chotai S, Parker SL, Sivaganesan A, Sielatycki JA, Asher AL, McGirt MJ, et al. Effect of complications within 90 days on patient-reported outcomes 3 months and 12 months following elective surgery for lumbar degenerative disease. Neurosurg Focus [Internet]. 2015 [cited 2018 Jan 14];39:E8. Available from: http://thejns.org/doi/10.3171/2015.8.FOCUS15302.
23. McGirt MJ, Godil SS, Asher AL, Parker SL, Devin CJ. Quality analysis of anterior cervical discectomy and fusion in the outpatient versus inpatient setting: analysis of 7288 patients from the NSQIP database. Neurosurg Focus [Internet]. 2015 [cited 2018 Jan 14];39:E9. Available from: http://www.ncbi.nlm.nih.gov/pubmed/26621423.
24. Parker SL, Asher AL, Godil SS, Devin CJ, McGirt MJ. Patient-reported outcomes 3 months after spine surgery: is it an accurate predictor of 12-month outcome in real-world registry platforms? Neurosurg Focus [Internet]. 2015 [cited 2016 May 12];39:E17. Available from: http://www.ncbi.nlm.nih.gov/pubmed/26621415.
25. McGirt MJ, Sivaganesan A, Asher AL, Devin CJ. Prediction model for outcome after low-back surgery: individualized likelihood of complication, hospital readmission, return to work, and 12-month improvement in functional disability. Neurosurg Focus [Internet]. 2015 [cited 2018 Jan 15];39:E13. Available from: http://thejns.org/doi/10.3171/2015.8.FOCUS15338.
26. Adamson T, Godil SS, Mehrlich M, Mendenhall S, Asher AL, McGirt MJ. Anterior cervical discectomy and fusion in the outpatient ambulatory surgery setting compared with the inpatient hospital setting: analysis of 1000 consecutive cases. J Neurosurg Spine [Internet]. 2016 [cited 2018 Jan 14];24:878–84. Available from: http://www.ncbi.nlm.nih.gov/pubmed/26849708.
27. Carreon LY, Glassman SD, Ghogawala Z, Mummaneni P V, McGirt MJ, Asher AL. Modeled cost-effectiveness of transforaminal lumbar interbody fusion compared with posterolateral fusion for spondylolisthesis using N(2)QOD data. J Neurosurg Spine [Internet]. 2016 [cited 2018 Jan 14];24:916–21. Available from: http://thejns.org/doi/10.3171/2015.10.SPINE15917.
28. Asher AL, Chotai S, Devin CJ, Speroff T, Harrell FE, Nian H, et al. Inadequacy of 3-month Oswestry Disability Index outcome for assessing individual longer-term patient experience after lumbar spine surgery. J Neurosurg Spine [Internet]. 2016 [cited 2018 Jan 14];25:170–80. Available from: http://www.ncbi.nlm.nih.gov/pubmed/26989974.
29. McGirt MJ, Parker SL, Chotai S, Pfortmiller D, Sorenson JM, Foley K, et al. Predictors of extended length of stay, discharge to inpatient rehab, and hospital readmission following elective lumbar spine surgery: introduction of the Carolina-Semmes Grading Scale. J Neurosurg Spine [Internet]. 2017 [cited 2018 Jan 14];27:382–90. Available from: http://www.ncbi.nlm.nih.gov/pubmed/28498068.
30. McGirt MJ, Bydon M, Archer KR, Devin CJ, Chotai S, Parker SL, et al. An analysis from the Quality Outcomes Database, Part 1. Disability, quality of life, and pain outcomes follow-

ing lumbar spine surgery: predicting likely individual patient outcomes for shared decision-making. J Neurosurg Spine [Internet]. 2017 [cited 2018 Jan 14];27:357–69. Available from: http://www.ncbi.nlm.nih.gov/pubmed/28498074.
31. Asher AL, Devin CJ, Archer KR, Chotai S, Parker SL, Bydon M, et al. An analysis from the Quality Outcomes Database, Part 2. Predictive model for return to work after elective surgery for lumbar degenerative disease. J Neurosurg Spine [Internet]. 2017 [cited 2018 Jan 14];27:370–81. Available from: http://www.ncbi.nlm.nih.gov/pubmed/28498069.
32. Asher AL, Kerezoudis P, Mummaneni P V, Bisson EF, Glassman SD, Foley KT, et al. Defining the minimum clinically important difference for grade I degenerative lumbar spondylolisthesis: insights from the Quality Outcomes Database. Neurosurg Focus [Internet]. 2018 [cited 2018 Jan 14];44:E2. Available from: http://thejns.org/doi/10.3171/2017.10.FOCUS17554.
33. Chan AK, Bisson EF, Bydon M, Glassman SD, Foley KT, Potts EA, et al. Women fare best following surgery for degenerative lumbar spondylolisthesis: a comparison of the most and least satisfied patients utilizing data from the Quality Outcomes Database. Neurosurg Focus [Internet]. 2018 [cited 2018 Jan 14];44:E3. Available from: http://thejns.org/doi/10.3171/2017.10.FOCUS17553.
34. Dixon-Woods M, Pronovost PJ. Patient safety and the problem of many hands. BMJ Qual Saf [Internet]. BMJ Publishing Group Ltd; 2016 [cited 2018 Jan 15];25:485–8. Available from: http://www.ncbi.nlm.nih.gov/pubmed/26912578.
35. Classen DC, Resar R, Griffin F, Federico F, Frankel T, Kimmel N, et al. "Global trigger tool" shows that adverse events in hospitals may be ten times greater than previously measured. Health Aff [Internet]. 2011 [cited 2018 Jan 15];30:581–9. Available from: http://www.ncbi.nlm.nih.gov/pubmed/21471476.
36. Makary MA, Daniel M. Medical error – the third leading cause of death in the US. BMJ [Internet]. 2016 [cited 2016 May 4];353:i2139. Available from: http://www.bmj.com/content/353/bmj.i2139.

Index

J. Ratliff et al. (eds.), *Quality Spine Care*,
https://doi.org/10.1007/978-3-319-97990-8

MIX
Papier aus verantwortungsvollen Quellen
Paper from responsible sources
FSC® C105338
www.fsc.org

If you have any concerns about our products,
you can contact us on
ProductSafety@springernature.com

In case Publisher is established outside the EU,
the EU authorized representative is:
Springer Nature Customer Service Center GmbH
Europaplatz 3, 69115 Heidelberg, Germany

Printed by Libri Plureos GmbH
in Hamburg, Germany